AF372102

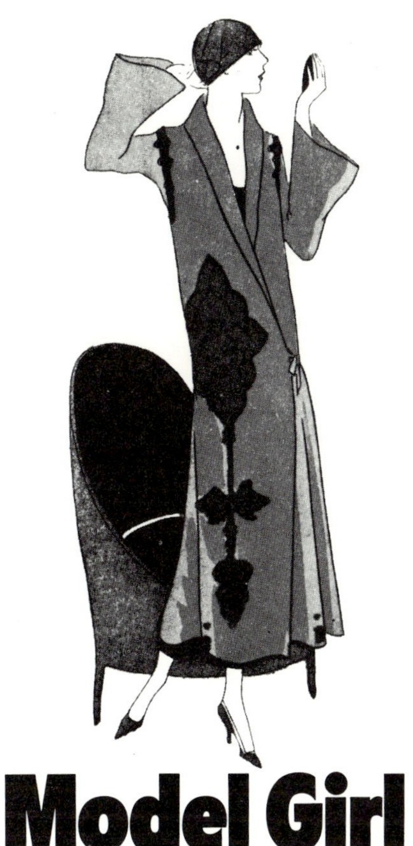

Model Girl

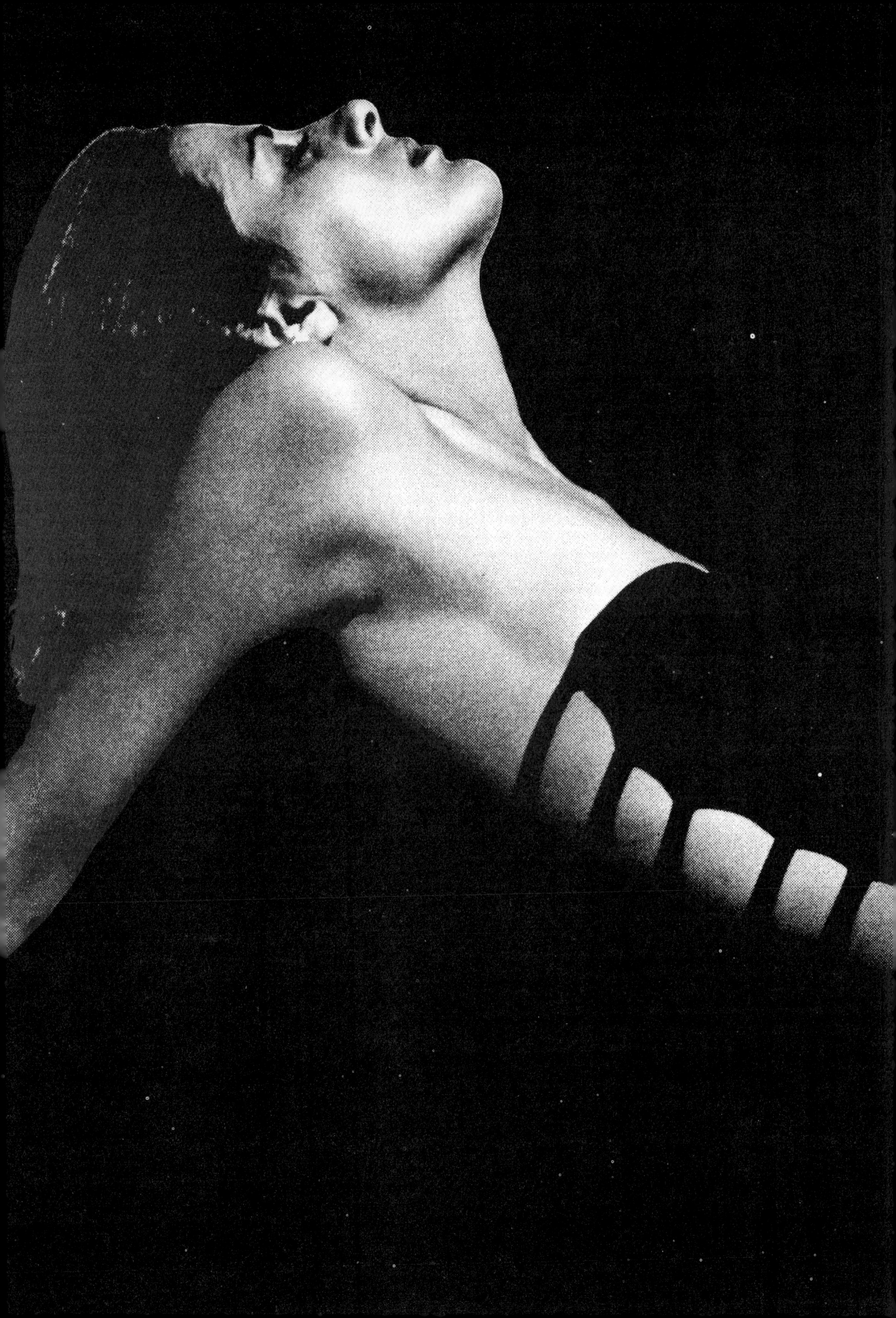

Model Girl

Charles Castle

David & Charles
Newton Abbot · London

Contents

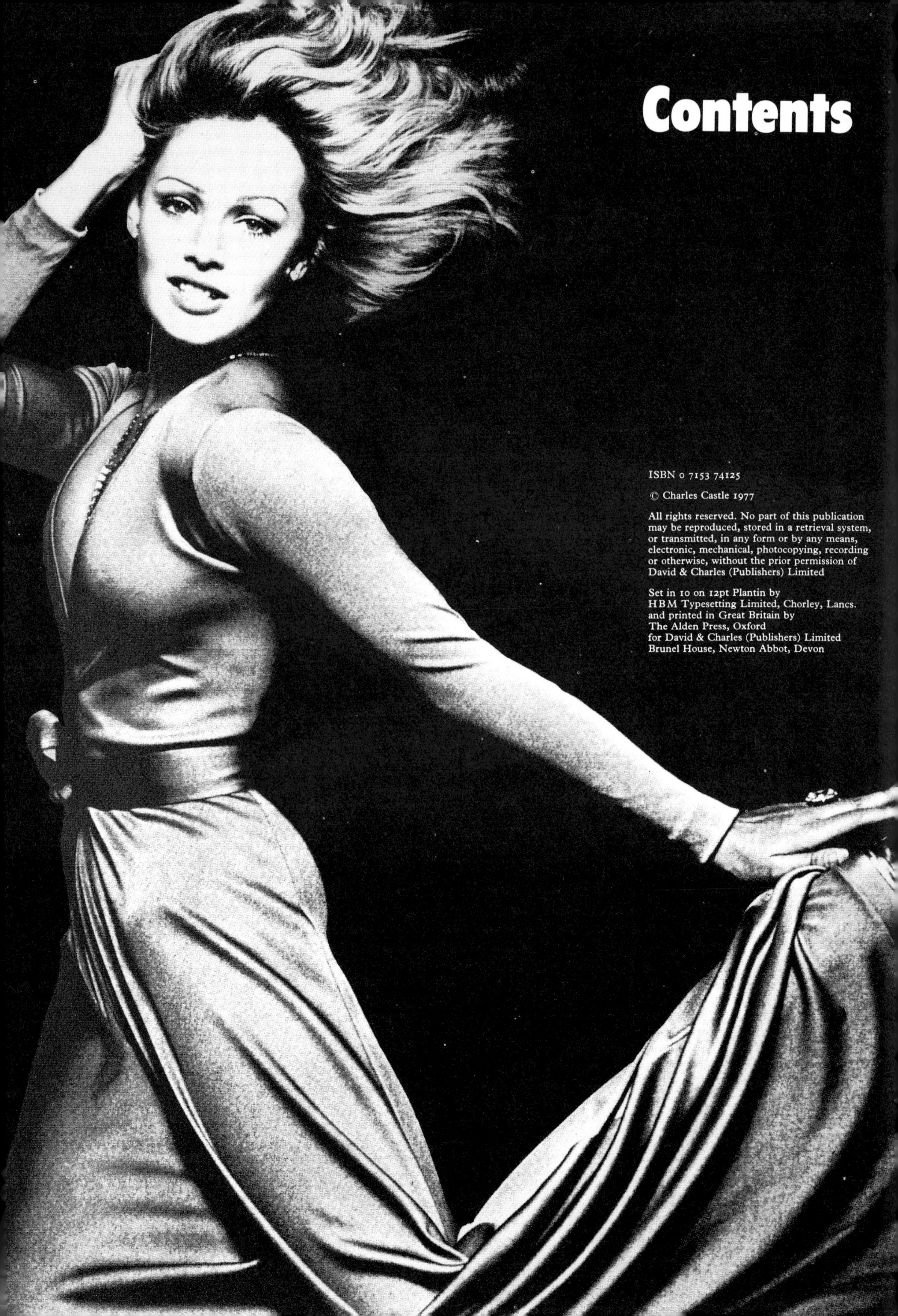

ISBN 0 7153 74125

© Charles Castle 1977

Set in 10 on 12pt Plantin by
HBM Typesetting Limited, Chorley, Lancs.
and printed in Great Britain by
The Alden Press, Oxford
for David & Charles (Publishers) Limited
Brunel House, Newton Abbot, Devon

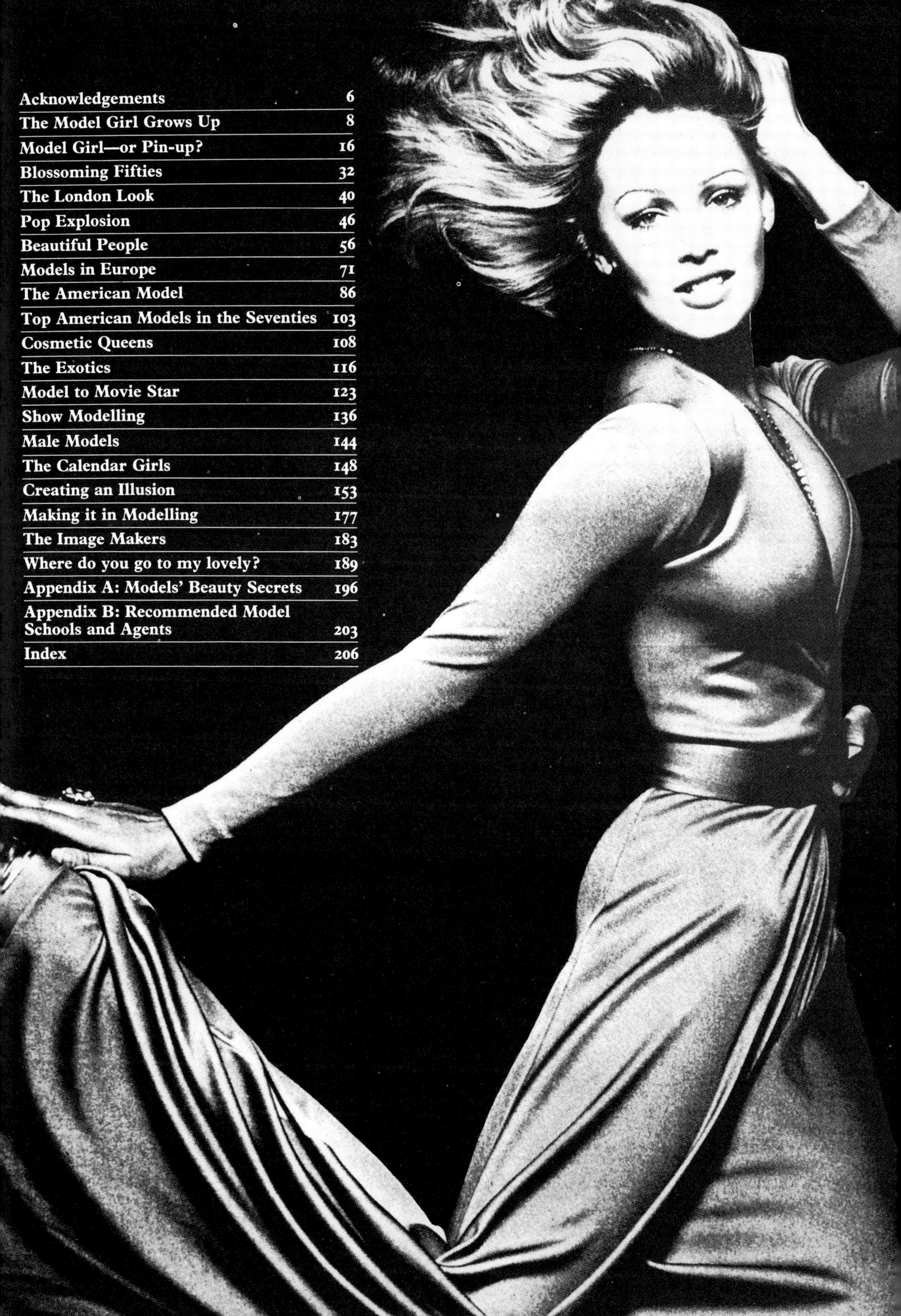

Acknowledgements

Although it has obviously been impossible to include all models and the work of every fashion photographer in *Model Girl*, I believe that the work included is indicative of some of the best of its kind in the world over the past five decades.

The research which has taken me to New York, Paris and back to London has brought me into contact with many models, agents, photographers, couturiers and fashion editors, without whom this book would not have seen the light of day. In particular, I would like to thank Stanley Hall, John Cavanagh and Peter Hope Lumley for their help and encouragement, and the many models and photographers for generously giving of their time and work; Lord Snowdon, Sir Cecil Beaton, Richard Dormer, David Bailey and Barry Lategan in London, and Condé Nast Publications publishers of English *Vogue* and *Brides* for permission to reproduce their work. Photographs are included from the John French Photo Library as well.

Henry Clarke in Paris has been extremely helpful and generous with his work, as have French *Vogue* in permitting the use of photographs by Clarke, Helmut Newton, Guy Bourdin, Sarah Moon, Barbieri and Bailey. In Milan, Barbieri himself has been most kind in providing some of his beautiful photographs.

In gratitude, too, to Condé Nast Publications publishers of American *Vogue* for work by Snowdon, Erwin Blumenfeld and Francesco Scavullo, and particular thanks to Scavullo for the use of so much of his fine work. Horst has been generous also, in allowing his exquisite work to be reproduced, as well as that of George Hoyningen-Huene. Also in New York, Eileen and Jerry Ford, Gene Barakat and Wilhelmina have been most helpful, as well as Sokolsky, Revlon and Avon.

With thanks to Dolores Gray whose advice and friendship in New York made all the difference, and to my editor Jonathan Martin, for his help and patience.

Model Girl is dedicated to all models, past, present and future.

Charles Castle

By the same author

This was Richard Tauber (with Diana Napier Tauber) W. H. Allen
Noël (biography of Sir Noël Coward) W. H. Allen/Doubleday
Joan Crawford: THE RAGING STAR New English Library

Jerry Hall, photographed by Richard Dormer

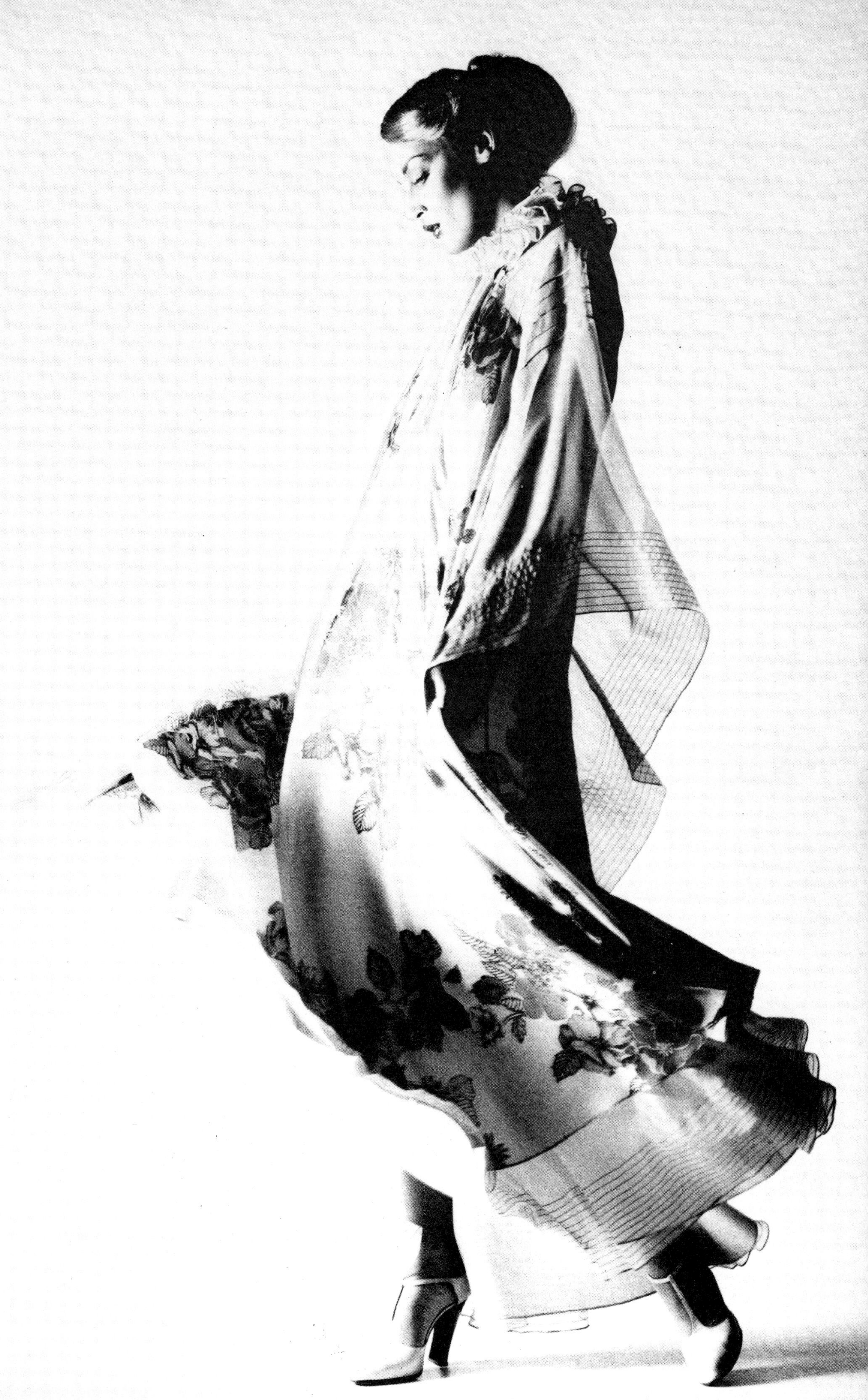

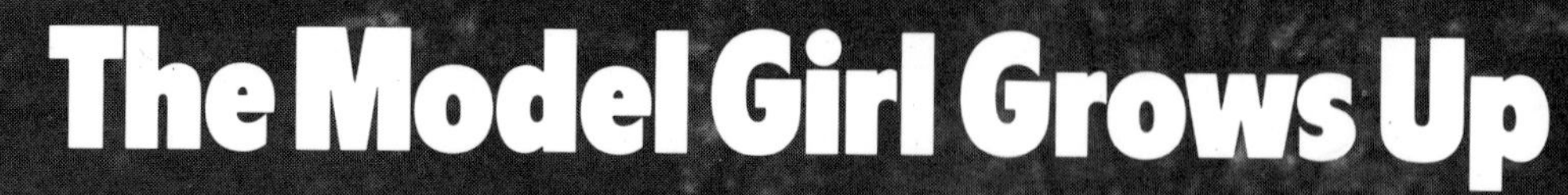

The Model Girl Grows Up

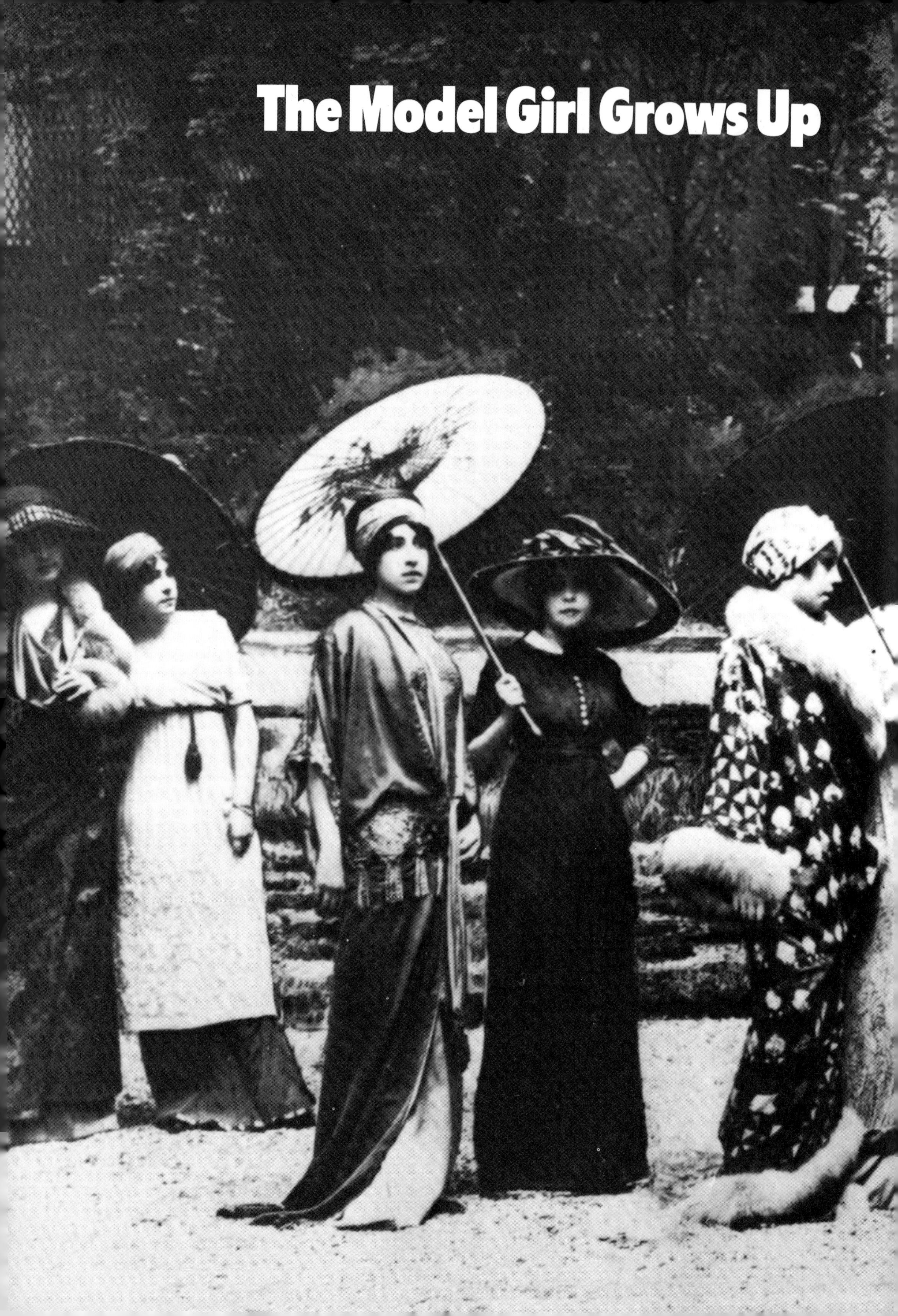

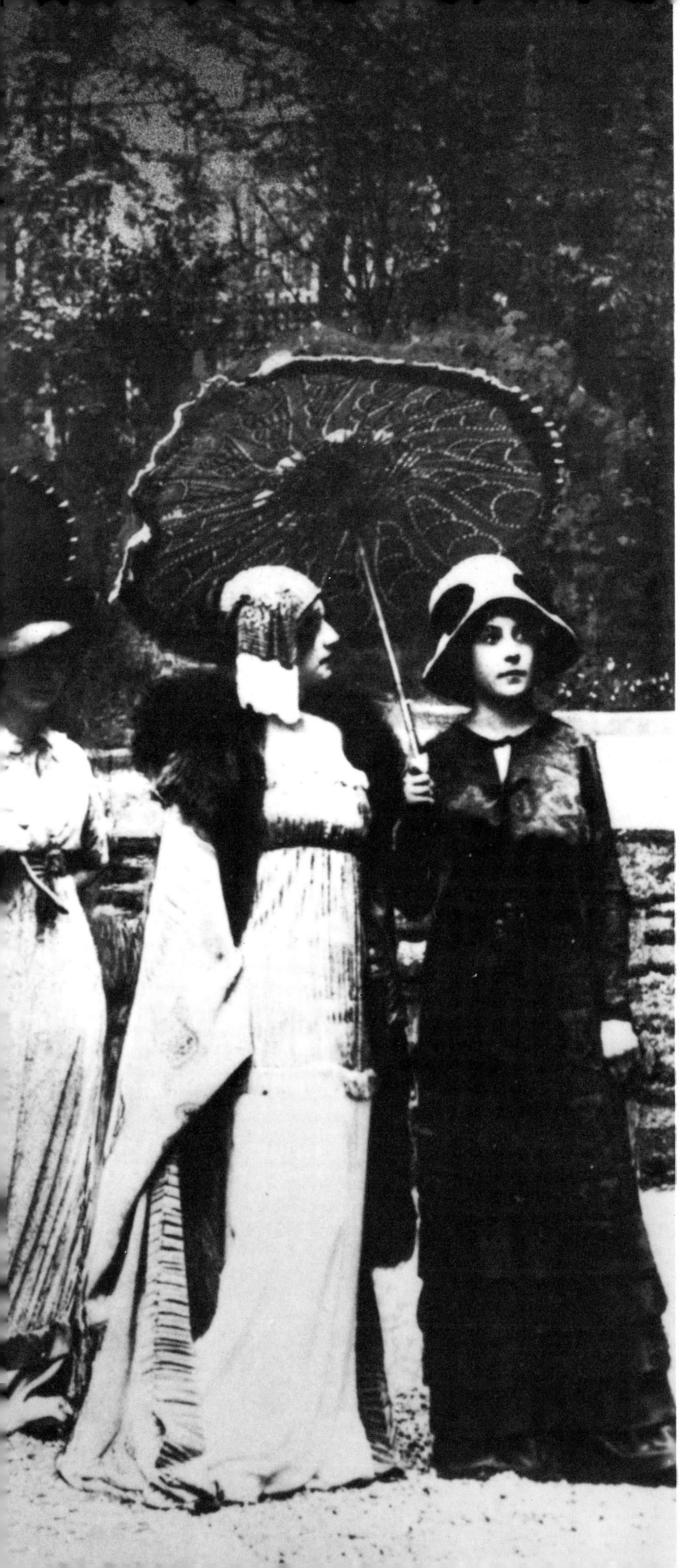

Today modelling is the most highly paid profession a young girl can enter. Top models in New York can earn up to a thousand dollars a day, and work all over the world. Some models have married into the aristocracy, others, such as Lauren Bacall, Jane Fonda, and Ali MacGraw, have become film stars. Grace Kelly began her career as a model, before moving on to become a movie star and then a princess.

But a century and a quarter ago it was very different. Models, or mannequins as they were first called, came from the ranks of shop-girls or sales assistants, and were treated as such. There was no place for them in society.

The very first mannequin was Marie Vernet, a sales assistant at one of the most fashionable Parisian shops, Gagelin et Opigez, of 93 rue de Richelieu, selling dress materials and shawls. An attractive girl with dark, curly hair and blue eyes, she was born in 1825—the same year as the Englishman she was to marry. When he was twenty-six, the Englishman, Charles Frederick Worth, joined Gagelin et Opigez as a salesman. They fell in love, and soon after, on 21 June 1851, married. A year later, she began modelling his clothes.

In order to describe the influence the mannequin had on her husband's career, one needs to explain a little about his background. Born in the hamlet of

Left: Poiret's mannequins as featured in *L'Illustration*, 9 July 1910

Below: Marie Worth in 1863

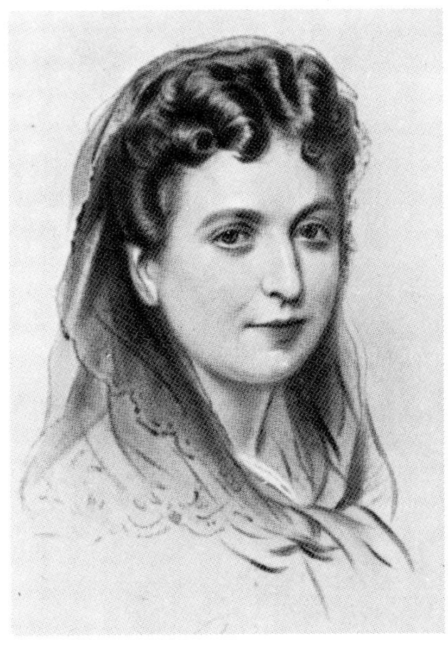

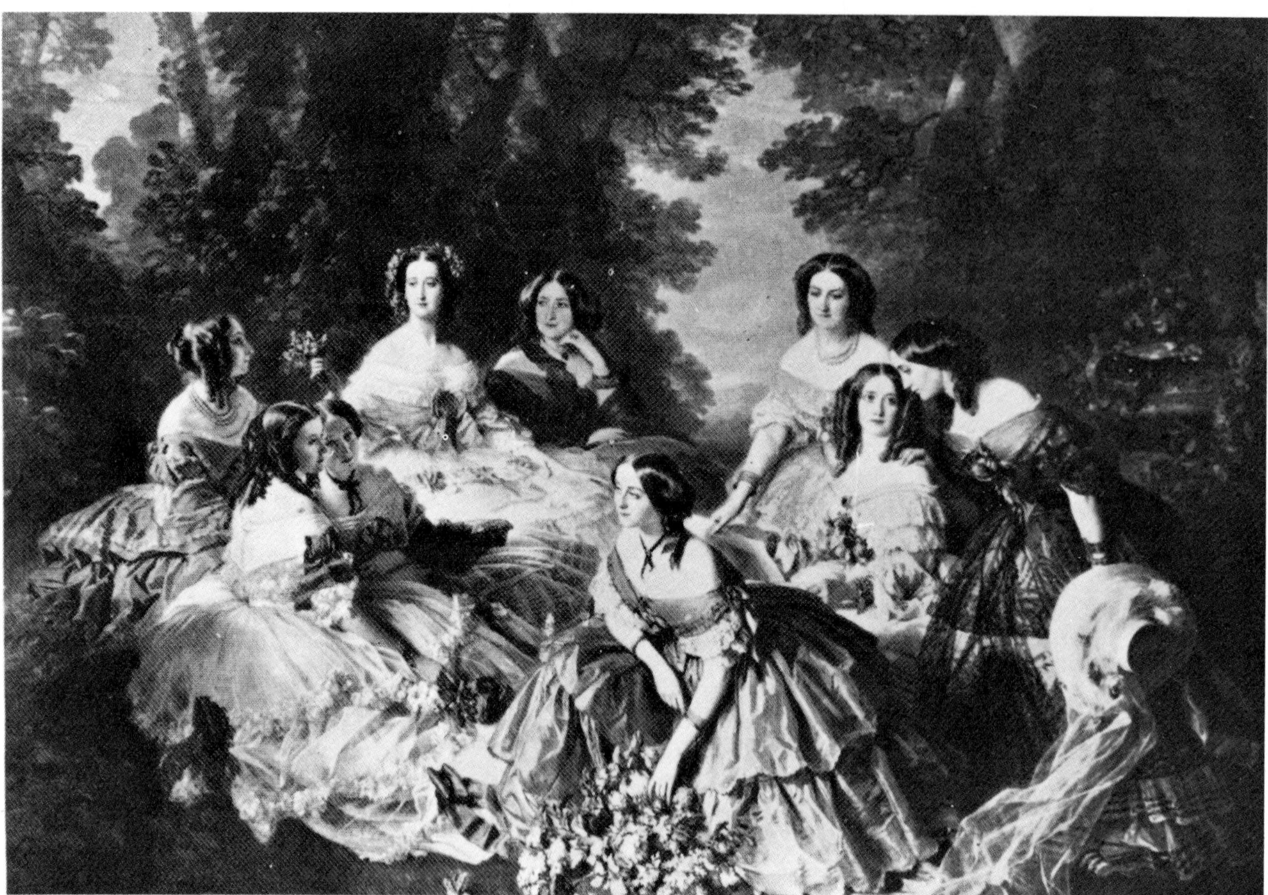

The Empress Eugénie, second from right, with her ladies-in-waiting, from the painting by Winterhalter at Malmaison

Bourne in Lincolnshire, Charles Worth began his apprenticeship in drapery and secured a job with Swan and Edgar in London. Had he been able to choose his own career, he might have become an artist but, instead, his future lay in dressmaking. Although surrounded by women's clothes at Swan and Edgar, he realised that mid-nineteenth century London had little to offer in the way of fashion, and so he set off in search of a future in Paris. He worked as a salesman for a year at the drapers La Ville de Paris and left to join the more fashionable Maison Gagelin, where leading dressmakers came to buy materials.

Worth was at the centre of the dressmaking fraternity, and now, with an attractive wife at his side, began designing clothes for the clients of his new employers. He sketched and made clothes he believed would suit Marie, and she, the possessor of an innate sense of elegance, wore—and modelled—the clothes in the shop. Dressmakers had, hitherto, made clothes for individual customers, but Worth was the first couturier to design individual high-class fashion. In 1851, Maison Gagelin took his designs to the Great Exhibition

in London, and there won the only Gold Medal awarded to France. This was the age of the crinoline, a style which Worth is said to have invented; he certainly established it as the only mode of the Second Empire.

In 1858 Worth left Gagelin et Opigez to open a business of his own where his mannequin wife became the instrument of his first great success. Marie approached the wife of the new Austrian Ambassador, Princess Pauline de Metternich, who had recently arrived in Paris, showed her Worth's designs, and secured an order for two crinolines, one for day and one for evening wear. So great was the impact of his clothes for the Princess that Worth soon became couturier to the most powerful and prosperous clientele of the Second Empire, which became known as 'the age of Worth'. At the age of thirty-five, he became the first *grand couturier*, supplying clothes for members of the court, but his most prized and influential customer was the Empress Eugénie, wife of Napoleon III, for whom he continued to create clothes for many years.

By 1865 Worth had several show-

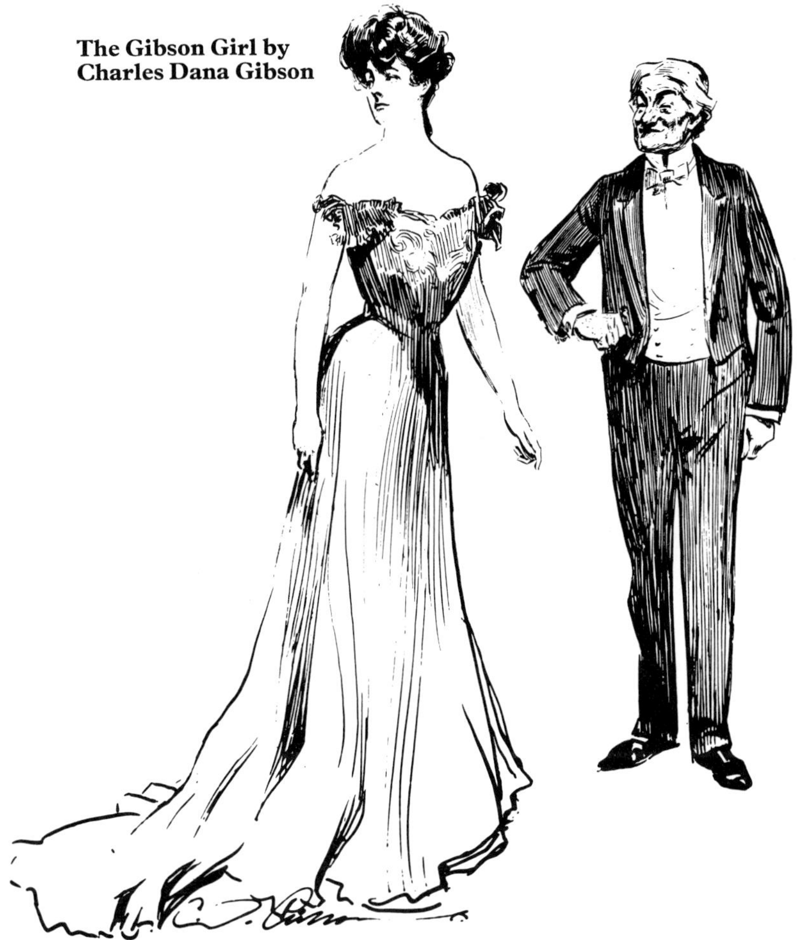

The Gibson Girl by
Charles Dana Gibson

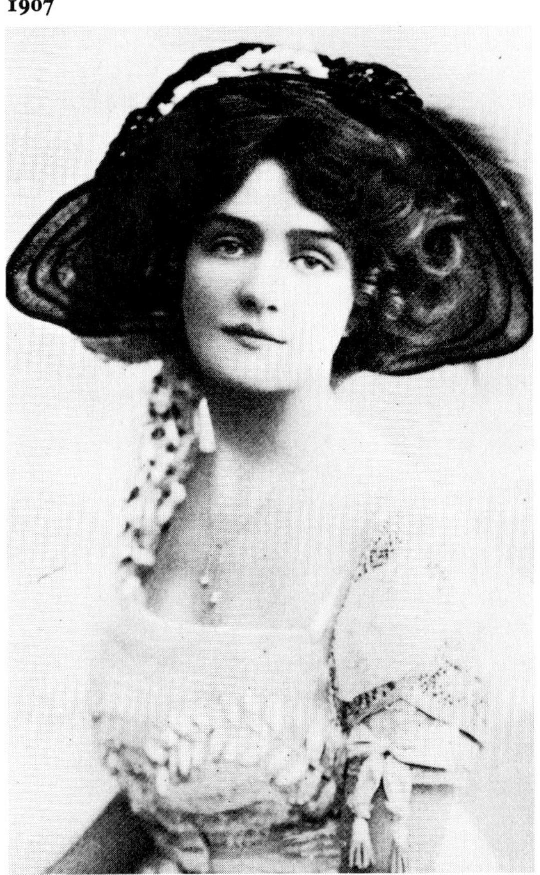

Lily Elsie as 'The Merry Widow' in
1907

rooms in his shop. 'Attractive young girls were much in evidence, the models of the establishment, many of whom were English', records authoress Edith Saunders. 'One of Worth's chief contributions to Haute Couture was the use of living models to show his dresses. It was an idea which had risen naturally from his collaboration with his wife. His models were always available to put on new dresses for the inspection of a client; but their own dresses, though in the height of fashion, were invariably made in black with long sleeves and high necks.'

Worth went on to lead and influence fashion in France, with his wife as his staunchest supporter, until his death in 1895; but his empire did not crumble with his death. His sons, Jean Philippe and Gaston, who had entered the business, carried the Worth tradition into the new century.

However, although it could be said that Madame Worth had secured for herself high regard in her capacity as wife of the creator of haute couture, her early profession as mannequin needed almost a century to be accepted by society.

With the death of Queen Victoria in 1901, the prudery and strict morals of the Victorian era were exchanged for modishness in the Edwardian style. At about this time the great couture houses of Paris came to dominate style and fashion all over Europe and America.

However, it was in America, at the turn of the century, that one of the earliest popular fashion crazes—the Gibson girl—was created by the society artist Charles Dana Gibson. Inspired by Irene Langhorne of Virginia, one of Nancy, Lady Astor's sisters, the Gibson girl, with her prominent bust, pinched-in waist, and saucy bustle, produced the S-line, or hour-glass figure. Gibson's art shaped the lives of a large portion of the American populace who tried to conform to the style of the people in his pictures—and occasionally succeeded, albeit with physical discomfort. The Gibson girl image was copied in Europe but this stiff look disappeared in 1907, when *The Merry Widow* with its waltzing star, Lily Elsie, took London by storm.

Dressed by Lucile (a Canadian who became Lady Duff-Gordon, and was sister of the sensationalist novelist Elinor Glyn), in chiffon and crêpe de Chine, Lily Elsie set London swaying and its women rushing to their dressmakers to copy her clothes.

The next spell to be cast upon the fashion world was the influence of the Ballet Russe in 1909; the French couturier Paul Poiret, who came to be known as the Sultan of Fashion, designed exotic and oriental creations influenced by the ballet, and liberated women from their corsets and whalebones, permitting them to move more freely.

His wife became the next model to be known by name. Poiret became engaged to nineteen year old Denise, daughter of a textile manufacturer, in June 1905, and before they married he began designing clothes for her. 'My wife is the inspiration for my creations', he explained. 'She is the expression of all my ideals.'

Although Poiret employed many mannequins, he was so proud of the way Denise showed his clothes that from 1910 she was frequently photographed wearing his creations.

Poiret's mannequins appeared in *L'Illustration* as early as 9 July 1910 and

Denise, Poiret's wife, in Paris, 1910

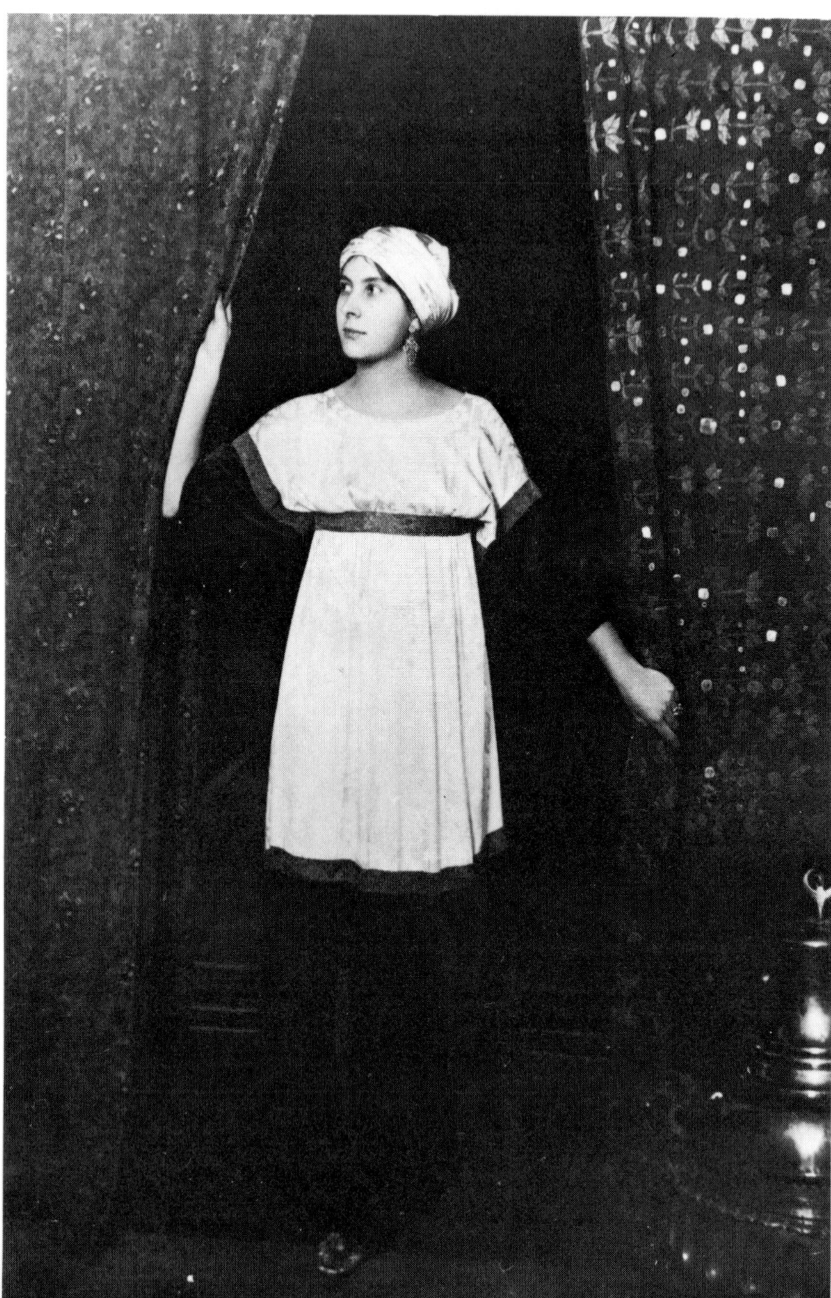

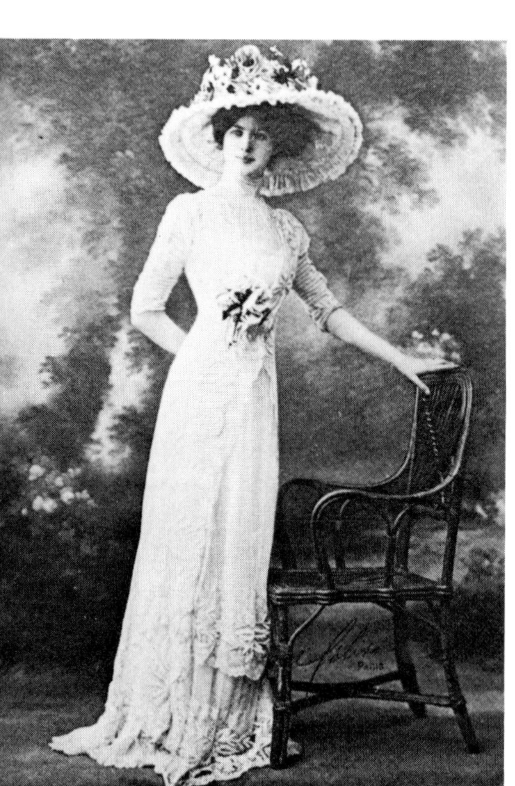

A mannequin photographed by Felix in Paris, 1907

again in February 1911, but the first fashion photographs to be published of models wearing his corsetless clothes were taken by the American painter Edward Steichen at Poiret's fashion house. These appeared in *Art et Decoration* in April 1911, and 'they were probably the first serious fashion photographs ever published', as Edward Steichen himself said.

Poiret was followed closely by Paquin, who designed clothes for women who wished to copy dancer Irene Castle's two-step and foxtrot, in 1912.

This same period saw the end of two of the great courtesans of all time—Forzane and La Belle Otero—who had held Paris in their sway. The latter, a Spanish dancer, was described at the height of her fame as 'the most scandalous person since Helen of Troy'. She married an Italian count, who ran off with her jewellery, but it was her fabulous succession of millionaire admirers that made her internationally famous. Caroline Otero was, as well, the most determined woman gambler of her time, and lost her fortune in Monte Carlo.

Cecil Beaton describes Forzane: 'An incandescent blonde of Swedish extraction, who appeared a short time before the First World War and had disappeared by the end of it. With her

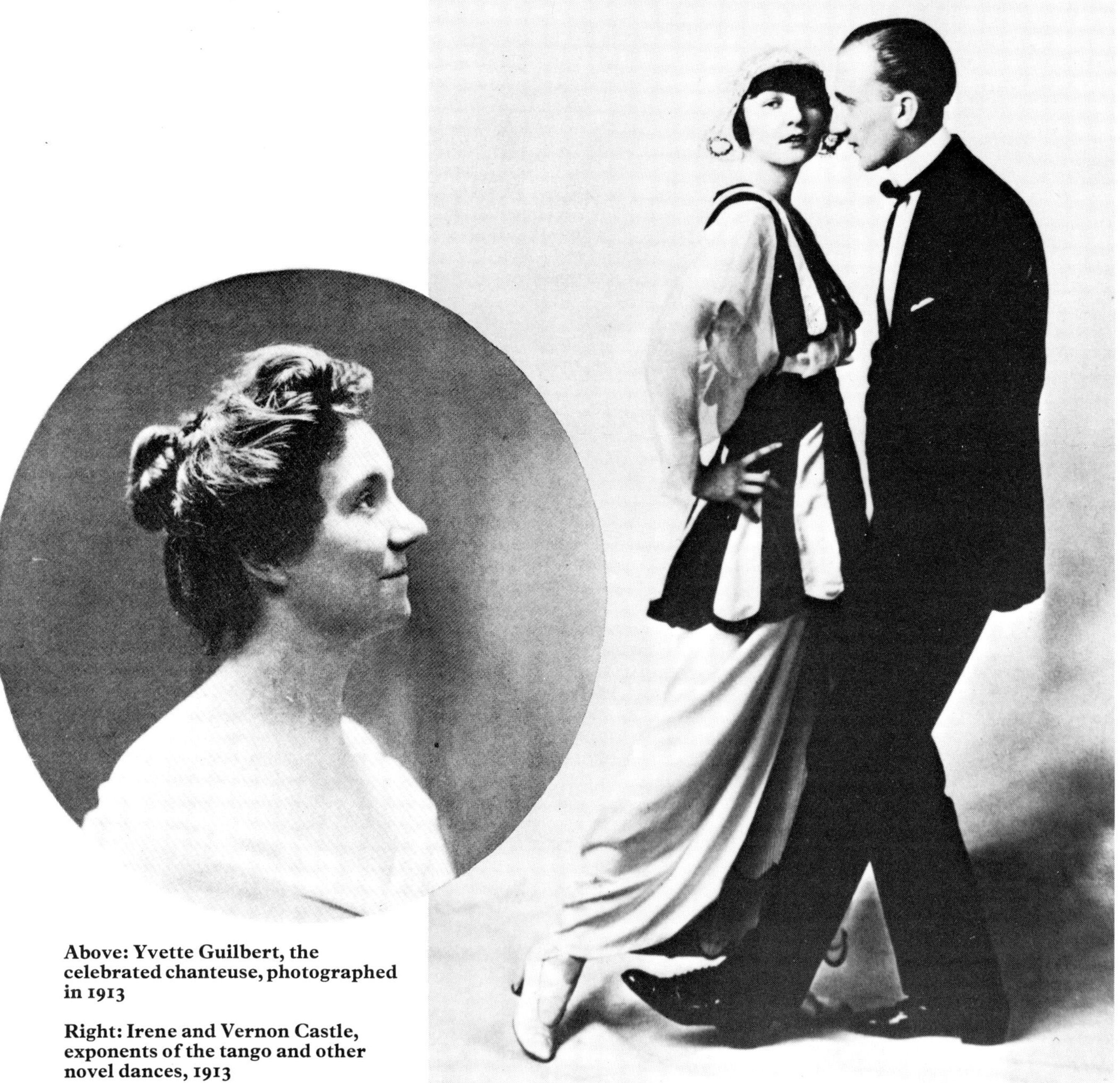

Above: Yvette Guilbert, the celebrated chanteuse, photographed in 1913

Right: Irene and Vernon Castle, exponents of the tango and other novel dances, 1913

exquisite grace and original line of body, her luminous pallor, her small chubby nose and fully fashioned, divided rose-bud lips, she was a clarion call to sex. Her Negroid eyes, set in a long pale face, had the same hot, somewhat queasy look that her rival, the actress Lantelme, possessed. But Forzane was more subtle, more restrained and ambiguous than her sultry blonde rival. Forzane's appeal was never vulgar. She seemed to breathe in the rarefied atmosphere of parma violets and gave the illusion of the un-attainable.

'Both Forzane and the *demi-mondaines* knew how to sustain interest, not only in their men but in their public. Perhaps it was easier to create a sensation in those days than it is today. When Forzane entered the restaurant of the Savoy Hotel in London, people stood on their chairs to get a better view.'

'The last of the truly elegant ladies', Poiret observed, 'was Forzane, who invented a new silhouette for women, with poses rather like a kangaroo. Do you remember her mornings in the Avenue du Bois, with her immense parasol? She could have been sketched as an ellipse. Since her, there has been nobody.'

Fashion, and as a consequence mannequins, suffered a set-back with the beginning of World War I. Chiffon and lace were replaced with the tailored suits favoured by suffragettes, and by the new 'George Bernard Shaw-inspired' free women. The French government banned evening-dress and jewels at the Opéra and theatre, and appealed to women to buy no new dresses until war had ended.

Nevertheless, some of the most notable beauties of the theatre were to be photographed modelling clothes. Amongst these were the famous Parisian dancer Ida Rubinstein who began modelling with a dress made by Worth in 1913; soubrette Gertie Millar (who became the Countess of Dudley), who was photographed by Rita Martin in

1916 modelling a fur coat: Yvonne Printemps, Gaby Delys, Alice Delysia, the exquisite dancer Florence Walton, and the delightful French musical comedy star Gina Palerme, who were all photographed wearing their favourite clothes from Vionnet (one of the greatest of all designers), Lanvin, Poiret, and the Callot sisters. The American show-girl Dolores, one of the most famous of all Florenz Ziegfeld chorus girls and one of the most beautiful young women of her day, was used as a model for a hat by Baron Gayne de Meyer in 1918, showing her exquisite profile, highlighted with back-light flooding onto her lovely features. In 1922 she was to be photographed modelling one of Lucile's elegant evening dresses, with long fringes trailing from the sleeves.

By the twenties, photographers had begun to play a major role in the presenting of fashion. Apart from Edward Steichen and Baron de Meyer, the finest photographers living in Paris were George Hoyningen-Huene and, later, in the thirties, his disciple Horst Boormann—who became known simply as Horst—and Man Ray, who contributed some of the finest fashion photographs to *Vogue* and *Harpers Bazaar*. Not least, in the twenties, in Paris, there was also the great innovator in fashion photography—Cecil Beaton.

Modelling had now been a profession for more than seventy years, but it was nowhere near to being accepted by society. For instance, Poiret's superlative taste in the clothes he designed hardly matched his treatment of his mannequins. After World War I, he took eight of his most beautiful mannequins on his fashion tours and, to prevent admirers from the various capitals from making off with his charges, dressed them all alike, rather shabbily, in blue serge uniforms, complete with belts, buckles, and epaulettes. Fashion writer Alison Settle went along to interview M. Poiret for *The Daily Mirror* in London in 1920: 'He invited me to lunch with him in the restaurant of the Carlton Hotel, even more chic than the Ritz, and when I joined him in the lounge, he and I marched in to a prominent table, at the head of four mannequins, by this era in uniforms of green and gold complete with peaked caps.

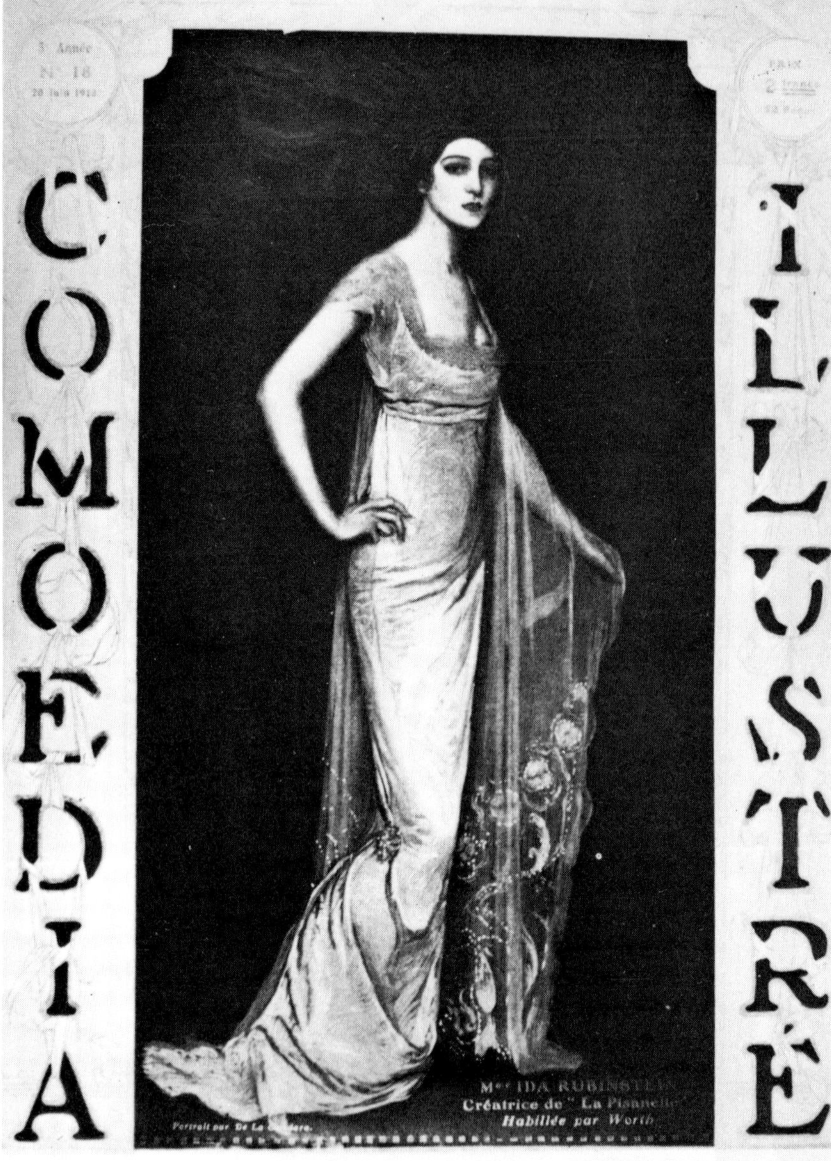

While he studied the menu, I turned to speak to the girl next to me. He put a hand on my arm, warningly: "No, mademoiselle", he said, "do not speak to the girls; they are not there." Quite definitely, they were, but not *socially*.'

Newly arrived in Paris in 1921 was an aspiring young American artist, Man Ray. He had taken up photography as a second string to his bow, in order to pay his way until his paintings sold, and managed to get an introduction to Poiret who allowed him to photograph his mannequins. Man Ray arrived at the salon and encountered several mannequins in negligees, getting ready to dress and go out for lunch.

They were beautiful girls with every shade of hair from blonde to black, moving nonchalantly in their scanty chemises, stockings and high-heeled shoes. Man Ray was introduced and his role explained, whilst he tried to seem as though he had not noticed their state of déshabillé. The girls were cool, almost forbidding, all, that is, except one black-haired, wide-eyed girl to whom he spoke in English—she did not look as French as the others. He told her that he was American, and discovered she too was from New York, studying singing and making her way by modelling. He explained that he was on an assignment from Poiret himself to take photographs and would like her to give him part of her lunch-hour to pose. She readily agreed and hoped the pictures would appear in one of the fashion magazines; it would be a great help for her. He assured her that he would do his best to get them published.

Looking around for a suitable back-

**Opposite: A portrait of Ida Rubin-
stein in a dress made by Worth for**
La Pisanelle

**Right: The great Florenz Ziegfeld
showgirl, Dolores, photographed
by Baron de Meyer in 1918**

**Below: Gertie Millar who became
the Countess of Dudley**

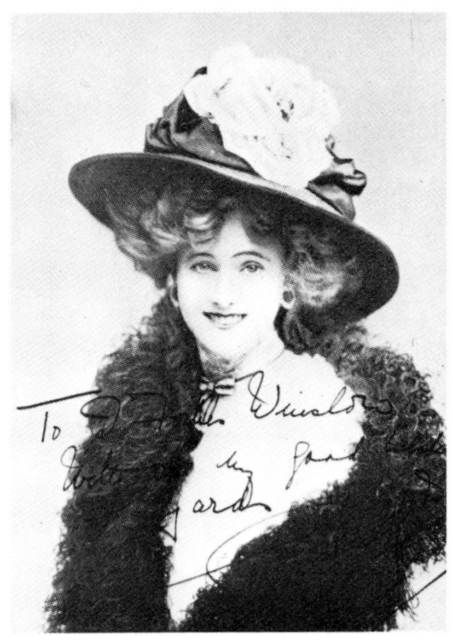

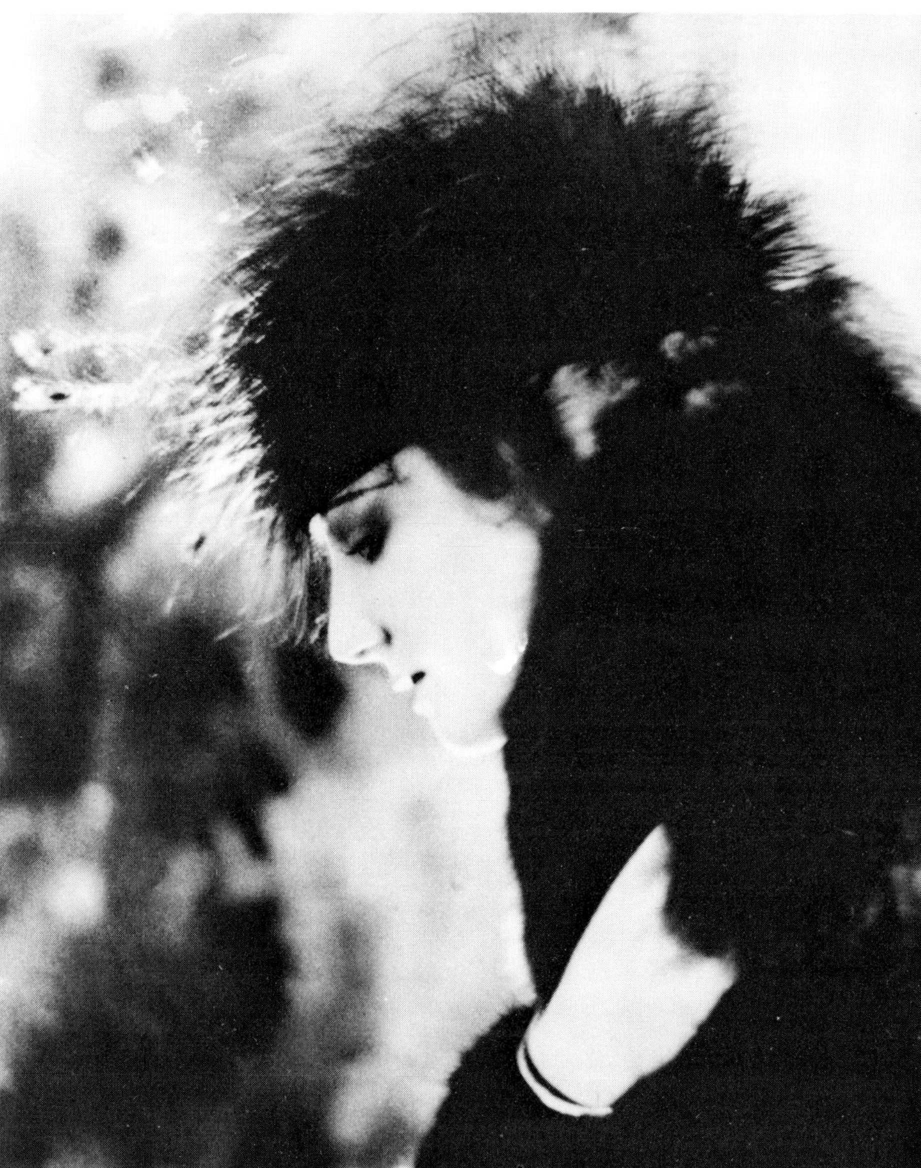

ground, he noticed the open door of
Poiret's office, the floor littered with
brilliant-coloured bolts of material. He
had an idea. He explained to his subject
that Poiret expected something original
from him, something different from the
usual fashion pictures. Pointing to the
disorder on the floor, he asked her to lie
down on the pile, taking a completely
relaxed pose. He had a practical reason
for this: the office was darker, would
require a longer exposure and she was
less likely to move in that position.

She looked at him with an amused
but doubtful expression; then went in
and dropped on the pile, with her arms
over her head, which she turned towards him with a coy expression. 'It was
ravishing, divine [as they say in fashion
circles]', he recalled. 'There was line,
colour, texture, and above all, sex-

appeal, which I instinctively felt was
what Poiret wanted.'

After focusing his camera, he walked
over to her, bent down to adjust a fold
in the dress, caught his foot in a bolt of
cloth and fell flat on top of the girl. She
made no abrupt gesture; he quickly
rolled over to the side and rose apolo-
gising profusely. She looked at him with
a smile; perhaps she did not believe it
was an accident, and he went back to
his camera. The girl rearranged herself
while he busied himself with his camera,
working quickly and seriously, making
a couple of exposures.

That night, as soon as it was suffi-
ciently dark in his hotel room, he pulled
the curtains, laid out his two trays on
the table, and, by the light of a candle in
a little red lantern, developed the plates.
They were not too bad as far as exposure

went, but nothing came out on the two
shots of the reclining figure—in his
distraction he had not pulled the slides
of the holders to make the exposures!

Man Ray went out with many beautiful girls, the most notable of whom,
Kiki, became both his model and his
constant companion. Kiki of Mont-
parnasse, as she was known, had been
rescued by him during a dispute which
arose between her and the owner of a
cafe because she wasn't wearing a hat.

Although, before World War I, there
was little activity in London as far as
haute couture was concerned, there
was one well known model, Madeleine
Seymour, who worked for Lucile before
becoming a George Edwards actress in
1910. Another model, Betty Stockfield,
also worked for Lucile, before turning
to the stage.

Model Girl-or Pin-up?

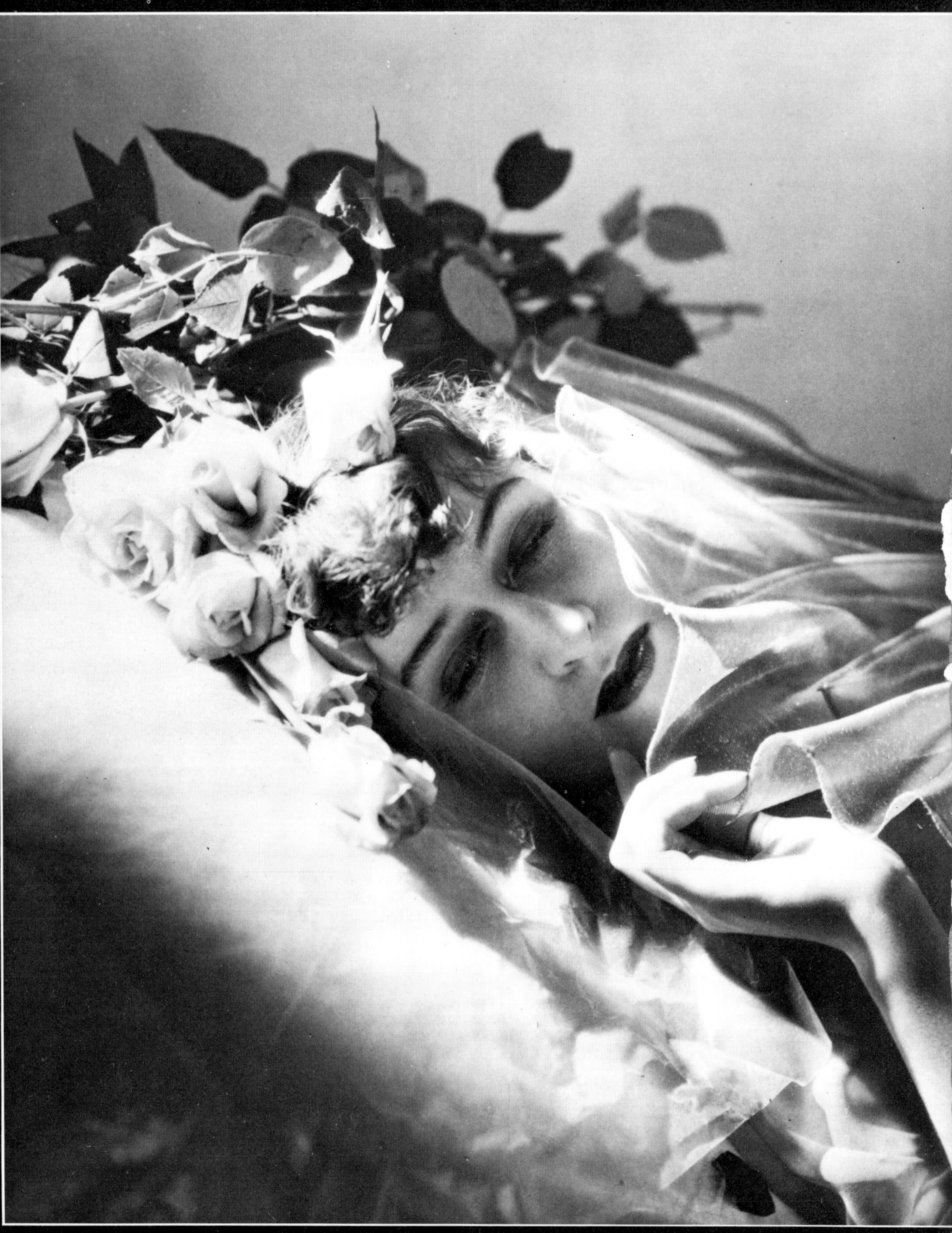

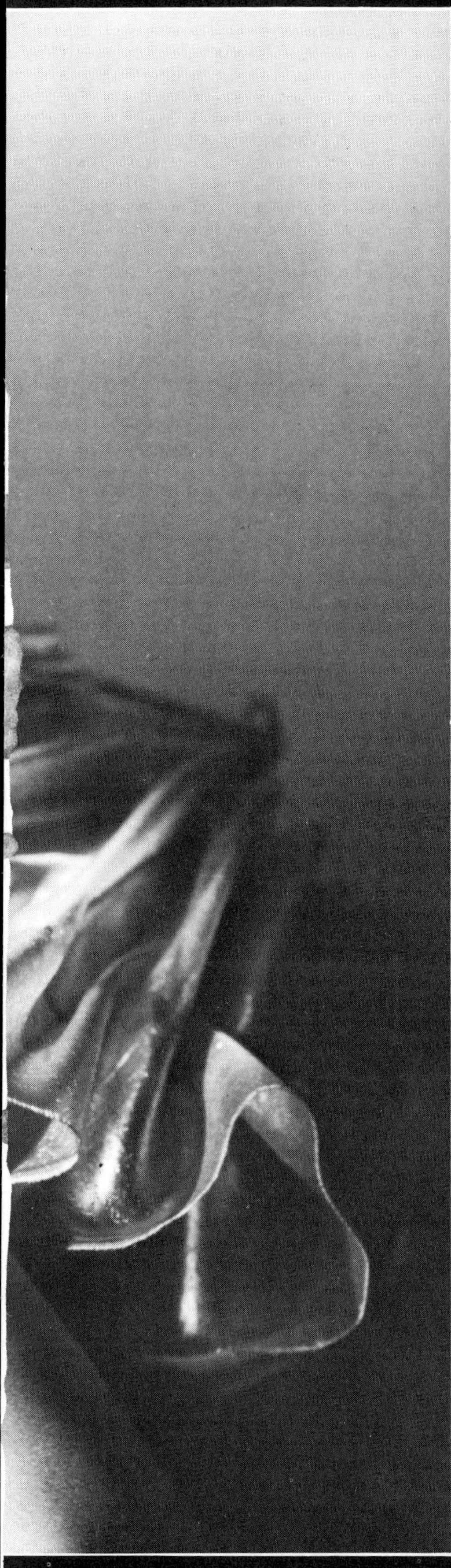

Marion Morehouse, photographed by George Hoyningen-Huene in Paris, 1933 (Copyright: Horst)

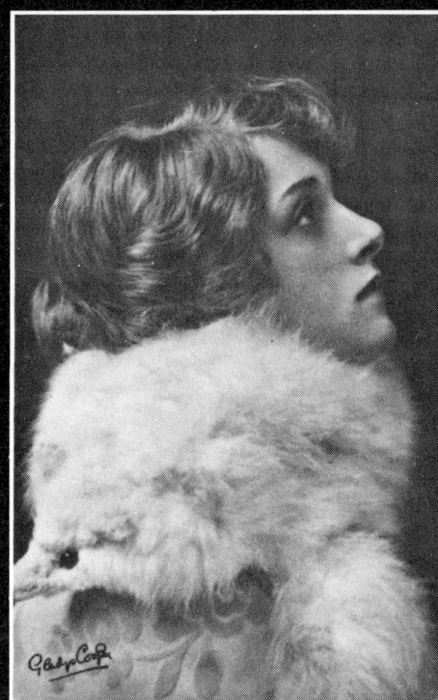

Gladys Cooper

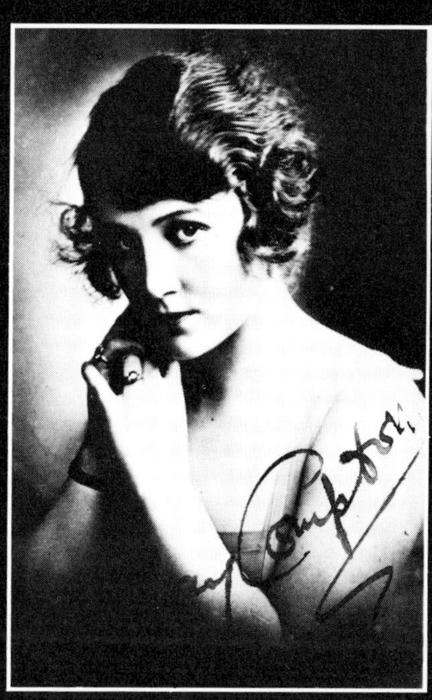

Fay Compton. Courtesy the Mander and Mitchenson collection

The twenties brought many innovations—in London, not only beauties but famous actresses faced the camera's lens, to be cast as pin-ups and sold as postcards. Gladys Cooper, Fay Compton, Zena and Phyllis Dare, opera singers, and dancers were all to reach a wider public through this medium.

In Paris, although mannequins showed the designers' clothes in sumptuous salons, it was the great society beauties and famous actresses and stars of the day who were, by and large, photographed in these creations for fashion magazines, thereby endorsing their favourite couturiers' clothes and encouraging readers to follow suit. Many well known figures were actually dressed by the famous houses for no payment whatsoever, and in return were seen wearing the clothes at Longchamps, the Opéra, or on stage. This habit did not die out until the fifties, when it ceased to be economical for the couture houses, and models began to be known by name to the general public.

However, the mannequin, or model, did not come into her own for many years yet, and throughout the twenties and thirties she would remain at best one of the selected mannequins known in the couturier's salon by first name alone, while little, if anything, was known—or cared—about her outside her professional duties.

Instead of models alone being seen in fashion magazines showing the couturiers' wares, aristocracy and stars alike assumed the role of model by allowing themselves to be photographed with suitable credit given to the 'tradesman' who supplied the garment—for the couturiers, or dressmakers, however much approved of by society for the design of the clothes, were suppliers nonetheless, and were regarded as such. Personifying fashion in the glossy magazines was the Duchess of Gramont, who became a famous Paris hostess, and of whom Madame Vionnet said: 'She is a real model, tall and beautiful. When I was making a dress I had only to ask her to come and try it on and I knew exactly where it was wrong'. Others who enjoyed the momentary limelight of the photographer's lens were the Duchess of Marlborough; the Queen of Spain; Mrs Dudley Ward, whose constant escort was the Prince of Wales; and the Duke of Rutland's daughter, Lady Diana Cooper, whose remarkable beauty has been revered for over fifty years, and who *Vogue* described as 'untarnishable, the loveliest young Englishwoman of her generation'.

'To enumerate Lady Diana's virtues is to risk being accused of exaggeration or prejudice', said Cecil Beaton. 'Yet

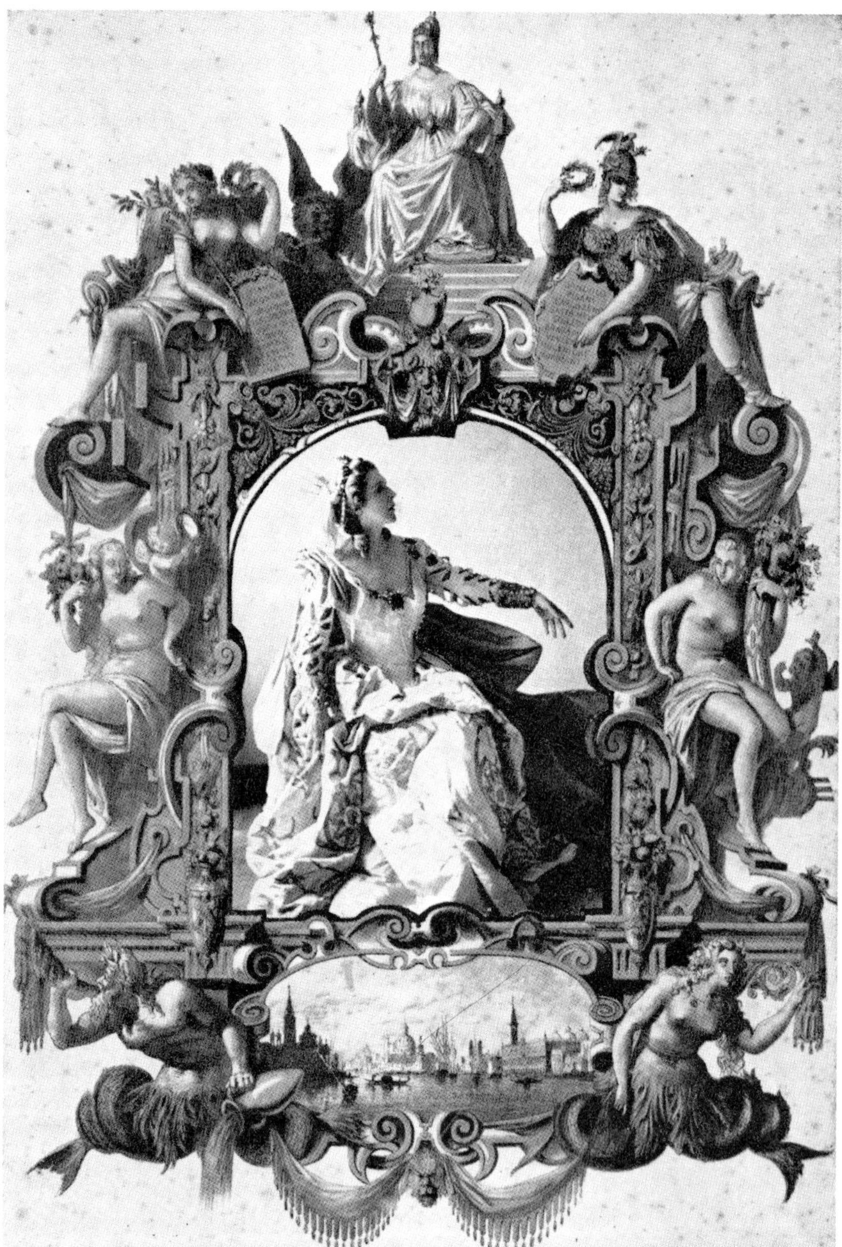

Left: Lady Diana Cooper as the famous eighteenth-century Italian painter Tiepolo's idea of Cleopatra, photographed by Cecil Beaton

Below: Lillian Gish as 'Romola' in New York, photographed by Edward Steichen in 1923

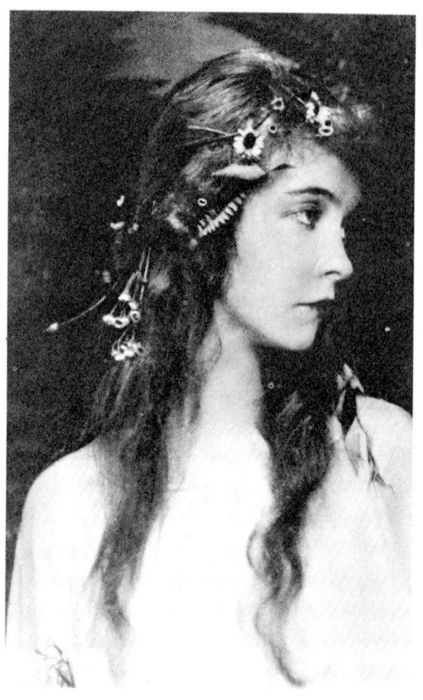

who does not warrant high praise if not a beauty who is a wit, an enlightening *raconteuse*, and a brilliant correspondent [it may well be that she will live in posterity by her letters]? She is an artist in life with countless artistic gifts, a friend with unswerving loyalties, at once business-like, capable, imaginative and full of heartbreak, an eccentric who is frank and outspoken with the knowledge of when not to mention any given subject.' Lady Diana, indeed, seems to have been a woman with most of the rare qualities.

Edward Steichen was the highest paid staff member on *Vogue*'s books before he was succeeded as top photographer for Condé Nast by Baron de Meyer. 'My first contribution to the fashion photograph was to make it as realistic as possible', Steichen commented. 'I felt that a woman, when she looked at the picture of a gown, should be able to form a very good idea of how that gown was put together and what it looked like. These photographs indicate how I carried out that idea.'

He also went to Hollywood, where for many years he photographed stars for *Vanity Fair*. Amongst these was Lillian Gish, in 1923: 'It was as if an angel had come into the place', he recalled. 'Every movement she made and everything she said seemed full of magic.'

Models who showed clothes at the great fashion houses, although hardly earning a decent living by showing the creations of the Lucile's, Paquin's, and Molyneux's, at least enjoyed the attentions of rich and titled young men as a form of compensation. They were fêted and pursued in true stage-boy-Johnny tradition, and once the curtain fell they scurried away from the public's adulation into private adoration. However, like actresses and courtesans of the period, theirs was an illicit, forbidden love. As they were neither invited into, nor accepted by, society; convention forced them into clandestine dinners-for-two in private rooms of fashionable restaurants, where they enjoyed the veiled attentions of their amorous, generous beaux.

One of the great mannequins of the twenties, Vera Ashby, had appeared as

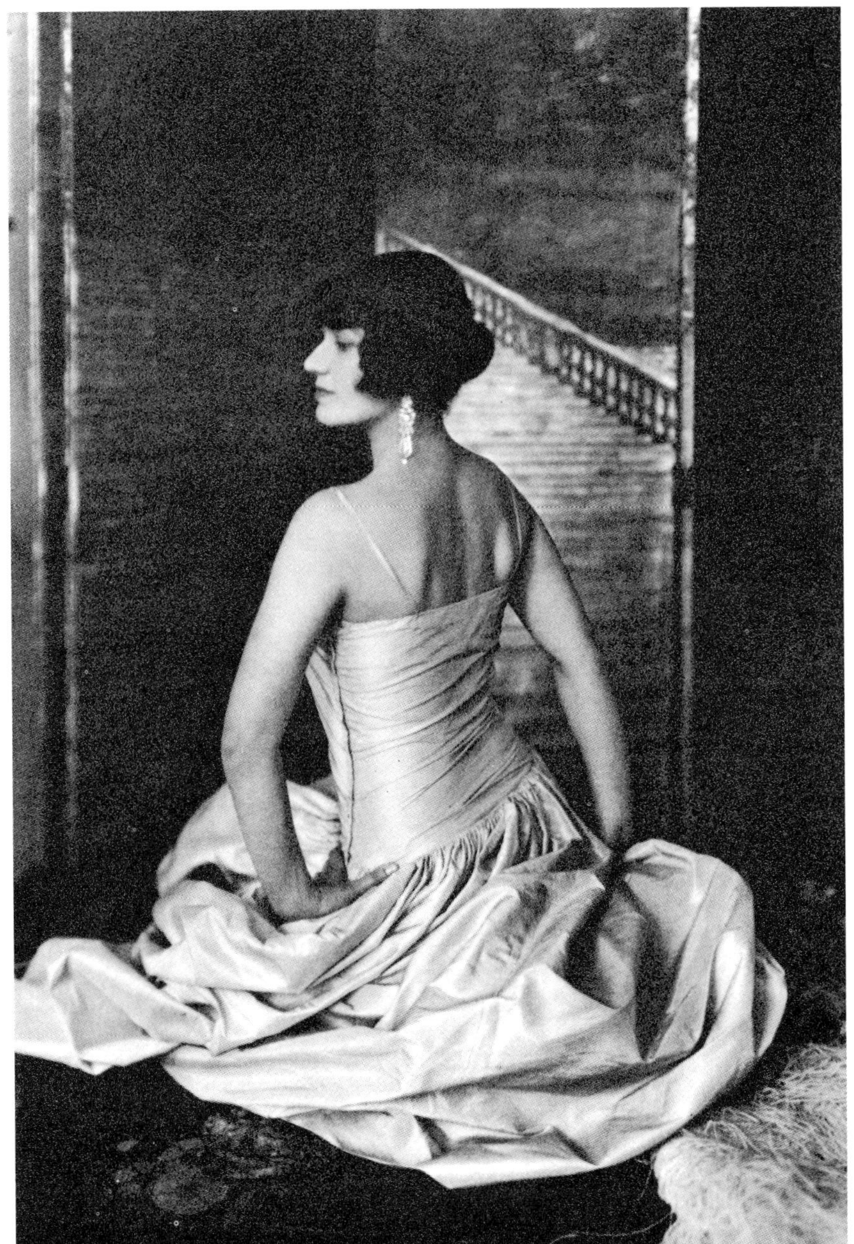

Left: The Duchess of Gramont, photographed in Paris by Edward Steichen, 1924

Bottom: Three fashion photographs for *Vogue* by Edward Steichen, 1923–5

Below: Zena and Phyllis Dare

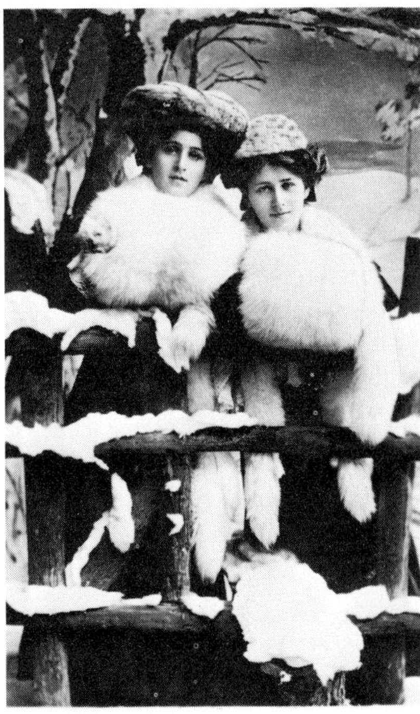

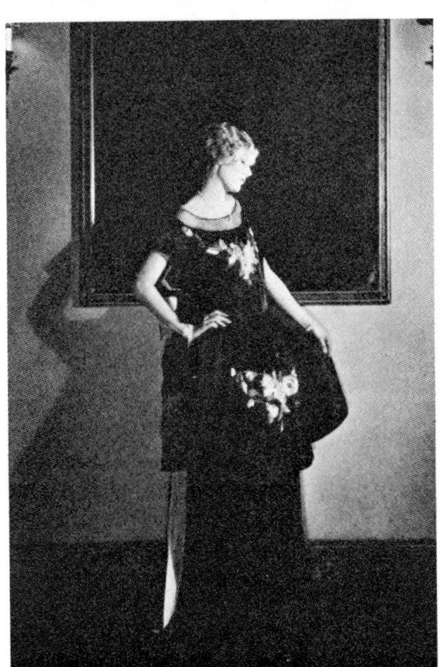

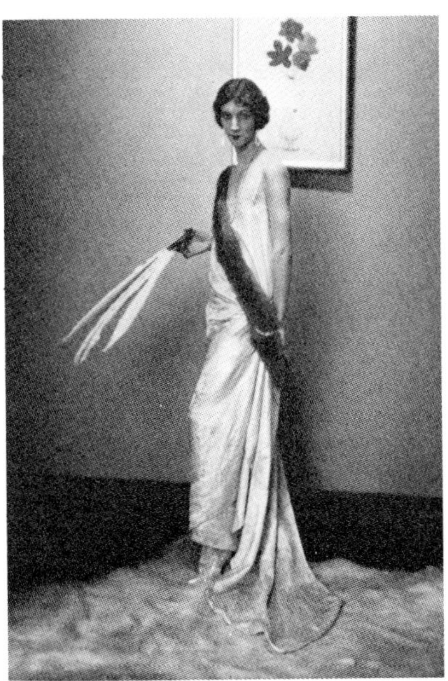

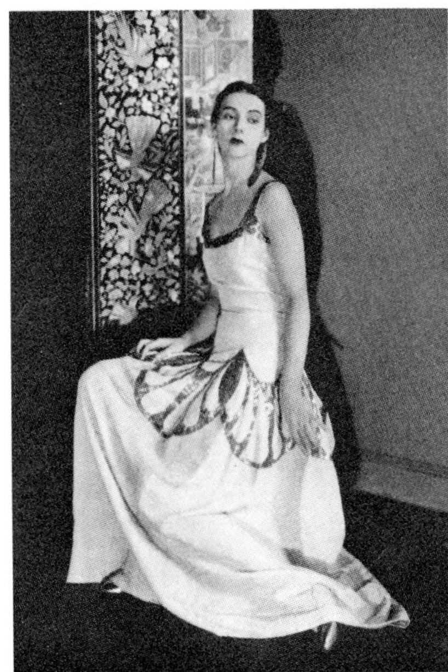

Sumurun at the *Bal de Petits Lits Blancs*

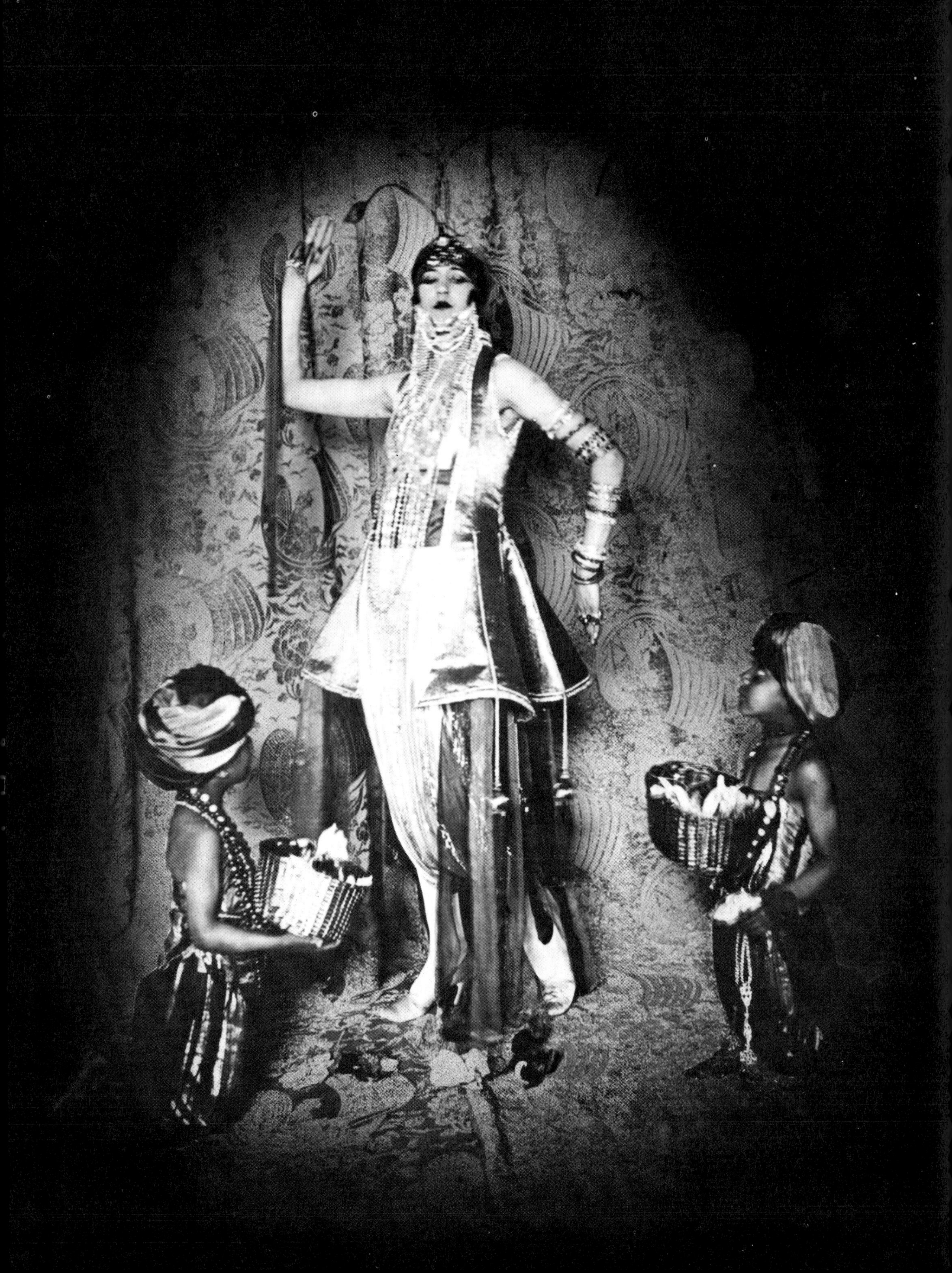

a showgirl in *The Bing Boys* during the war, but gave up the stage to work for Molyneux as a mannequin. Molyneux, at that time, was employed by Lucile as her designer, and both he and Lucile created some clothes by designing and draping them on Vera. When Molyneux decided to open his own fashion salon in Paris, he asked Vera Ashby to join him as his head mannequin, but, since he considered that her name, Vera, was too plain, he re-christened her Sumurun.

'I went to a show at Molyneux', recalls the Queen's couturier, Sir Norman Hartnell. 'Sumurun was in a pink dress and coat and gave out a sort of vamp. I never thought she'd be working for me one day', but, much later, she was to be employed by Sir Norman as a vendeuse, until her retirement.

Sumurun worked with another model whose name was Constance, but as her name wouldn't do either, she became known as Hebe. 'She was half-English and half-French', says Vera Ashby, who is an attractive white-haired eighty year old today. 'She had lovely wavy brown hair, cut short. She was very beautiful and had the most marvellous eyes, rather like Princess Marina's, and like Princess Marina, too, she was very nervous and shy. Hebe married very well. She had "a friend", as they put it, for many years; a rich American called Arthur Kingsland. They finally married and went to live in America.'

'I remember Hebe', continued Sir Norman jovially. 'She wore a picture hat dripping with lilac and wisteria, and she was sozzled all the time!'

Sumurun was later described as 'enchantress of the desert, the world's most famous mannequin, courted and fêted by many men, proposed to by at least a score'.

Sumurun herself remembers being taken to dinner in private rooms just by the Madeleine in the rue Royale: 'Those were the grand days of fashion shows, but there was no money in it, and modelling was considered very fast and loose in France. We were not received in society, but the young men adored to be seen out with us. I was always out. I went everywhere. I lived in a hotel bedroom, and a cheap one at that, but Captain Molyneux lent me beautiful clothes to wear. Sometimes they were

sewn on to me and I'd have to unpick myself before going to bed.

'I suppose I was such a success with the boys because of the clothes Captain Molyneux used to lend me. I was the "rags to riches" girl of all time. I used to have four or five boys after me at a time. There was the Comte de-this and the Vicomte de-that. There was even a Duc among them, the Grand Duke Dimitri. Whatever mannequin or young woman was fashionable at the time, they always wanted her.

'I was the highest paid model in Paris, but even then the money was very poor, 3,500 francs a month—today, the equivalent would be £50 to £100 a month. I lived in a nice little hotel attic room in the Rond Point, but it was really a come-down after all my marvellous evenings at all the best places. We went to the races, to the South of France, to Deauville, saw everything, but I was a working girl and was always very poor. I remember one winter when I really didn't have a coat warm enough for me. In France it was considered that you had to have someone "looking after you". The French girls used to say, "Well, haven't you found anyone yet?"'

During the twenties, the *Bal de petits lits blancs* (ball of the little white beds), in aid of a children's charity, used to be held in Paris, whereas these days it is held in the South of France. Mannequins from the top couture houses were dressed by the famous couturiers as a spectacular finale. Sumurun, as Molyneux's head mannequin, had pride of place, and entered last. 'I wore an exotic costume, in golds and rich oriental colours, encrusted with jewels. There was another large jewel in my turban. These little jewels had little electric light bulbs in the centre connected to a battery which was concealed on me. I was preceded by two little black boys who scattered rose petals for me to walk on. At a certain point the lights were lowered, and I pressed the battery-light. All the jewels on my costume and my turban lit up, and there was such excitement among the aristocracy and famous, that they rushed forward to gather up the rose petals strewn before me.'

'Marion Morehouse was the greatest fashion model I ever photographed', said Edward Steichen of the model he

photographed for *Vogue* in New York in the twenties. 'Miss Morehouse was no more interested in fashion as fashion than I was. But when she put on the clothes that were to be photographed, she transformed herself into a woman who really would wear that gown or riding habit, or whatever the outfit was.' She was also frequently photographed by three other great photographers who had begun working in Paris in the twenties—Cecil Beaton, Horst, and Hoyningen-Heune.

One of the most famous models in thirties' Paris was Swedish-born Lisa Fonsagrieves, whose first and second husbands were photographers. She was

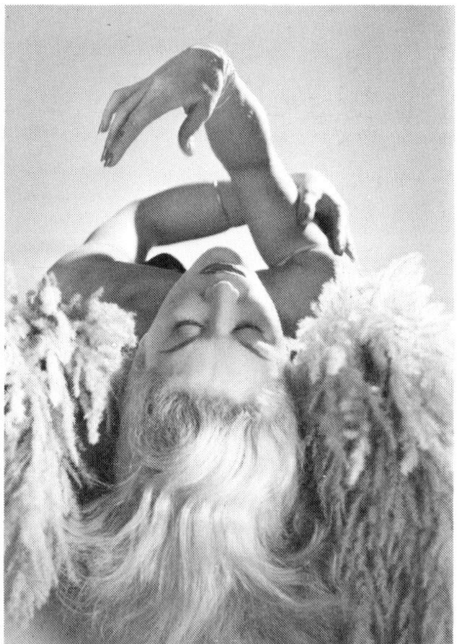

Lisa Fonsagrieves, photographed in Paris by Horst, 1939

a fine model, sweet and adorable. 'The only trouble with her,' Horst recalls, 'was those days we had those big cameras, and the exposure took a second or two. And she always shook. She couldn't stand still! But she was divine, and always turned up. Some of those girls just didn't turn up. There were no model agents to complain to.'

Lisa Fonsagrieves continued her successful modelling career into the forties, later marrying the great photographer, Irving Penn.

Horst's admiration is shared between Lisa Fonsagrieves and the Russian Princess Natasha Paley whom he believes to be related to the last Tsar. With the advent of the Revolution, her family settled in Paris, and she completed her education in Switzerland.

She later returned to Paris where she

met and married the great couturier Lucien Lelong. Her second husband, the late John C. Wilson, was an American, Noël Coward's business partner and life-long friend. Preferring to be known as Mrs John C. Wilson, she has now settled in New York.

'She had such elegance', Horst enthuses. 'We walked into Maxims, which at that time was in its prime, and everyone turned to look at her. The elegance and noblesse! She was astonishing, sweet and charming at the same time.'

In the thirties, as in these days, the top models were anything but French. Although the French models were ravishingly beautiful, and very smart, they had short legs and large behinds. 'The American girls had this beautiful long line', Horst said, 'and were free and easy, like the Germans and Swedes. There were some good English girls like Mickey Hood, but they didn't move. At that time they were taught to stand erect, very lady-like. They were

too inhibited.' Today they move more.

Both Beaton and Horst photographed another great model of the thirties, the Russian-born Lud, who was discovered by Horst. She was a penniless young messenger girl by the name of Ludmilla who lived on a barge with her brother. One day she delivered some dresses to Horst at the *Vogue* studios in Paris, and the photographer, thinking that she was marvellous looking, persuaded her to pose for him. When Condé Nast, the owner of *Vogue*, saw the photographs, he told Horst that he did not want her. Her nose was too short, and she didn't look like a lady. Horst, however, continued to photograph her, and then Mr Nast fell madly in love with her, and wanted to marry her. War broke out, and Horst joined the army. When he returned to Paris, he found that she had married a lion-tamer in a circus instead. 'One night at a party given by Molyneux', Horst added, 'Schiaparelli came up and said to me, "You can't have Lud.

No. No. No. She is mine, now."' She had hired Lud to model her clothes, and didn't want her photographed any longer.

Among the other models in Paris in the thirties, the American models who worked consistently were Helen Bennett, Anne Weatherburn, Betty MacLaughlin, Bettina Jones and Muriel Maxwell. A German girl, Agnetta Fisher, who lived in Paris, was considered very good too, as well as another German girl whose name was Muth.

Muth had married a Jewish boy in Germany and, when Hitler came to power, they escaped to Paris where Muth became George Hoyningen-Huene's favourite model. However, her husband was killed by the Nazis when they got to Paris—and Muth was killed by the French. In order to protect her Jewish husband in German-occupied Paris, Muth had fraternised with the Germans, and became the mistress of one of the German officers. She was a

Right: The great Russian model, Lud, photographed by Horst in Paris, 1936

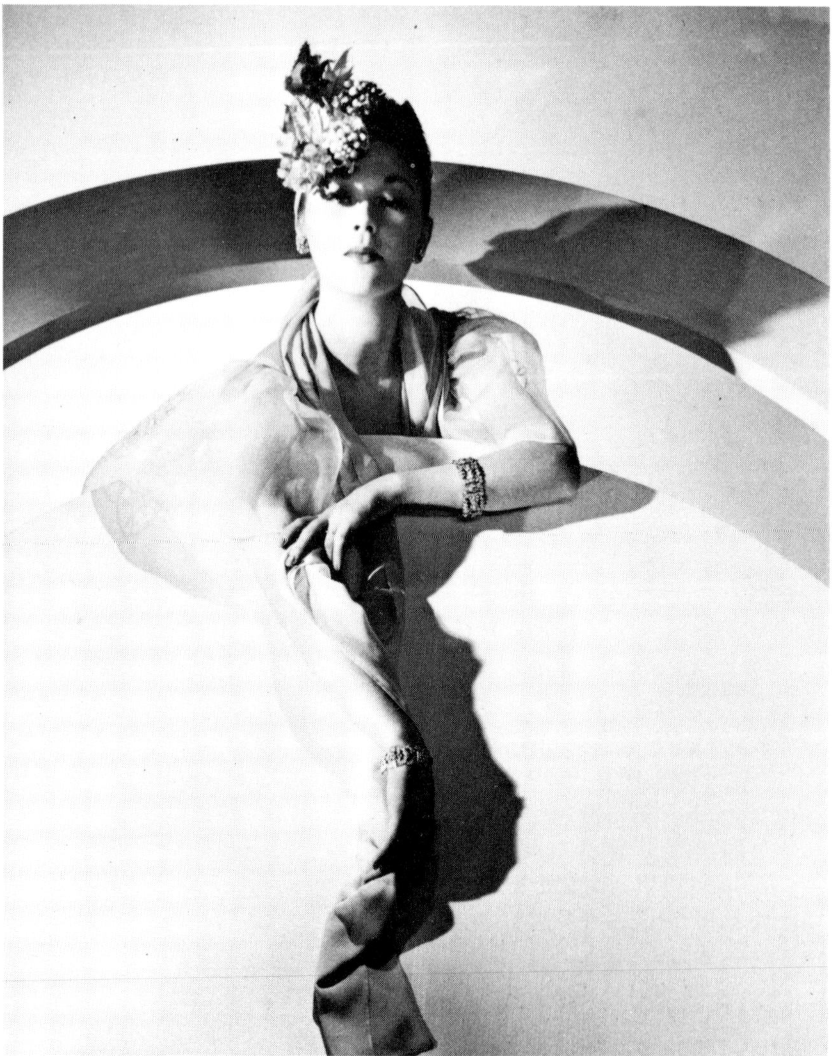

Opposite: Princess Natasha Paley, photographed by Hoyningen-Huene in New York, 1934 (Copyright: Condé Nast Publications Inc)

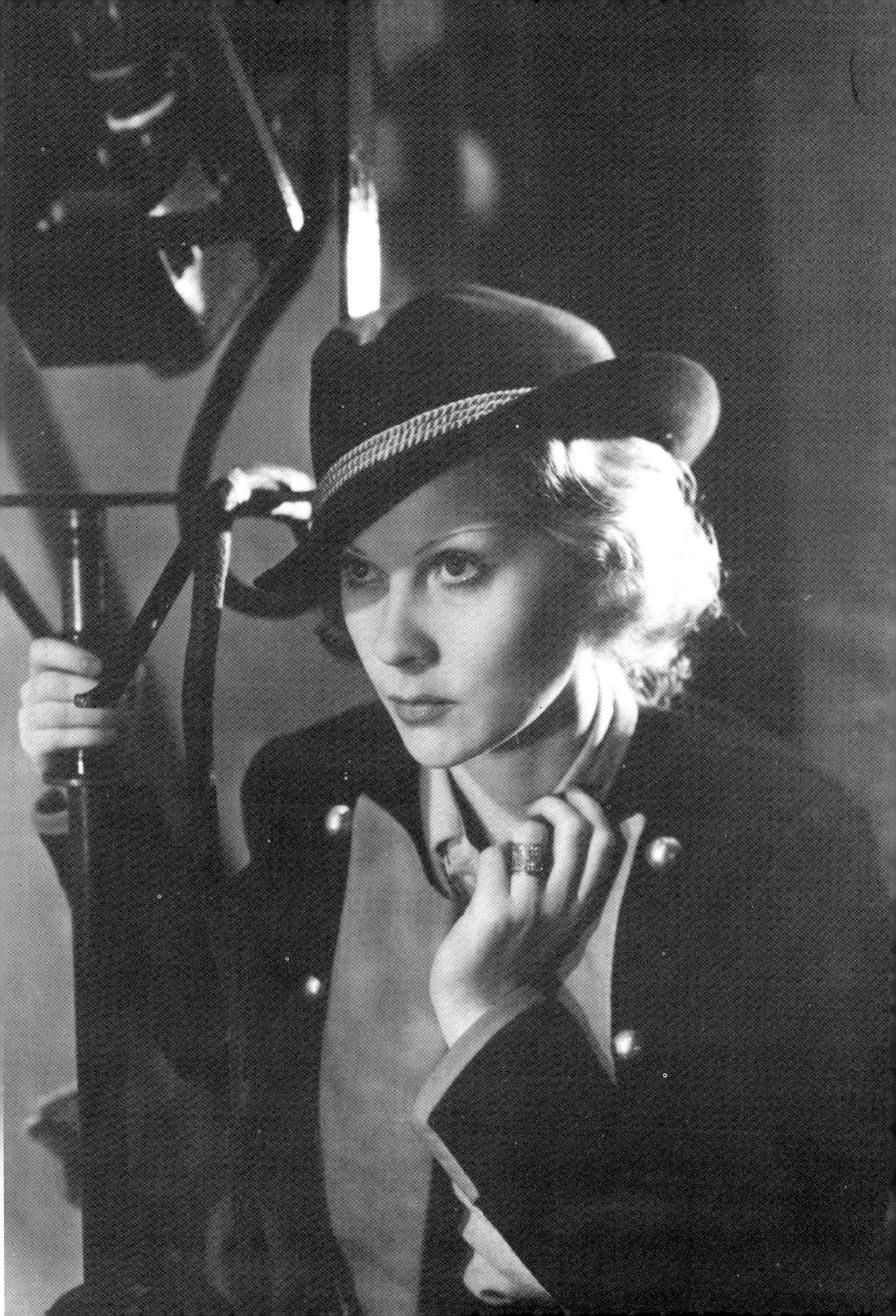

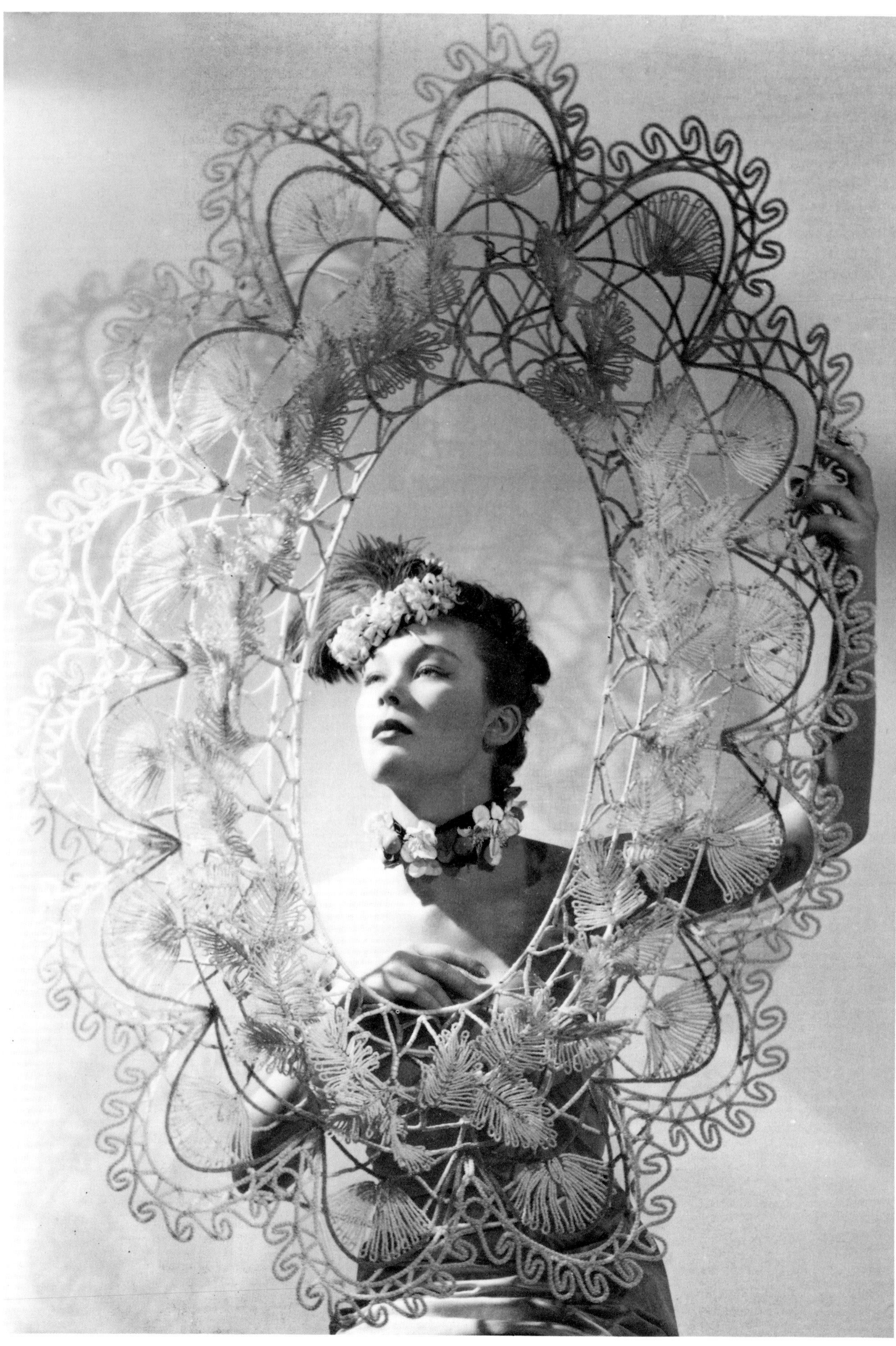

Opposite: Another photograph of
Lud, this time by Cecil Beaton

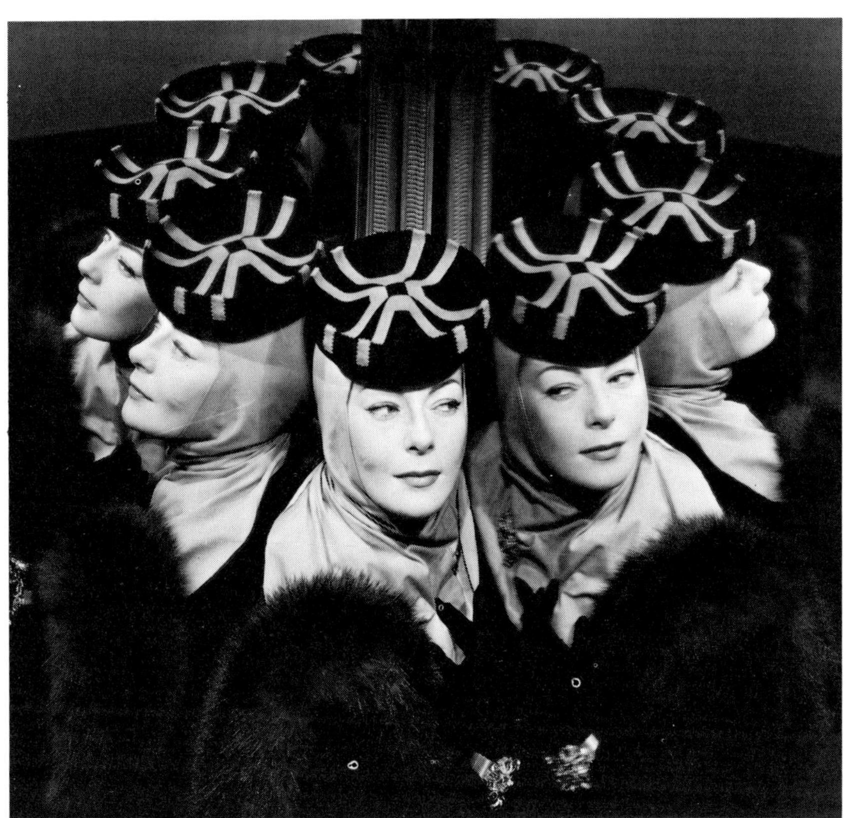

Right: Muriel Maxwell, photographed by Horst in New York, 1940

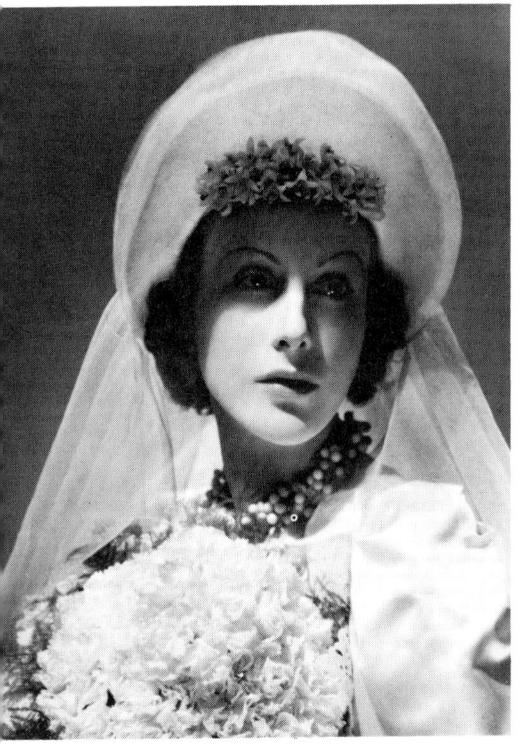

Above: Cora Hemmet, taken by
Hoyningen-Huene in Paris, 1934
(Copyright: Horst)

Right: Helen Bennett, by Horst, in
New York, 1938

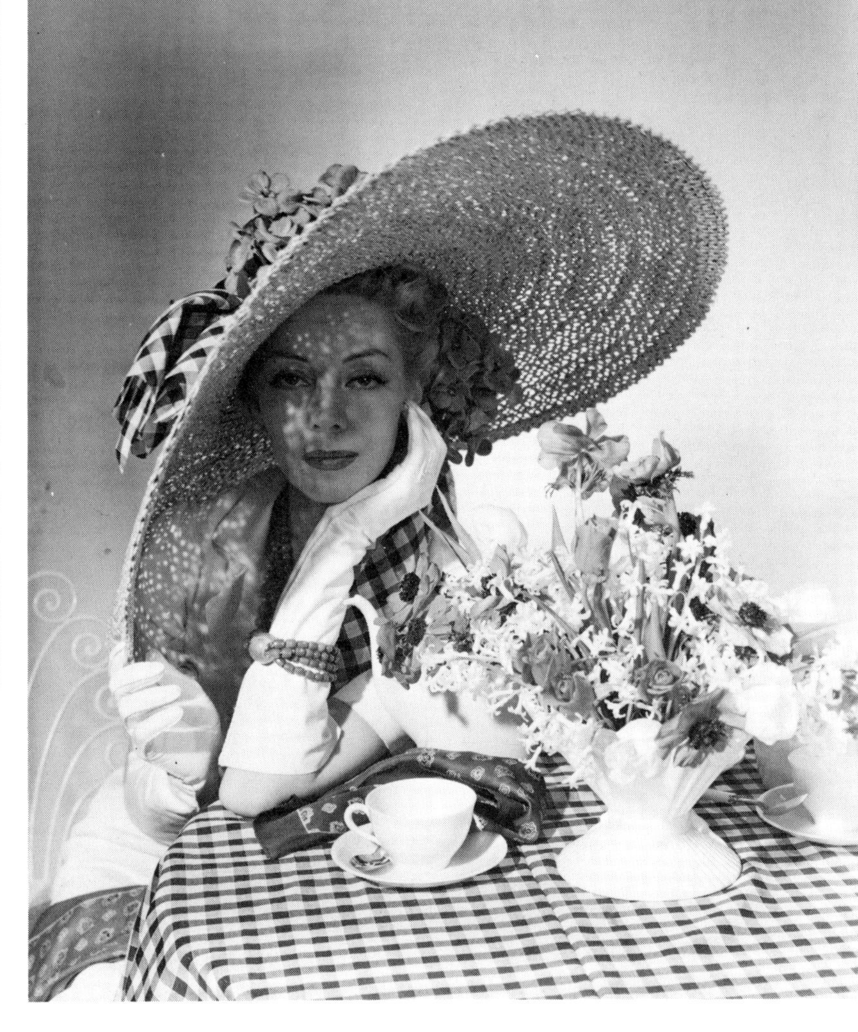

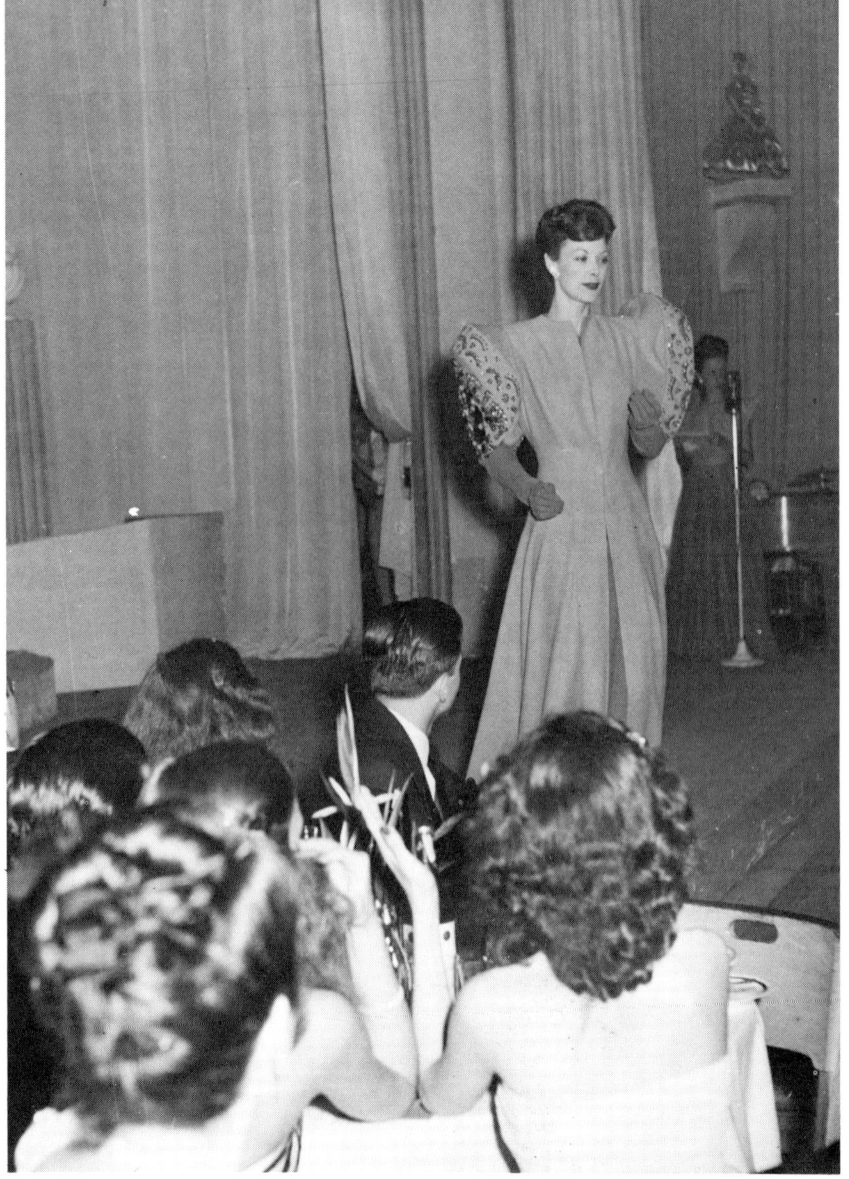

Below: Iris Lockwood showing Norman Hartnell's collection in Buenos Aires, 1946. Photograph by Kurt Paul Klagsbrunn

Opposite: Toto Koopman, photographed by Hoyningen-Huene in Paris, 1934 (Copyright: Horst)

sweet girl, and frequently took food and stockings to the secretaries at *Vogue*, secured through her lover; but she was careless. The German officer discovered the identity of her husband, and the French Resistance discovered her liaison with the Nazi officer.

The half-Dutch, half-Indonesian model Toto Koopman was another favourite of Hoyningen-Huene's. She had a marvellous elegance, and was extremely popular about town. She lives in London these days, assisting in the running of an art gallery.

Of the English models working in London in the thirties, Iris Lockwood, who later married impresario Robert Nesbitt, was photographed by Cecil Beaton, Horst, John Rawlings, John Everard, and Peter Clark. 'In those days they used the most enormous sort of camera with three slides that went through, and you had to keep still the entire time', recalls Iris Lockwood. 'You couldn't move between the three shots otherwise the picture would be out of focus. Often we had what was called a "model-stand". It was a stand with a bar across which was shaped so that it went into your waist, and as long as you had it there, you knew whether you were still or not.' Iris Lockwood, however, was a showgirl in the theatre, an ex-Cochran Young Lady, and like Joan Richards and Tarlin, who were on the stage as well, did modelling as a sideline.

Irene Williams, who modelled at trade shows, was 'bridesmaid' for five years running, until 1934, when she married and gave up modelling. Lorna Sinclair was another girl who modelled at the Ideal Home Exhibition occasionally, and Dorothy Walker modelled dresses for the larger sizes, working from the thirties through to the fifties. She had been a Gaiety Girl at one time and knew how to handle her audience. 'Beautiful and elegant', recalls fashion entrepreneur Michael Whittaker. 'She knew how to get the applause, and if she didn't, she'd wait until she did. Everybody waiting to go on would wait for the applause, and say, "Dorothy hasn't got it yet. *Wait*." And then the dressing room would go silent until the applause rang out, and everyone backstage would shout, "She's done it!" And then the show would go on.'

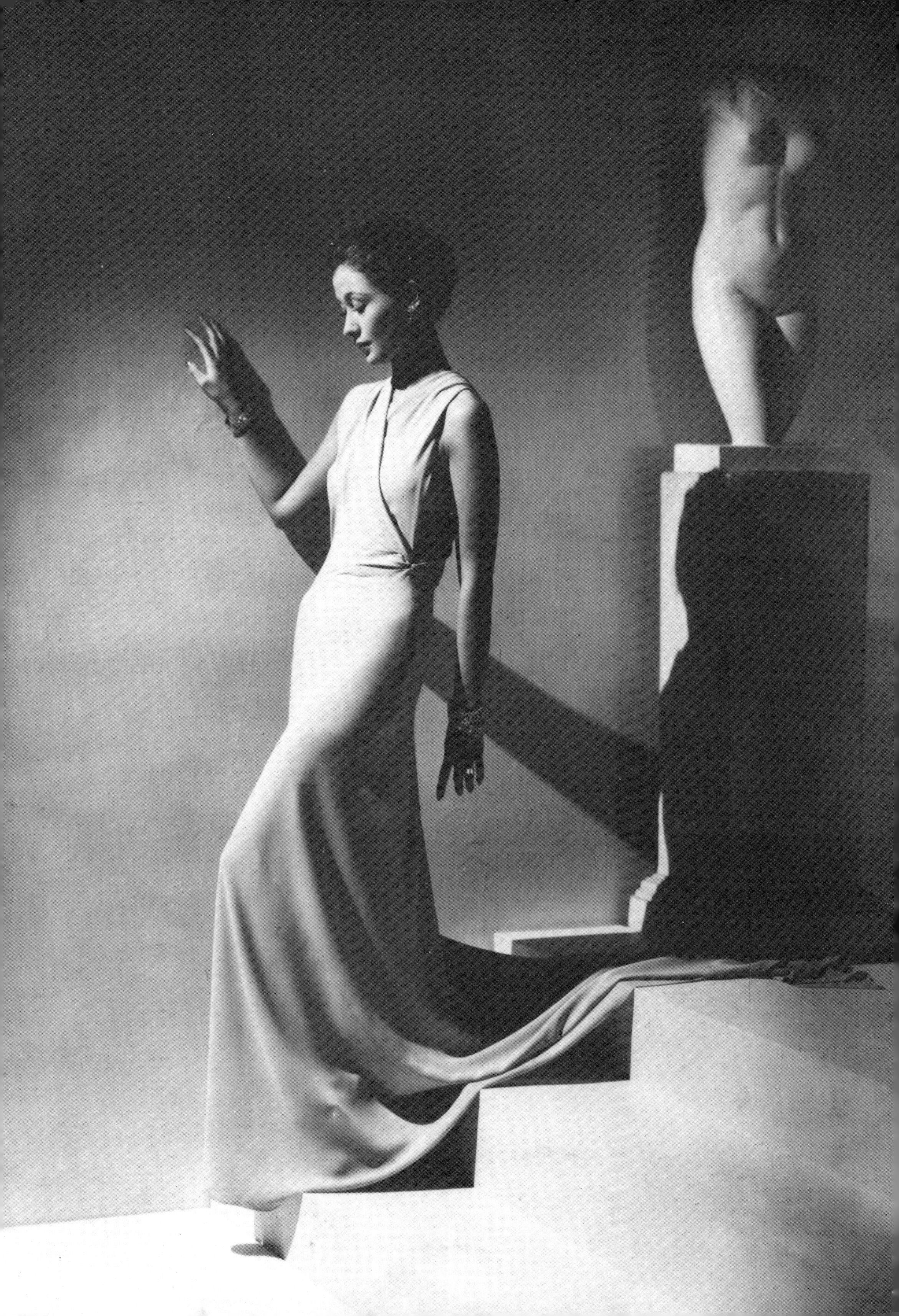

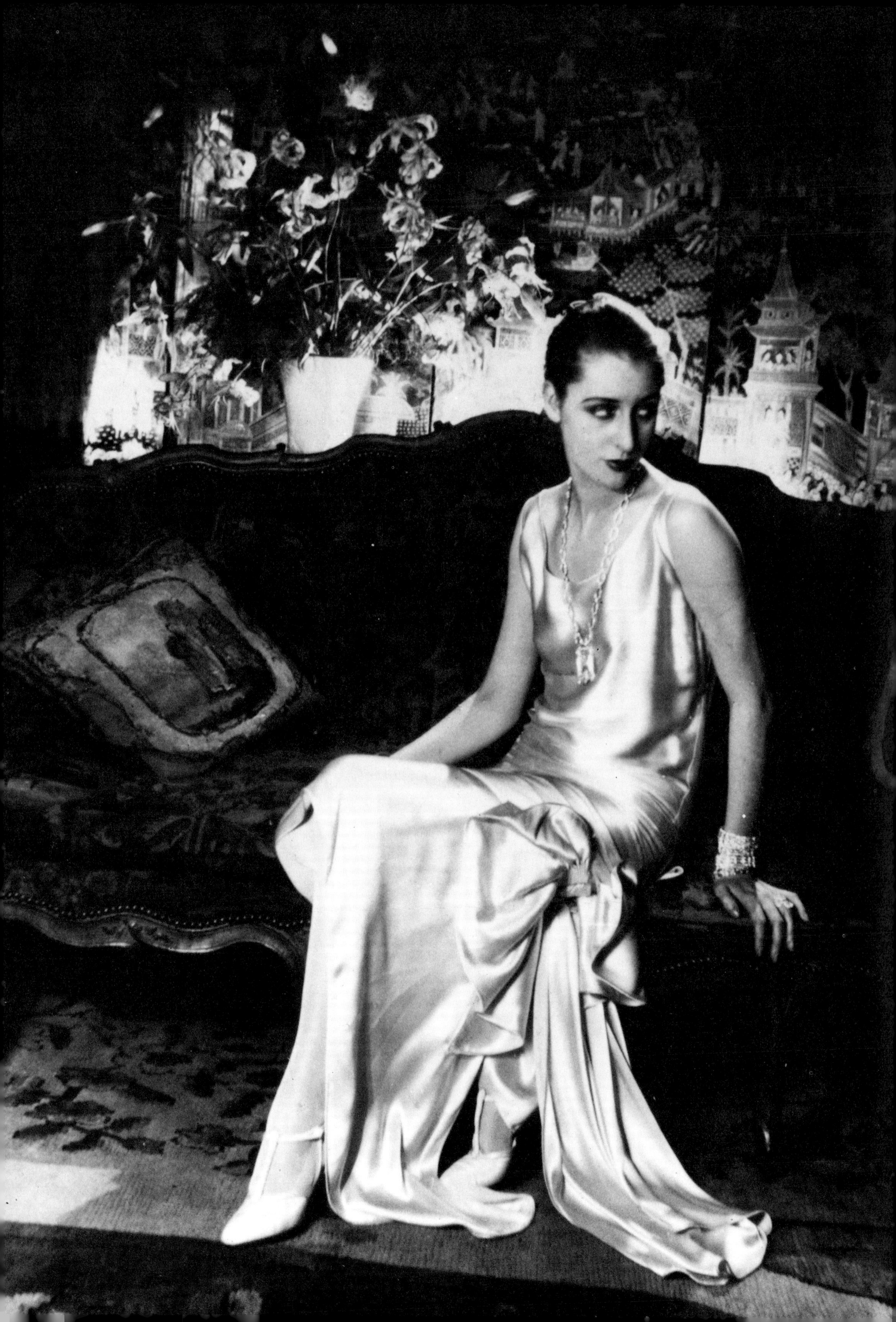

Lilly Christine was another famous model in 1938, together with Irene Williams and Penny Gillard, who continued working in the forties and fifties.

'Penny was a tremendously hard worker', recalls Michael Whittaker. 'She did a show for Princess Muna in the morning at Ronald Paterson's, and then another show from one to two o'clock at Marshall and Snelgroves Restaurant, rushed along to do the Matita Collection in the afternoon at three and four-fifteen, and then hurried along to do a show for the Queen at Norman Hartnell's afterwards.' These days she works as one of the top managers for Wallis dress shops in Marble Arch.

Whittaker's mother, Elsa Whittaker, was another well known model in the thirties and forties. She was a maturer woman, and did photographic as well as show modelling. 'Even though, like all English women, she was pear-shaped', says Whittaker, meaning she had narrow shoulders and wide hips.

Other well known models in London in the thirties included Hannerli Dane, Jane Chorley, Joan Francis, Isabel Babianska, Jill Pengilly, and Audine Honey.

Throughout the thirties, however, modelling was not regarded as a full-time profession by the few girls who worked, but more like a pin-money job for part-time actresses. Merle Oberon, too, modelled periodically in the days before she became Lady Korda, and afterwards the wife of the Mexican multi-millionaire Bruno Pagliai, and more recently wife of Dutch-born American actor Rob Wolders.

In 1932, Edward Steichen even managed to get Marlene Dietrich before his camera in New York, wearing a black feathered hat. 'The first time I photographed Marlene Dietrich, the job was supervised by Joseph von Sternberg', complained Steichen. 'The Sternberg-Dietrich method of working was a sort of Svengali-Trilby arrangement. She never would pose for anybody unless Sternberg was present, watching and telling her what to do. That afternoon, I had spent two hours and made about forty exposures, but I was not getting anywhere. Finally, I resorted to pretending I had taken a picture and then trying to steal a shot, for, the moment I was through with a picture, Miss Dietrich relaxed and commenced to talk and was really quite charming. But under Sternberg's gaze she was about as exciting as a wooden cigar-store Indian.'

Other successful models of the thirties who continued working into the fifties were Julie Beresford, who was elected 'Miss Art in Commerce' and also 'Miss Venus' in 1936, Eleanor MacDonald, an outdoor type, a champion fencer who specialised in health and beauty studies, and Peggy Chester who, perhaps, was the most familiar face from the past. Starting as a mannequin in Schiaparelli's London salon in 1937, she then had a ten-year run as top model and cover girl of the era, during which time she must have worn more knitting-pattern sweaters than Lana Turner ever dreamed was possible.

The late, long-legged, musical comedy star Hy Hazell began her career as a model in the thirties, as Hyacinth Higgins, and Evelyn Spilsbury, daughter of the late Sir Bernard Spilsbury, graduated from modelling to running her own model agency. Katie Hinton was the outstanding John French photographic model of 1939.

The glamour of the thirties was brought to an end by World War II. France was occupied, while in Britain the emphasis on total war brought drabness and a growing revulsion for fashion by design rather than by desire. Not only were materials and embellishments impossible to obtain, but they were also forbidden by law after the war. The occasions at which to wear them became non-existent; neither opera, ballet, diplomatic receptions or theatrical parties were the order of the day.

'I had collections during wartime', recalls Sir Norman Hartnell, 'but the Board of Trade instructed us to show utility clothes. We were terribly restricted. Embroidery was immoral and pleats were forbidden.'

Postwar austerity was quickly transformed by Dior with his famous New Look in 1947 that captivated the world and made his name a household word overnight. Never had a designer's name become instantly known to so many outside the fashion world and society hostesses' drawing rooms before.

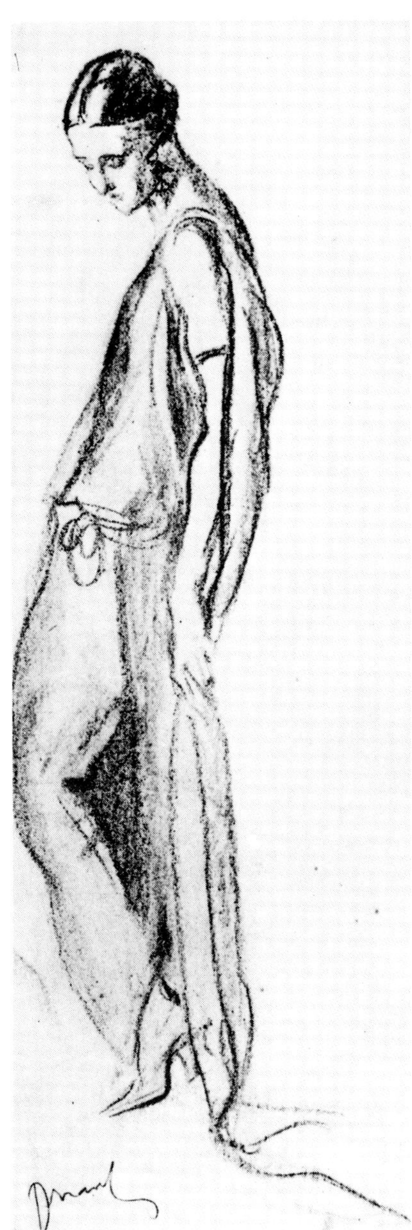

Above: A drawing of Sumurun by Drian

Below: Gertrude Lawrence, Noël
Coward's great leading lady, as
she appeared in the role of Amanda
in the original production of
Private Lives, 1930

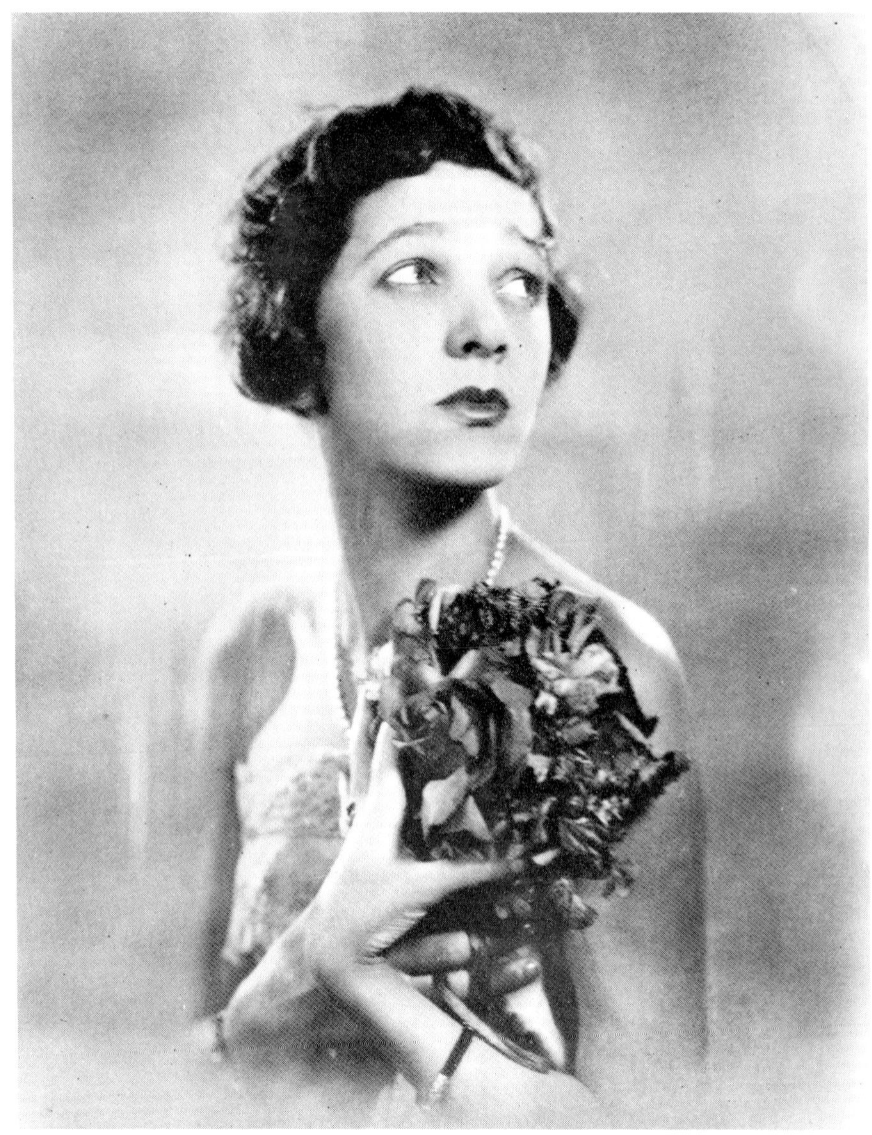

Opposite: Marlene Dietrich, by
Edward Steichen in New York,
1932

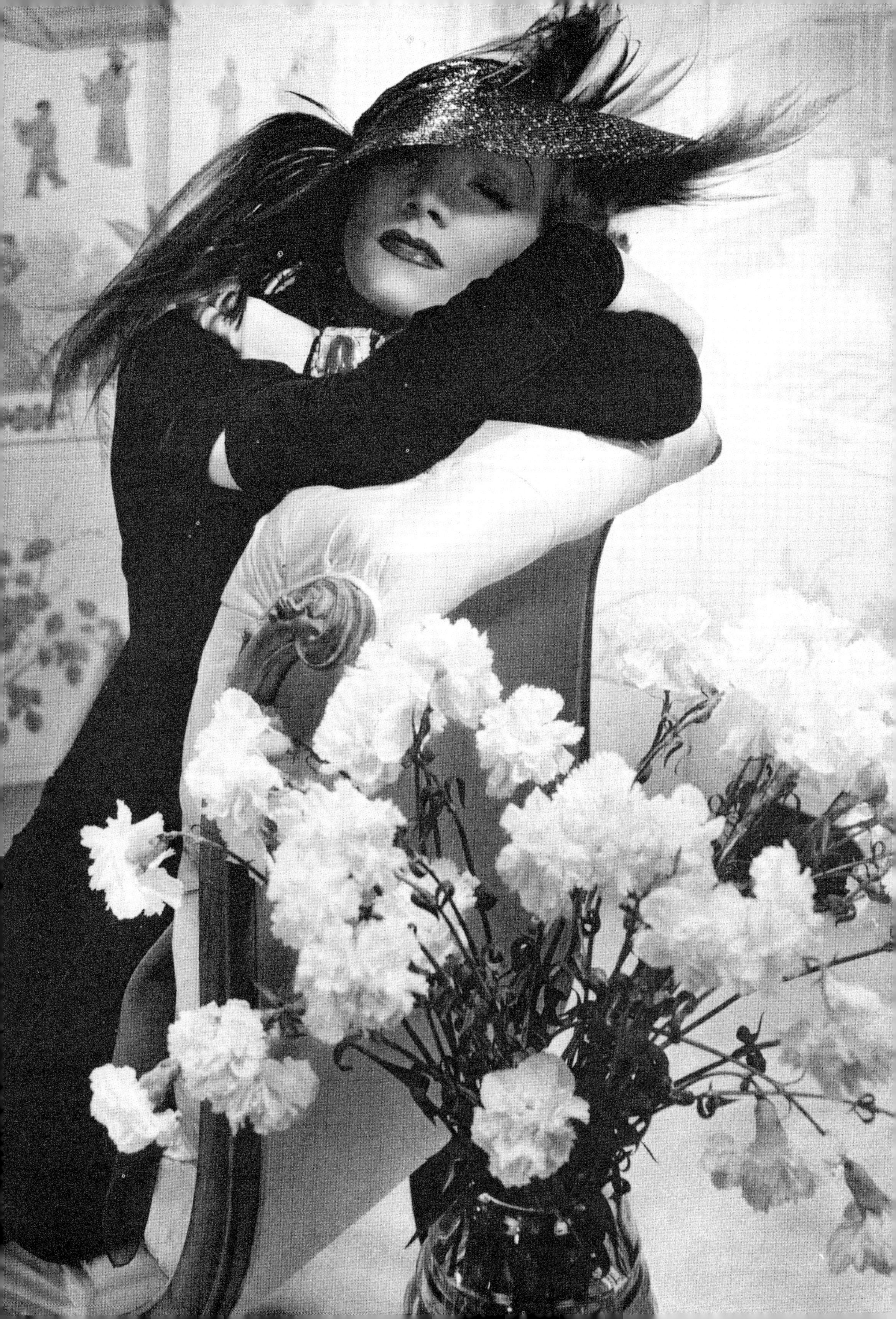

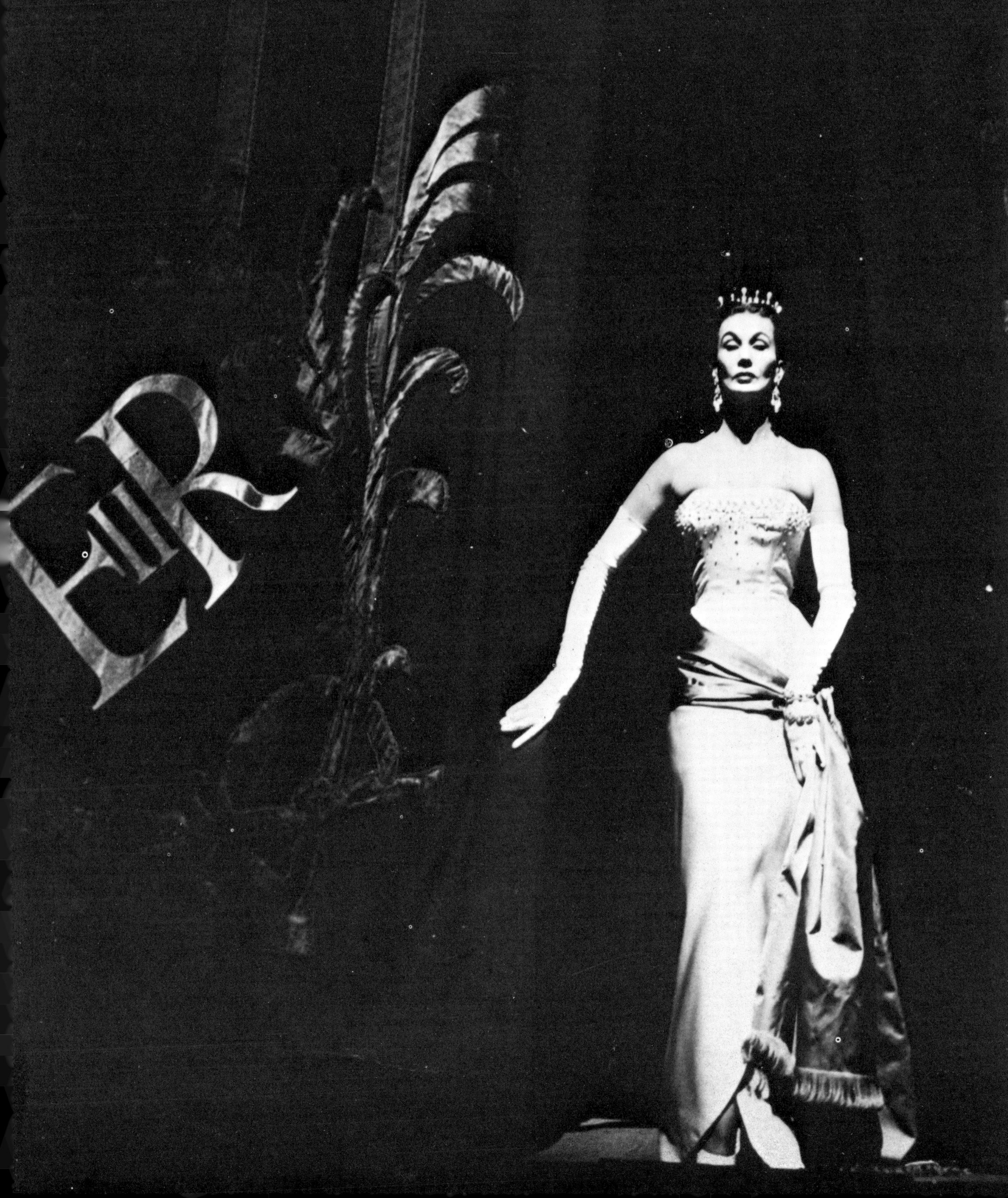

Blossoming Fifties

Mannequins had shown the creations of the great couturiers since 1852, but it only came to be considered a profession for ladies in the 1950s, a century later. Suddenly, English models, with their haughty look, cultured backgrounds, and elegant turn-out, began marrying into the peerage; they were, at long last, not only accepted by society, but welcomed into it.

Whereas modern fashion, and as a consequence the model girls, has had to move with the times, developing rapidly over the past three decades, World War II seemed to provide the first great stimulus for change. Ernestine Carter is one of the most widely influential fashion writers of recent times. Her career has included posts as a curator at the Museum of Modern Art in New York, and on the editorial side of *Harpers Bazaar* and *The Sunday Times*. She suggests that just as the thirties ended abruptly with the advent of war, the forties, in the sense of civilian life, did not really begin fashion-wise until 1947, with the debut of Christian Dior and his New Look.

With the rebirth of haute couture in the fifties after wartime austerity came a demand for glamorous models to show the new and exciting creations. Whilst Paris led the field in fashion, America provided some of the best models who were photographed in these new and wonderful clothes. American models such as Lisa Fonsagrieves, Dorian Leigh, Suzy Parker, Jean Patchett, Sunny Harnett, Dovima, Carmen, and Dolores Hawkins dominated the fashion modelling scene in New York in the fifties.

The fifties in Britain boasted a handful of leading models, namely Barbara Goalen, Anne Gunning, Fiona Campbell-Walter, Sue Abrahams, and Shelagh Wilson, but these did not achieve the same international recognition as their American sisters, with the possible exceptions of Goalen, Gunning, and Campbell-Walter. They were, however, photographic models as opposed to show models.

There is a broad distinction between photographic and show models—the money they are paid being the least of it. Whereas these days a photographic model in Paris doing an editorial for *Vogue* is paid 300 francs a day, the show model might be paid that same figure for a week's work, in one of the top salons. It was rare for dresses to be photographed on the show models, the girls employed by the large couture houses, because they were seldom photogenic and photographers had little time to acquaint themselves with models they did not know. Bronwen Pugh, for instance, the Welsh-born model who reigned as Balmain's top model, was rarely photographed. Whilst she was supreme on the cat-walk, photographers found her doe-eyed looks and angular proportions too exaggerated for readers of *Vogue* and *Harpers Bazaar* who could hardly identify with the individuality of this exceptional model. The famous French model, Bettina, on the other hand, was highly regarded as both a photographic *and* show model.

Photographers who were sent along by the top glossies arrived for the collections with their pet models who knew how to pose for them. They had to work quickly because the clothes had to be photographed out of business hours as they were needed for the buyers during the daytime. This is, of course still the case nowadays, but with the demise of the high-fashion tradition and the rapid rise of *prêt à porter*, or ready to wear, the pressures and prizes aren't as great. The photographers and their models worked into the early hours—closely supervised by fashion editors, who selected the clothes and chose the accessories to be photographed, with runners from the studios calling for the dresses from the fashion house, to be photographed and returned by morning. There used to be a month-long embargo on the reproduction of the couturiers' original designs in the press, in order to prevent piracy, or copying, and it was estimated that, within a month of the collections, the buyers would have made their selections and had the orders made up and delivered into the shops before copiers could beat the couturiers at their own game. Since the monthlies *Vogue* and *Harpers Bazaar* took so long to get into the bookstalls because of the time it took to print their magazines, this embargo hardly affected them in the same way as the dailies and weeklies.

The best known of all British models in the fifties, the first to give the profession prestige and the first to become a celebrity, heralded by the press as *La Goalen*, was Barbara Goalen. Her well bred, haughty look gave an aristocratic air to modelling, and women, for the first time, identified the fabulous clothes she showed with the model. She gave the impression that the Balenciaga and Norman Hartnell creations in which she was photographed actually belonged to her, rather than to the houses for whom she was selling them.

'I happened to be the right shape at the right time. I weighed 105lb and my measurements were 33–18–31', says Barbara Goalen. 'I always did high fashion and I never touched anything that wasn't top quality', she continued, 'because in those days if you *did*, you were finished. You had to be very careful of your image. At one time I would only be photographed by John French, who was one of the best. But the worst of it was that the glossies paid you nothing; I was the highest paid model and I got only five guineas an hour. At *Vogue*, I used to get only two guineas a day! So you never made any money out of it.

'However, they were vintage years. One was treated like a queen. We were taken everywhere in chauffeur-driven Rolls. I loved every minute of it, so much so that I dreaded the weekends. I longed for it all to start again on the Monday!'

This photograph by John French, of Barbara Goalen and male model Tommy Kyle, revolutionised fashion photographic techniques when it appeared in the *Daily Express* in April 1950

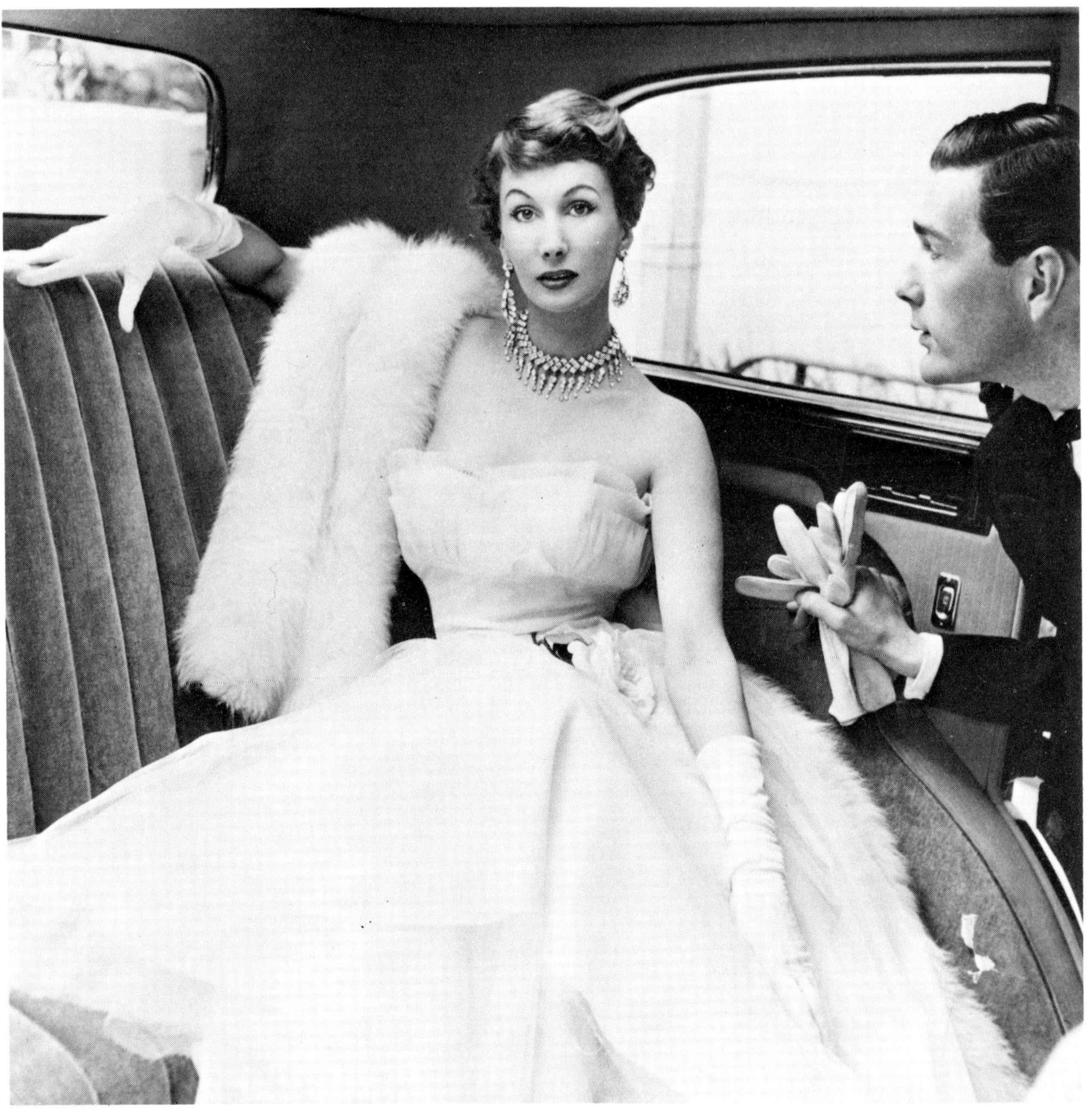

Surprisingly, although Barbara Goalen became one of the world's best known models, she worked for only five years before retiring at her peak. Her greatest contribution to modelling was when she and John French revolutionised fashion photography. 'Fashion, in the daily newspapers', Barbara Goalen continued, 'had always been rather static and hard in presentation from the photographic point of view. But we really put the type of photography that we did in the *glossies* into the *Daily Express* and revolutionised the whole concept, because they had never seen anything like it before in the dailies. They thought the photographs would be too soft on the paper—but they weren't.

'One of the high points of my career was being sent to Paris to be photographed for *Vogue* for the French collections. It was quite an honour because I was the first English girl to be sent by *Vogue*.

'People always used to say I was snooty, but I'm not a bit. It was the image that I seemed to create from the camera's point of view. Even when I was seventeen, my friends used to say, "Oh, beside you, we feel like country cousins!"'

'Barbara was very professional', said Paris-based American photographer Henry Clarke, 'and she had an innate sense of chic. For example, when we were doing clothes for an advert, terrible little shirt-like dresses, and Barbara could make them look marvellous. You put the dress on Barbara and she made it sing. She knew the angles, how to make this thing really live!'

'Barbara was one of those extraordinary people', confided Richard Dormer who photographed her many times, and who became associate editor on *Harpers Bazaar* for five years. 'The first time I met her, we got on like a house on fire, and I think Barbara made me a photographer. I think the best pictures I took at that time of my life were of Barbara. That was about 1954 when Barbara was at the top. She was *the Vogue* model. She was terribly amusing, and had the most fabulous sense of clothes; and this is very important with a model. Unless they really like wearing clothes, and, as their job, can make anything look good, then they

can't make it. She used to wear some ghastly creations, but she had the knack of making everything look terrific. And this is a gift.'

This is what makes modelling a career. It isn't enough to have a pretty face and stand like a stick. What is necessary is a sort of star quality; to click in front of the camera; then something happens.

'You wouldn't look at a lot of these models before they've got their faces on', Dormer laughed. 'You simply wouldn't think many of the top models I've worked with were models before they've gone into the dressing room and started making up.'

One of the essentials of an interesting face is large, expressive eyes. There are few female film stars, for instance, with tiny eyes; the possible exceptions being Norma Shearer, Greer Garson, and Barbra Streisand, but, for the most part, big stars tend to have large eyes. Witness Joan Crawford, Bette Davies, Greta Garbo, Vivien Leigh, Elizabeth Taylor, and Liza Minnelli. But Richard Dormer believes that this does not apply to model girls: 'Barbara didn't have very large eyes, but she knew how to make them up. Quite a few models don't have big eyes, but by the time they're made up, the eyes become very big—that's part of their craft. It was easier in the fifties, because artificial eyelashes were very much in fashion, and it was a much heavier make-up.'

'I went to Australia for a whole month, which fascinated me', Barbara Goalen continued. 'I did a one-woman tour and about two thousand people turned up at the store. I had to stand on the counters and just talk, ad-lib, to them, which I rather enjoyed. When I was in Sydney, it was like being the Queen. All the streets were lined with people. I just couldn't get through. My car had to be guided through. And when I got back to Britain, the same thing happened in the North of England and Scotland.'

With her cool looks it might be suggested that Barbara Goalen was a bit of a cold fish, caring for nothing but her beauty and her figure, but her haughty exterior belies her cosy nature. 'I had a lot of rough nights out', she confesses disarmingly. 'In fact I used to go dancing at the 400 until four in the

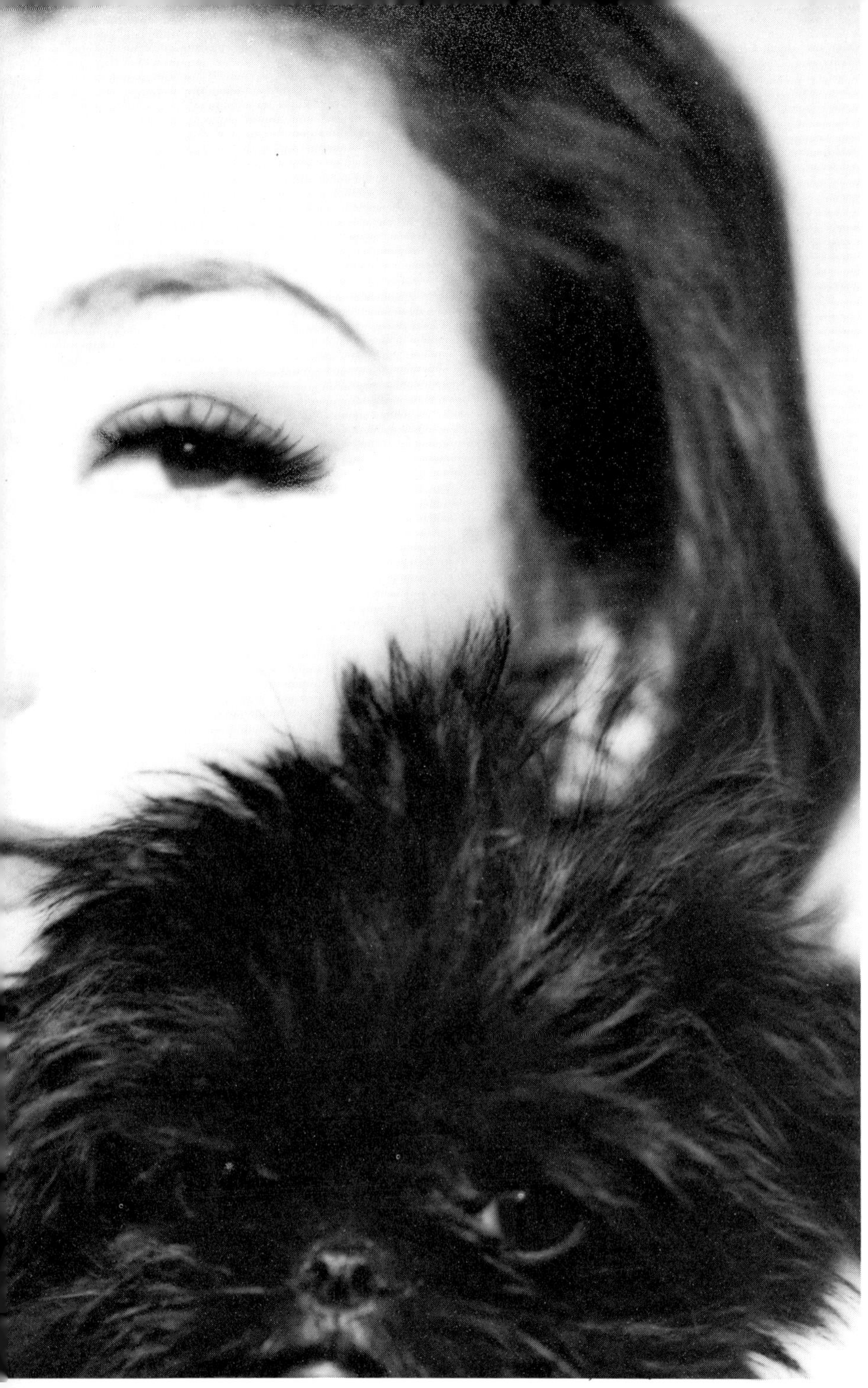

Florence was emerging through the fashions created by Pucci, Simonetta, Fabiani, and Galitzine, who were establishing themselves in Rome with Capucci close on their heels. Yves Saint Laurent, Dior's successor, whirled into the headlines with his Trapeze line, and the great names of fashion, Chanel, Fath, Piguet, Lelong, Schiaparelli, and Molyneux dropped into second league.

In Britain, the fifties saw top models catching top men with their haughty disdain; their aloof, striking looks appealed to politicians and aristocracy alike. Bronwen Pugh became Lady Astor; Fiona Campbell-Walter, Baroness Thyssen; Anne Cumming-Bell, the Duchess of Rutland; Shirley Worthington became Lady Royle; Jean Dawnay, Princess George Galitzine; and Nina Dyer, Princess Saddrudin Khan. Anne Gunning married Anthony Nutting and later became Lady Nutting, and, amongst lesser-known models, Jane McNeill was soon Countess of Dalkeith, now the Duchess of Buccleuch and Judith Roberts, Lady Birdwood.

If it could be said that Barbara Goalen's name is linked with photographer John French, Suzy Parker's with Richard Avedon, and Jean Shrimpton's with David Bailey, then Anne Gunning and Richard Dormer were the model/photographer partnership in the fifties to achieve success together. A great beauty, with extraordinary film-star features; high cheek-bones, a perfect profile, her face was faultless. She did, however, have rather large hands and feet, but she was well aware of her shortcomings and managed to conceal them with cunning care.

Anne Gunning's career as a model began by chance. She had neither given thought to, nor wished to, become a model. But one evening, whilst dining in a restaurant in the Kings Road, she was visited at her table by the American photographer Henry Clarke, who lived and worked in Paris but made periodic visits to London to work for English magazines. To her complete surprise, Anne, who was only eighteen, was asked whether she would be interested in being photographed for *Harpers* by Clarke. She agreed.

'Henry Clarke worked with me for about a week', said Anne Gunning, 'and was marvellous because he gave me

Anne Gunning, by Richard Dormer

morning and come back as high as a kite, and then I'd have to work the next day. But I was very lucky because I didn't get bags or dark circles under my eyes. It didn't show. It was pure luck. I combined business with pleasure very much! Sometimes I don't know how I managed to work at all, really! I was a terrible flirt. I feel I lived very hard and worked very hard. And as I get older, I'm damn glad I did, what's more!

'They were the happiest years of my life. I wouldn't have missed them for anything in the world. I feel I had a unique experience. A glorious time!'

Leading the modelling field, Barbara Goalen projected the fashion-house mannequin image. She didn't move very well, though, and, as her hips at thirty-one were too slender for stock-sized dresses, fashion photography became her forté. In fashion photography, the clothes can be pinned and pegged at the back to be made to fit.

Little had changed by 1957, although Dior promoted the new length of skirt. New names emerged. In 1950 Pierre Cardin opened his couture house followed by Givenchy in 1952. Though Paris was still the fashion leader,

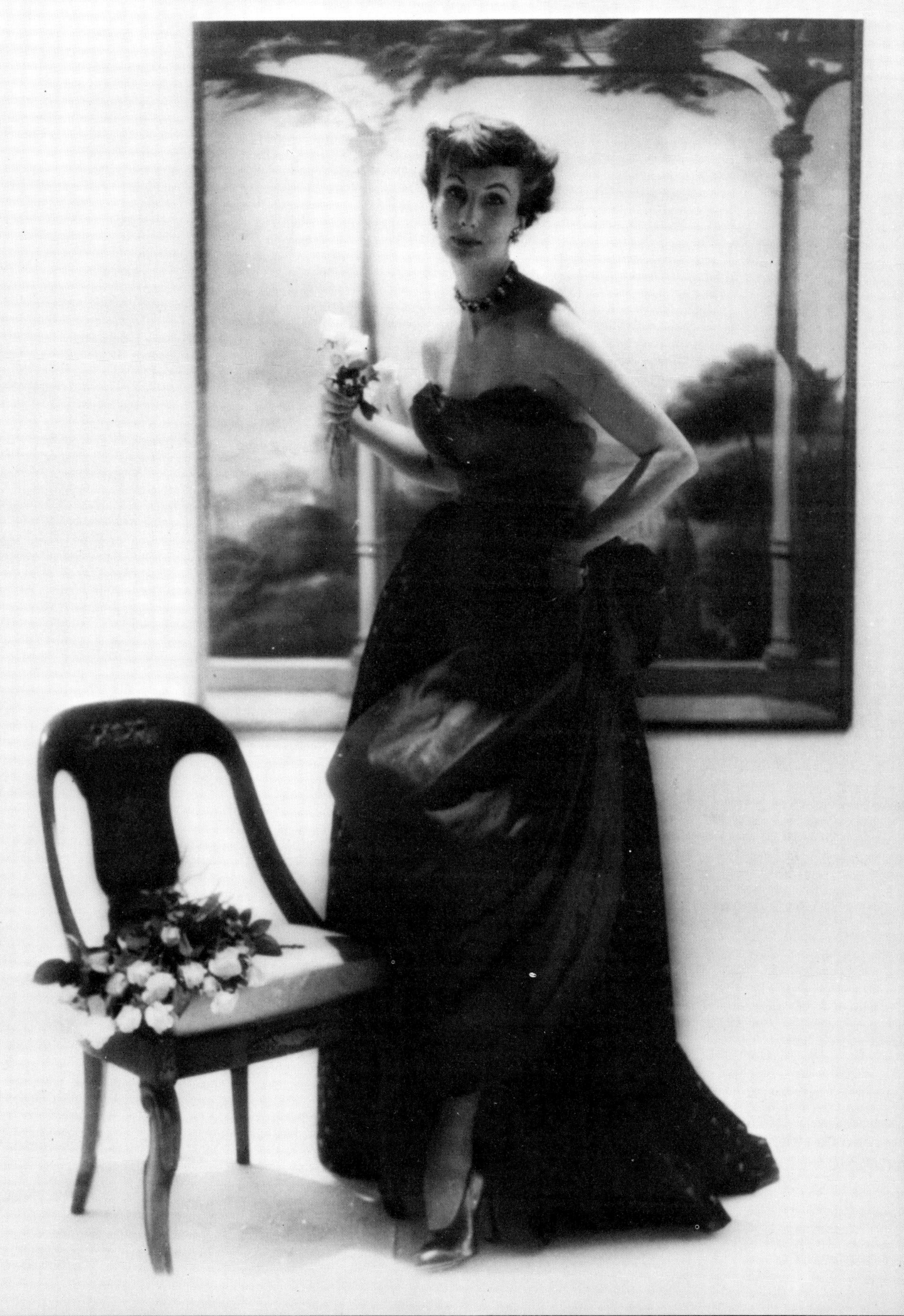

Barbara Goalen, who is married to Lloyds' underwriter Nigel Campbell, photographed by Richard Dormer for *Harpers Bazaar,* 1952

Right: Fiona Campbell-Walter at the height of her career. Photograph by Henry Clarke
Opposite: The beautiful Anne Gunning, who became Lady Nutting, in a photograph by John French

tremendous encouragement. Then I did an advertisement for Marshall and Snelgrove with John French, and his wife Vere recommended me to Richard Dormer; and from then on, I worked enormously with Dick. I felt I really "made it" when I started working for *Harpers*. But I was very lucky.

'I started bang off, no training, no model schools. And this was really due to meeting Henry and Dick, being taken up by two very, very good photographers. I didn't have to do that awful thing of taking my photographs around, knocking on studio doors for work. I could never have done that.'

Anne Gunning specialised in photographic modelling. The only time she did a fashion show was for Sybil Connolly as a favour, but she disliked doing it because it made her feel self-conscious. 'I used to panic about getting down to the end of that cat-walk, turn around and come back, without falling over. And that sea of faces glaring at me was too daunting. Chanel asked me to model a collection for her, but I knew I couldn't do it. She gave me a photograph of herself, taken by Horst, and said to me, "You know, you could have been my daughter, you look so much like me." I realise now I should have done it. I might have got all my Chanel suits for nothing if I had!'

Clothes set the style for a model's work. 'If you were wearing Balenciaga, there was a way of wearing Balenciaga. You had to be formal. That's what you're employed to do; to show the clothes to the best advantage!'

Her worst feature was her hands; they were too large, and she had to keep them away from her face, which is small. 'And my nose goes a little crooked— and I squint, sometimes!'

Although she preferred modelling clothes, she did beauty advertisements for Max Factor and Helena Rubinstein. She was careful not to over-expose herself and became selective about the type of work she would undertake, and the photographers with whom she would work. The trips were the high-

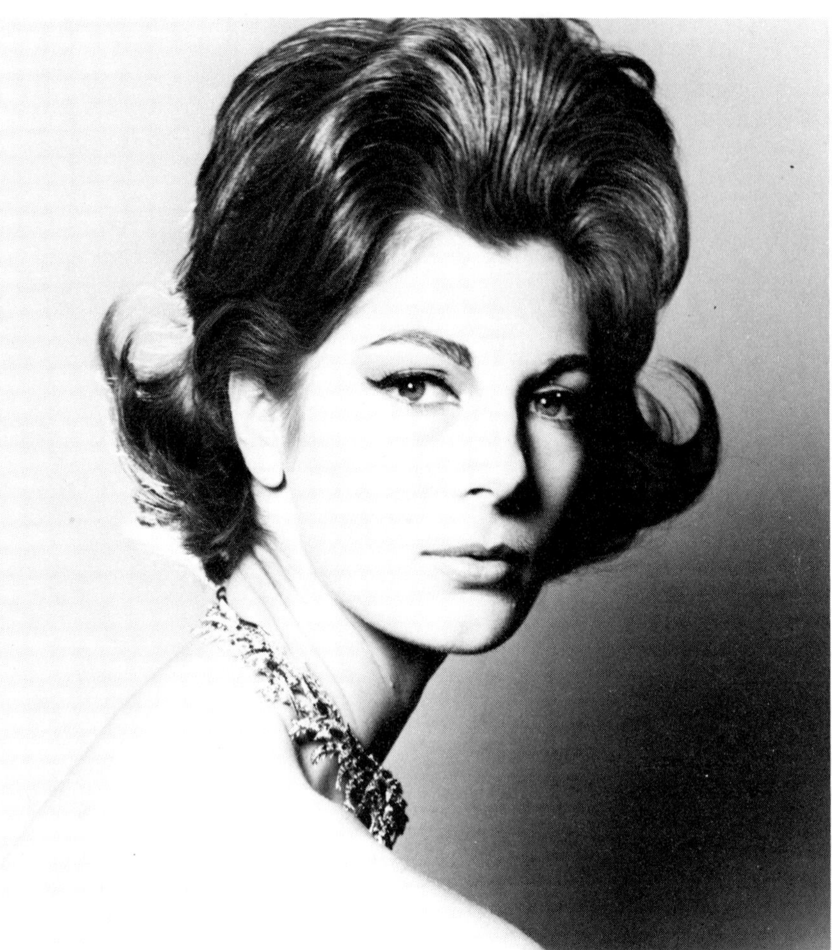

lights for her because of her love of travelling. 'But there was no time for parties at night because I would be up at five in the mornings and come back absolutely exhausted, have to prepare my accessories and reset my hairpieces for the next day's work, have a bath and go to bed.

'I smoked and drank a bit, and occasionally got podgy, but I was awfully sly, unlike Barbara [Goalen] who was always out at social gatherings and nightclubs, but she *talked* about it.

'She told everyone that she was wobbly because of what she'd been up to the night before, and then they'd say, "We don't think we can use Barbara, she's been out rather a lot this week." I had been out a lot too, but I would never tell anyone. I'd think, "Silly girl. You shouldn't have mentioned it."

'Barbara was so nice and generous. She was sort of like the Queen to us, and she never felt her position or career was being threatened when the new young models came along. She was equally charming to them.'

Fiona Campbell-Walter was another top model in the fifties. By the time she was twenty-two, she was one of Britain's most photographed models. She worked with industry and concentration, and achieved success with the help of her ambitious mother. A beautiful young girl with an ambitious mother behind her can rise to undreamed-of heights. Fiona Campbell-Walter married a German millionaire, steel magnate Baron Thyssen.

Henry Clarke took Fiona's first photographs when she was a very young girl in London. They did some work in the studio, and then went on location to Ware, in the north of England: 'She was so young then that the make-up wouldn't stay on her face', recalls Clarke. 'Her skin wouldn't support make-up. She was so fresh, and so beautiful, and so lovely. She had great style. Even at the beginning when she was amateur, and her movements weren't perfection, she had that marvellous profile and great allure; she was very mature for her age—she was a girl with almost a woman's body, which was perfect for the clothes of that time. She was a great trooper; always on the dot. Of course, she was of the old school!'

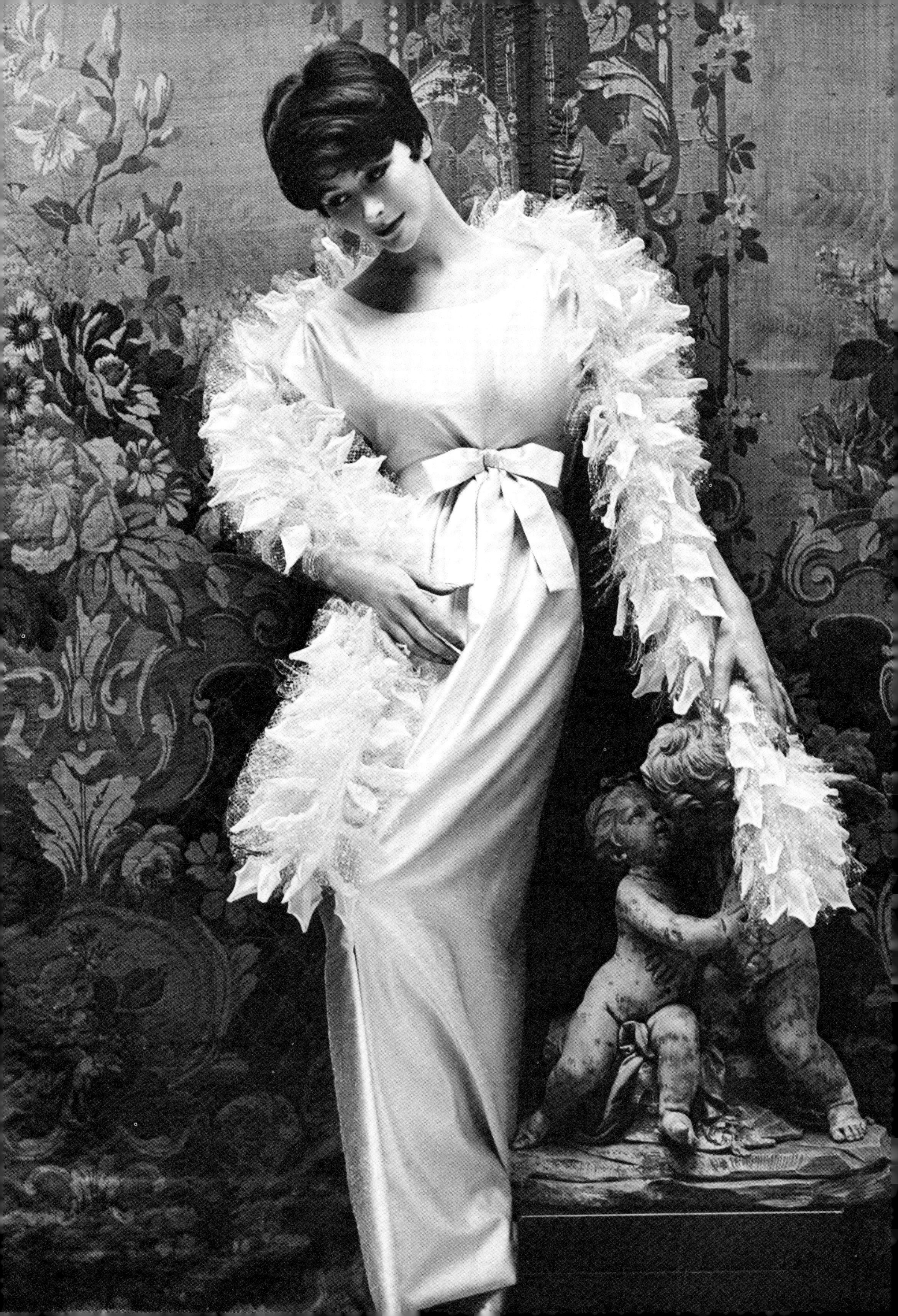

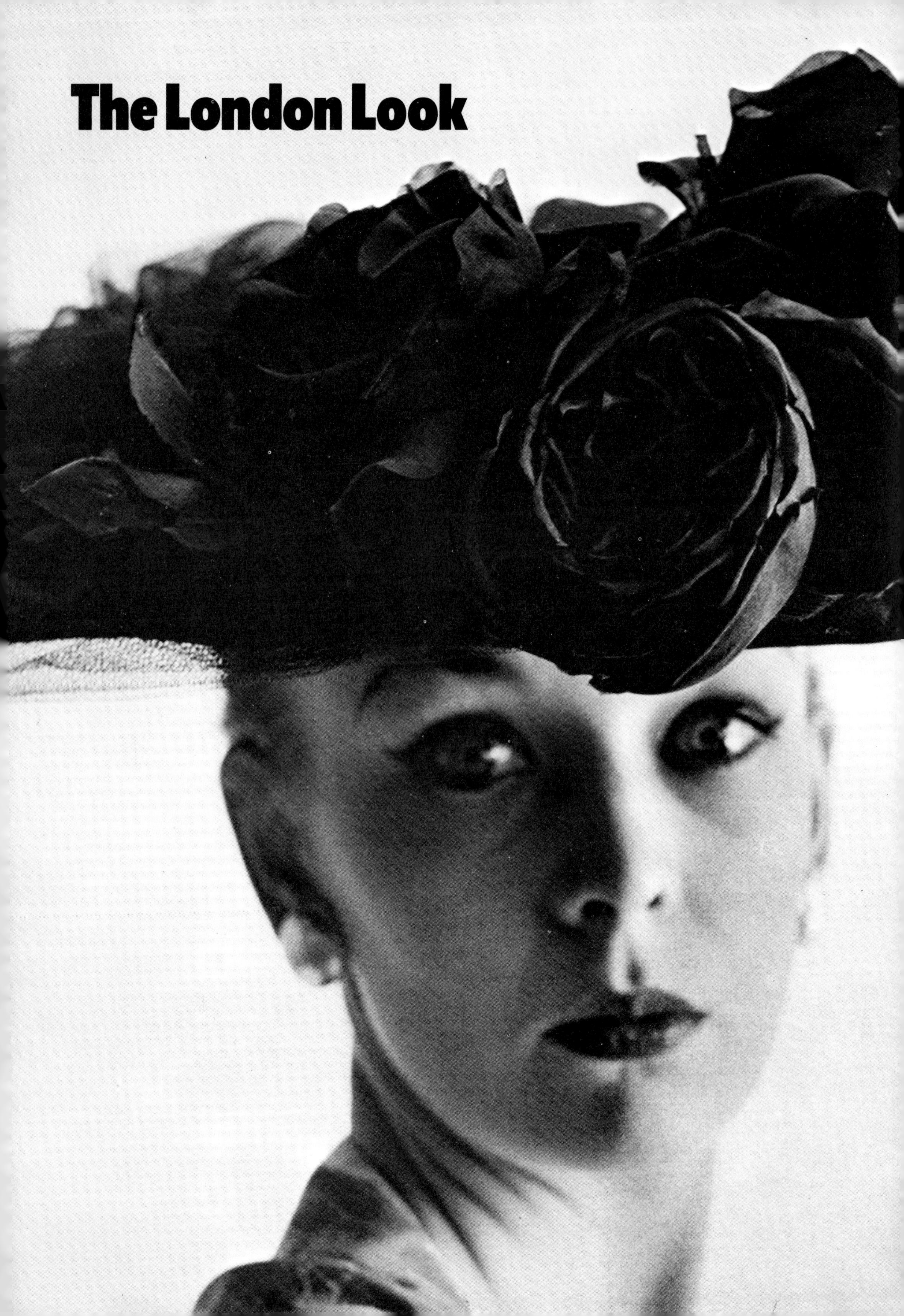

The London Look

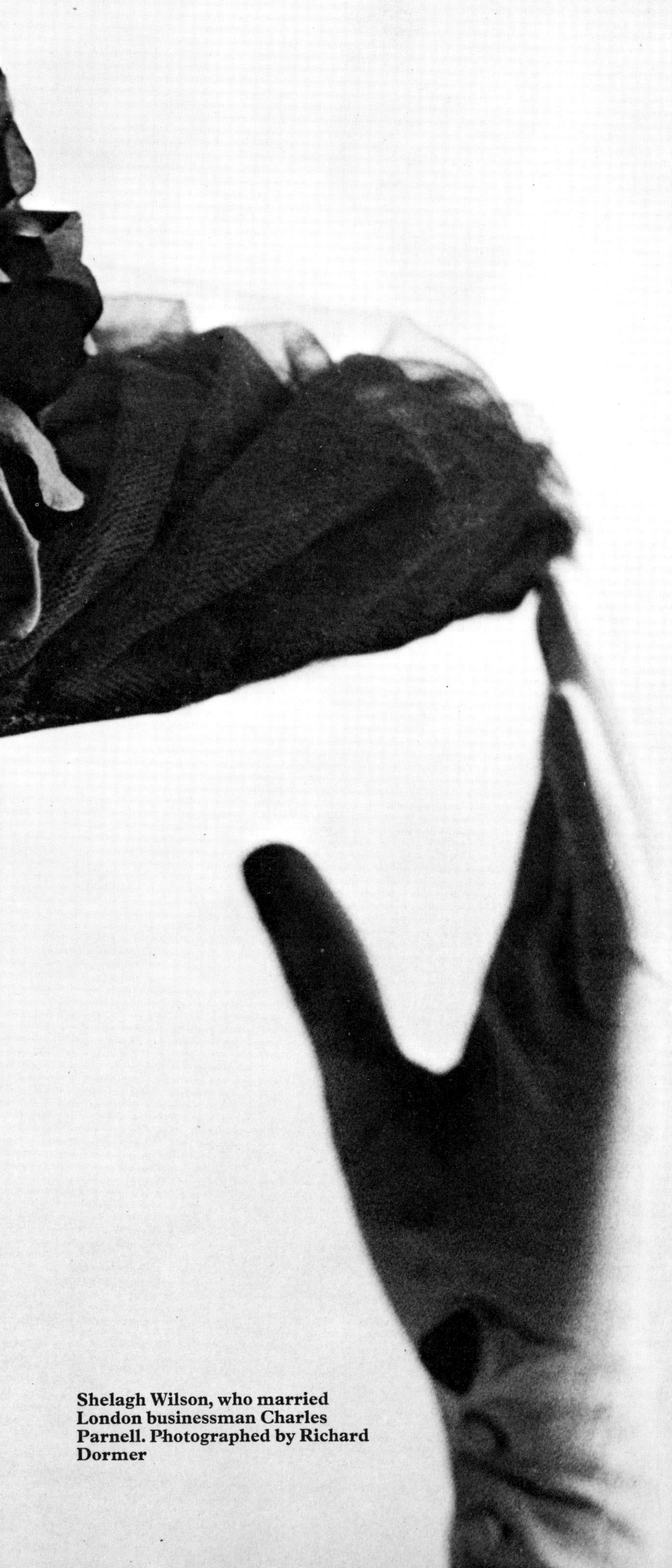

Shelagh Wilson, who married London businessman Charles Parnell. Photographed by Richard Dormer

In the fifties, the three British models to reach international status were Barbara Goalen, Anne Gunning, and Fiona Campbell-Walter. There were at least a dozen others, however, whose faces became known to the public—even though their names did not. They worked consistently, some of them preferring, or being more suited to shows than to photographic modelling, and as a consequence they were not so much in the public's eye as the photographic models.

Sue Abrahams was a first rate model, and seemed only to like the profession because of the rewards she could reap from it. She was a girl who carried her make-up practically in a matchbox, she used so little.

She had the most extraordinary camera flair, but until she was in front of the camera, she projected very little. She was very much an outdoor girl, and although somewhat gawky, she emerged as a glamorous model with substance.

June Clarke had a waif-like look, not unlike Jessie Matthews. She was youthful, and rather special, almost sparrow-like. She was charming with typical English looks, but never reached the top league.

Anne Cumming-Bell did very little photographic work because she was essentially a show model. In the fifties, models specialised more than they do today; show models seldom did photographic work, and photographic models did not always care to do shows. These days many photographic models do shows because it adds glamour to see those fabulous girls who appear in glossies in the salons. Whereas they were not well paid before, these days they are.

Anne married the Duke of Rutland, but was later divorced. Now she lives in Gloucestershire where she breeds show ponies.

Jean Dawnay became a model in 1947, worked for Dior in Paris, and later compèred fashion shows. She was short-sighted and as she could not see the stairs to the ramp for a fashion show, show director Michael Whittaker insisted she wear glasses. 'When a girl like Jean wears glasses', the compère announced when she came on, 'gentlemen always make passes.' The papers picked it up, and she never stopped

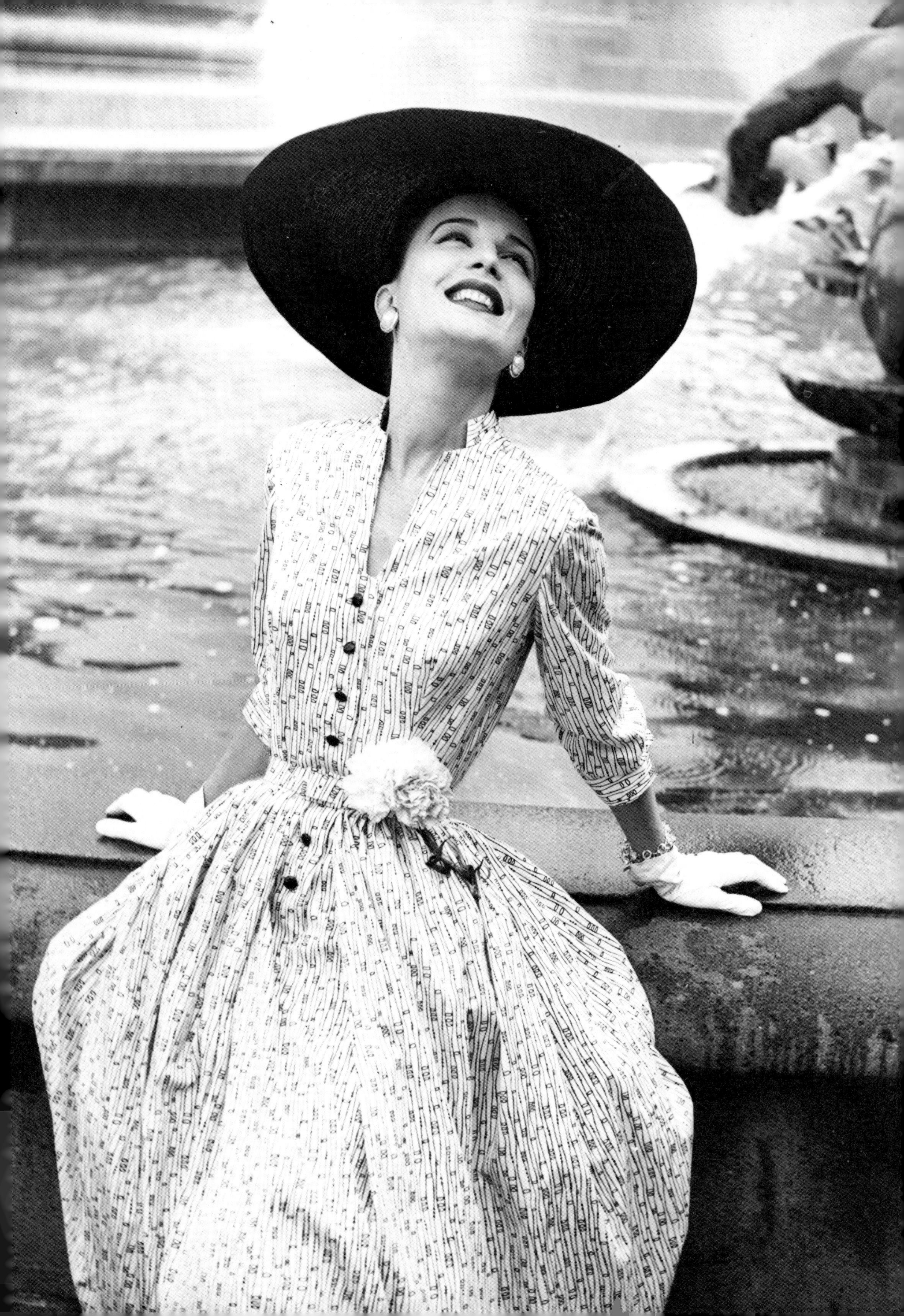

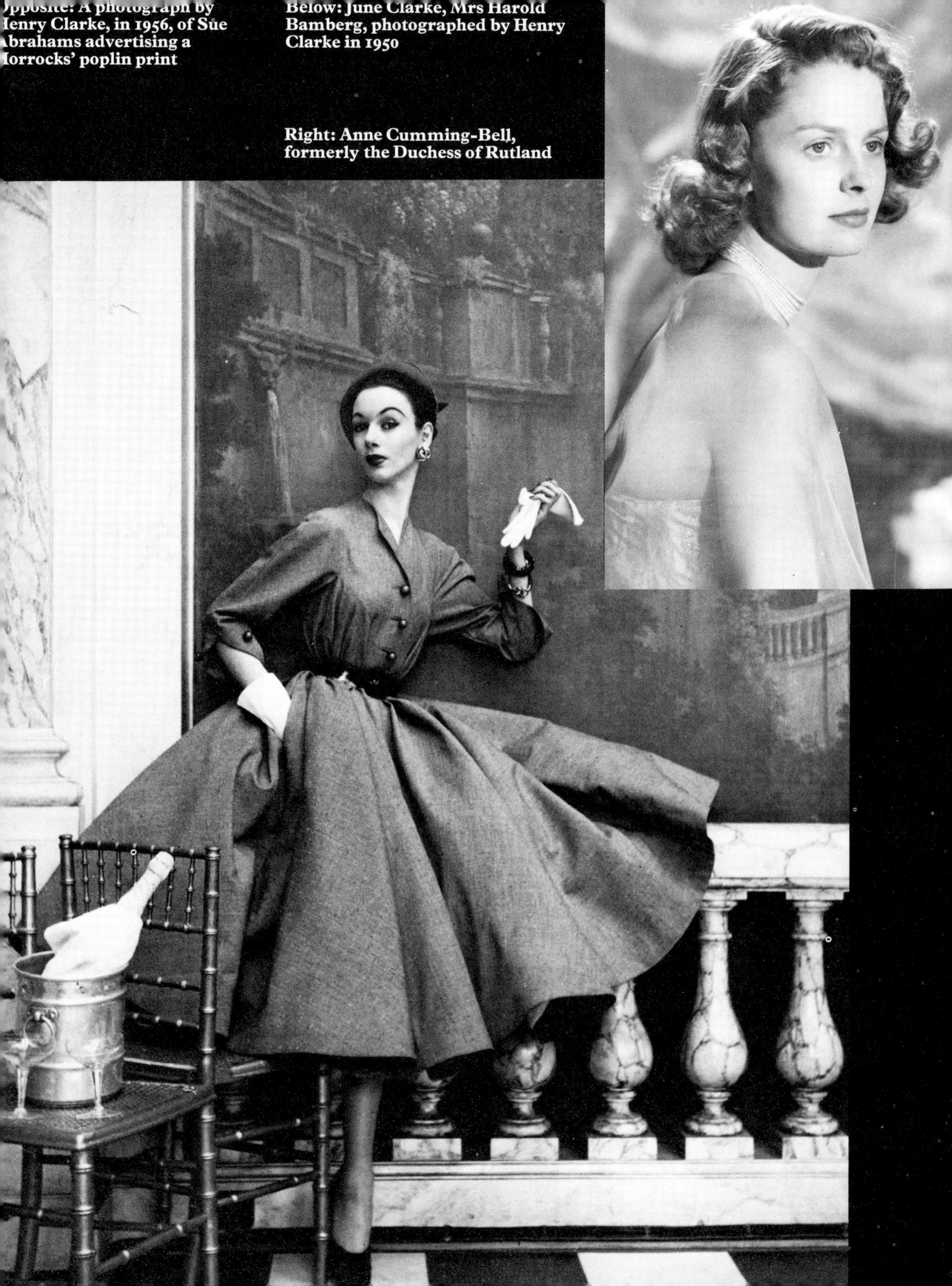

Opposite: A photograph by
Henry Clarke, in 1956, of Sue
Abrahams advertising a
Horrocks' poplin print
Below: June Clarke, Mrs Harold
Bamberg, photographed by Henry
Clarke in 1950
Right: Anne Cumming-Bell,
formerly the Duchess of Rutland

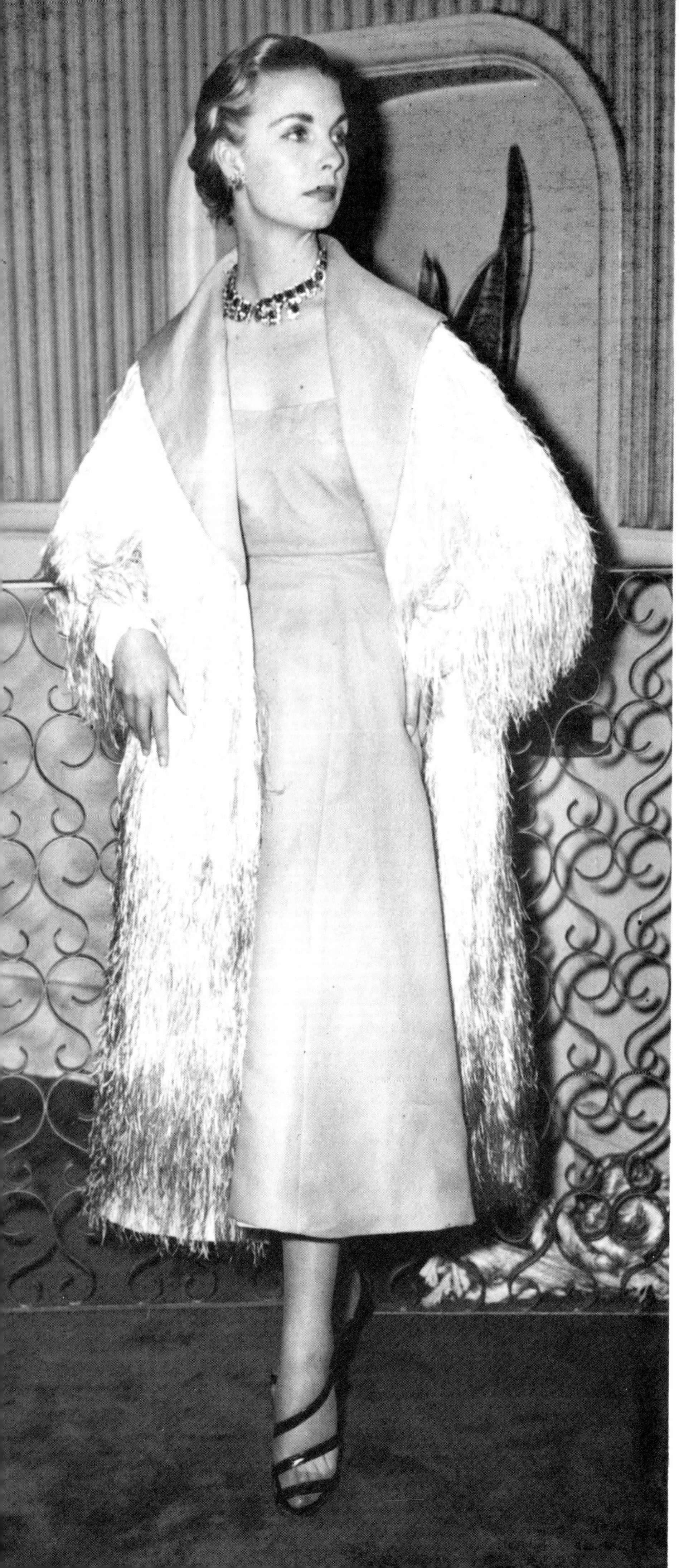

working after that. She was always punctual, very professional and had everything in her favour except her diminutive height, which nobody ever realised because she moved so effectively.

Maggie Eghardt was the best of the models to come from Australia. She was discovered by Sir Norman Hartnell who brought her over to London. 'She was terribly beautiful,' recalls Sir Norman, 'and looked like Elizabeth Taylor'. She had tremendous style and an individual look. She fell in love with a photographer who only liked thin girls, and so she thinned down, 'like a razor-blade dressed up'.

Jennifer Hocking, also an Australian, started off as a show model and became a top photographic model. She had an ability to make anything look good, but lacked an individual style since she, and many others, copied the look of the top American model, Anne Saint Marie. Jennifer had aloofness and sophistication, yet basically she was the most down-to-earth person imaginable.

Enid Munik was born in South Africa and went to London where she became a much sought-after model. She was very good, but limited because of her height. She was rather small, but had an individual look, being a most beautiful woman with an extraordinarily attractive tip-tilted nose, and absolutely washed-blue eyes. Unlike the other models at the time who were terribly sophisticated, she remained totally natural.

Pat O'Reilly, known as 'Mad O'Reilly', was youthful and tempestuous, with a typical Irish temperament. A very charming girl, she made the maximum out of very little. She was versatile and had enormous vitality, with her own, individual look. She modelled evening gowns with sophistication, although she was basically the out-of-doors type, specialising in modelling sweaters and skirts.

Shelagh Wilson was one of the top five models in the fifties who, with Anne Gunning and Sue Abrahams, took up where Barbara Goalen left off when she gave up modelling. She was a healthy looking English girl with fair hair and blue eyes, possessing perfect looks that suited tweeds, cashmere, and pearls, but showed evening clothes equally well.

Opposite: Shirley Worthington, wife of Sir Anthony Royle

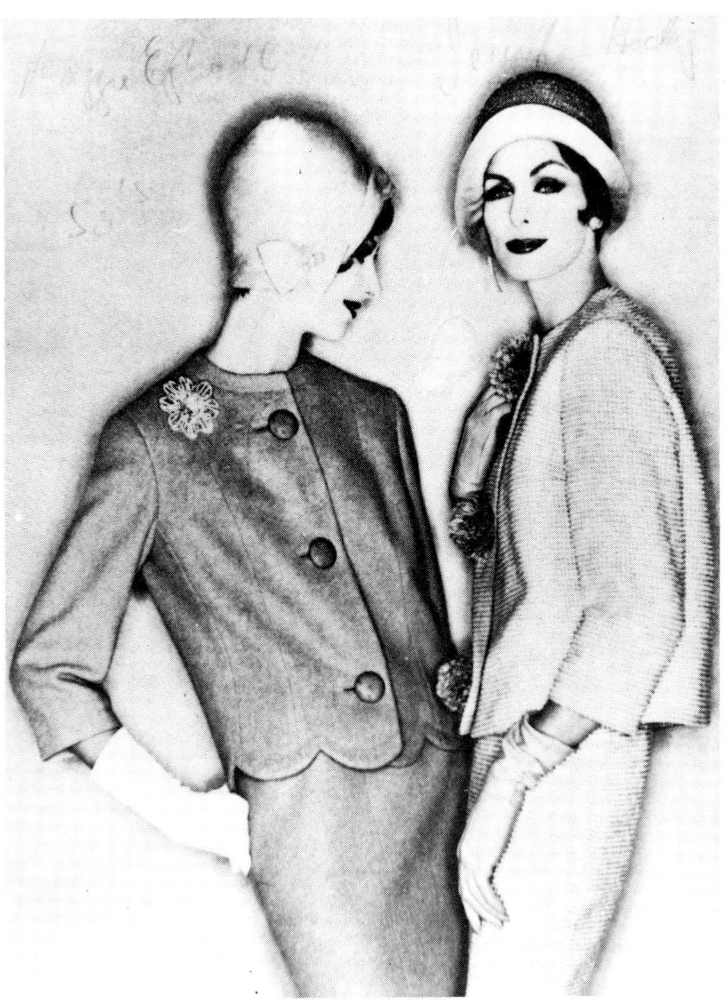

Right: Maggie Eghardt and Jennifer Hocking, by Richard Dormer

She was a photographic as well as a show model. If one had to equate her with a movie star, she was the Margaret Sullivan type who would have committed suicide for love!

Born in Cheshire, Shelagh Wilson was evacuated to America during the war, where she completed her education. She began modelling in London after the war when she was seventeen, doing shows for couturiers Sir Norman Hartnell, Digby Morton, and Michael, and on occasions appeared on the covers of *Vogue*, *Harpers Bazaar*, and *Elle* simultaneously.

Shirley Worthington who had a lovely, cool, marble look, was regarded as the 'sporty type' in modelling. She worked consistently, continuing to be photographed longer than almost any other model. She represented the English rose, slightly fading, but never quite. 'The real English beauty always looks as though she is about to drop her petals', comments fashion entrepeneur Michael Whittaker wryly.

Of the other models who worked in London in the fifties, Zoë Newton, who became the Milk Marketing Board's model, was first photographed by Lord Snowdon, then known as Antony Armstrong-Jones. Perhaps one of the most well known faces of the period because she appeared on posters throughout Britain, she was first photographed by him in 1955 for a small job for Crooks Laboratory. Shelagh Bligh, who had begun modelling in the forties, continued into the fifties. She and Sylvia Shelley worked consistently, and so did Jane McNeill of the fair hair, blue eyes, and typically English look. Joy Weston did a great deal of photography, and Valerie Thurlow, another well known model, made her mark. Sheila Whetton was a marvellous house model at Molyneux for years and became one of the most highly regarded of women; she is now working as a fashion editor for English *Vogue*.

The well known Mrs Exeter, the fictional name given to Margot Smyly by *Vogue*, appeared on its fashion pages throughout the fifties. Mrs Exeter gave hope and encouragement to fashion-conscious readers in their fifties. Because she hated her hands and became self-conscious of them, Margot Smyly was invariably photographed wearing long suede gloves.

Whereas the fifties saw the model on the cat-walk, slithering along from one end to the other, perhaps pulling on a glove—or taking one off, in order to find something to do with her hands—the sixties and seventies were to change all that. These days, the models act and dance. The latest music is played through stereo-speakers, and choreographers or show-directors are employed to stage the shows.

The 'woman of the world' personified by the models of the fifties disappeared with the advent of Mary Quant who opened her first Bazaar shop in the Kings Road in 1955. The Beat Generation was around the corner; soon photographer David Bailey would arrive on the scene with his discovery, Jean Shrimpton, and introduce a new, natural, young style into fashion photography.

Pop
Explosion

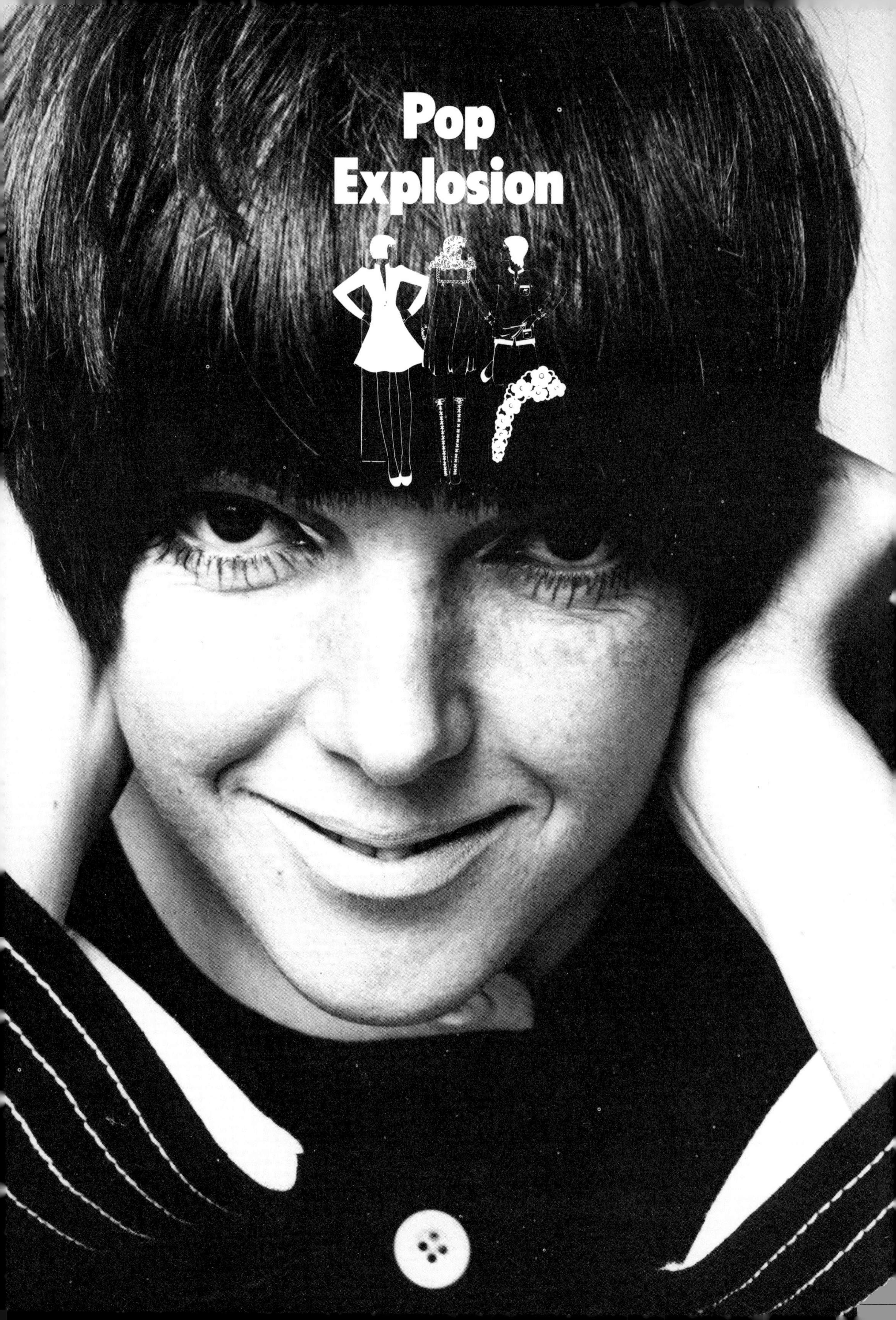

Revolution came in the early 1960s in London with Beatlemania, Carnaby Street, and the youth cult. Mary Quant exploded on the fashion world, shortening the skirts Courrèges had couragously slashed to the hilt, and the mini-skirt was born. New designers applied sweeping new standards to all aspects of fashion; and these new standards of beauty and modelling meant that the model girl would never be the same again. Gone forever was the woman of the world look, traditional conventions were anathema, the dated look was death—but for all that, the model's lofty status proved immortal.

The sixties did not swing until 1965, and when they did fashion was in a quandary; it did not know in which direction it was heading. On one hand was the ordinary, girl-next-door look, culminating with Twiggy, and on the other, the way-out freaky look with weird women—models like Veruschka for *Vogue* and Donyale Luna for *Harpers Bazaar*, fantasising, showing clothes no woman could wear. Nostalgia began creeping in under the label of Biba in London, but, in contrast, astronauts inspired Courrèges and Cardin with space-age cuts. New designers John Bates, Gina Fratini, Ossie Clark emerged, followed in the late sixties by Bill Gibb, Zandra Rhodes, and Yuki, while a new generation of photographers David Bailey, Norman Eales, Brian Duffy, Terence Donovan, and Barry Lategan in London rivalled America's Richard Avedon, Irving Penn, Melvin Sokolsky and Britain's Norman Parkinson.

For the traditionalist, the changes were hard to accept. Sex in the sixties provided a new idealism in permissiveness. The model became the mistress; the photographer came from behind his camera to take her to bed. It was bad for the profession, not only because the photographers used the models to improve their own reputations, but they would tie a very good girl down and stop her working with other photographers.

In the end, the model's career suffered and the fashion editors turned

Opposite: Mary Quant, by David Bailey. Her development of the mini-skirt revolutionised fashion in the sixties

Right: Twiggy, one of the faces who epitomised the sixties, at the height of her career as a model

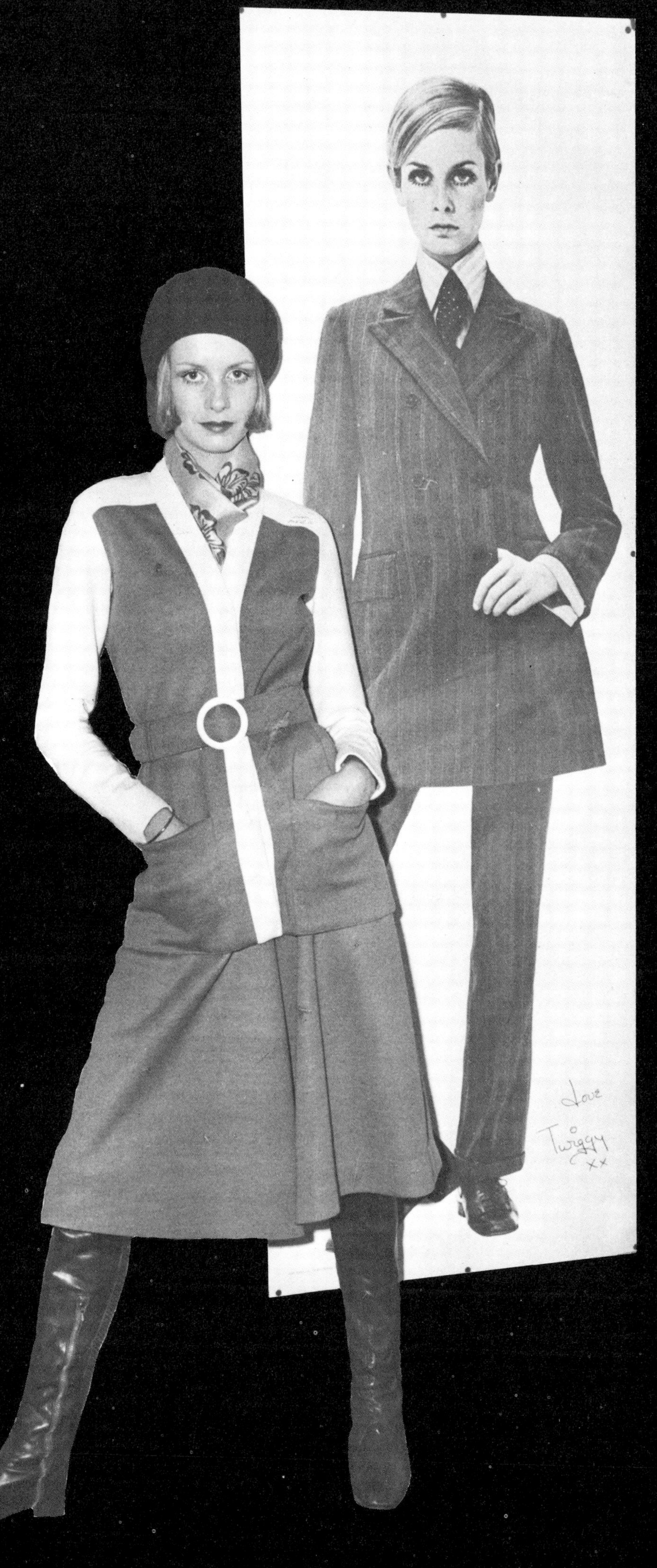

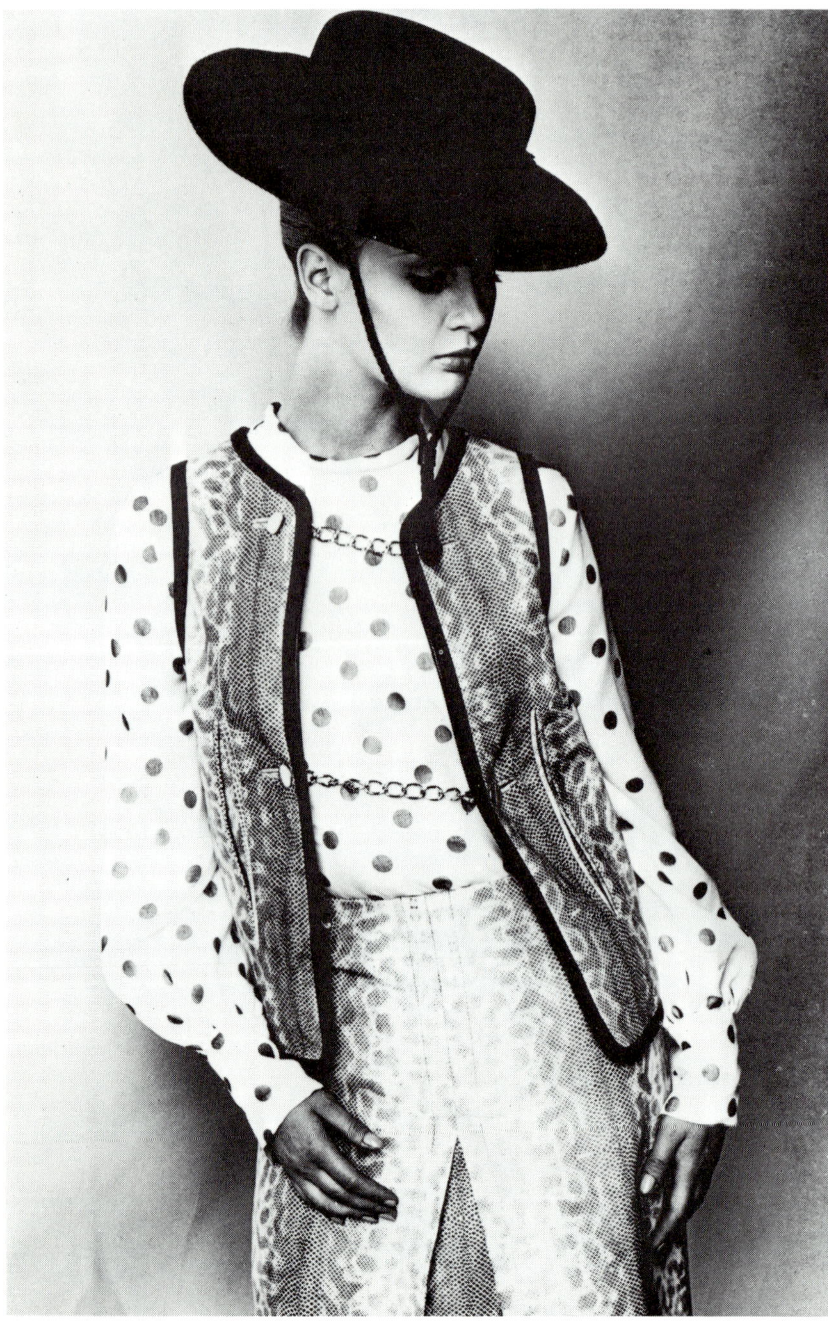

Above: Celia Hammond, whom David Bailey considered one of his top six models. Photographed here by Terence Donovan, one of the other leading British fashion photographers

Opposite: The classic *Vogue* cover by Erwin Blumenfeld which appeared in 1950 (Copyright © 1949, 1977 by The Condé Nast Publications Inc)

against the photographer as well. Magazines were being blackmailed into using a particular photographer, when what they really wanted was the model. They realised that their advertisers and subscribers were tiring of seeing the same face shot in the same way by the same photographer.

'It wasn't like that in the old days', complains a photographer of the old school. 'Alright, if you liked the model, you'd go off to dinner together. It wasn't associated with sex. I think most professional models prefer to have a relationship with a photographer which has nothing to do with her private life at all.

'I know photographers who work on pot, and it's rather similar to being drunk; you think you're saying the most marvellous things, you think you're being terribly clever; you think you're taking the most marvellous pictures when you're high, but when they're developed, what this hallucination has produced in your mind hasn't come over on the film at all.

'I've only known one model who was definitely drugged when she worked, but it had no effect on her. She was always fabulous. Now, I'm told she's fully hooked on heroin—and that's the beginning of the end.'

This revolution in looks and modelling which typifies the sixties was begun through the camera lens and genius of David Bailey. He describes how he discovered Jean Shrimpton— the catalyst who changed everything: 'I found the girl that I had always dreamed of finding. I had ideas of what I felt the perfect woman should be in that area, but she was actually the caricature of what I wanted to make girls look like; and suddenly there she was. Jean Shrimpton. *Vogue* will tell you that they discovered her, but in fact, I did. They claim to have discovered me, too, but they didn't.

'Jean and I were very well established before the Beatles appeared. We started roughly at the end of 1960 and the beginning of 1961. We were established by 1963, then the whole Carnaby Street syndrome started late '63, and by 1966 it started fizzling out because all the Chelsea cowboys started jumping on the bandwagon.' She started modelling at seventeen and by the time she was twenty-one Jean Shrimpton was an

VOGUE

1950

MID-CENTURY
FASHIONS
FACES
IDEAS

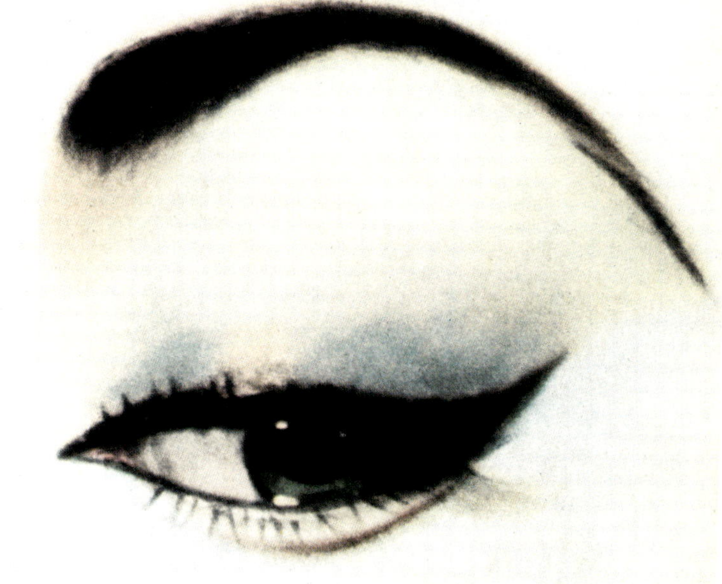

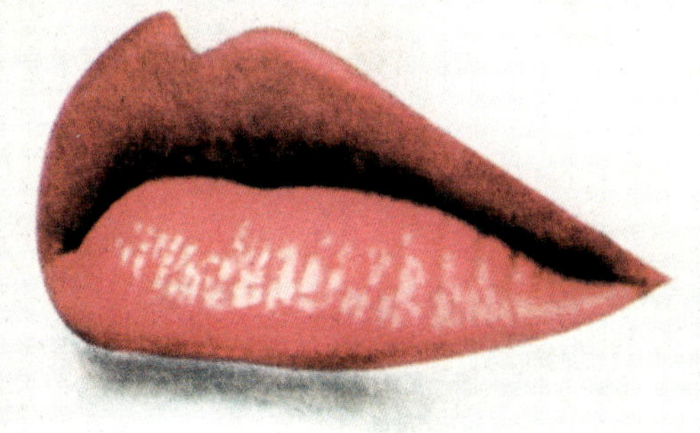

**ADVANCE
RETAIL
TRADE
EDITION**

TRAVEL

HANDBOOK

Incorporating Vanity Fair

January 1950

Price 50 Cents in U. S. and Canada
$1.00 All Other Countries
COPYRIGHT 1949 THE CONDÉ NAST PUBLICATIONS INC.

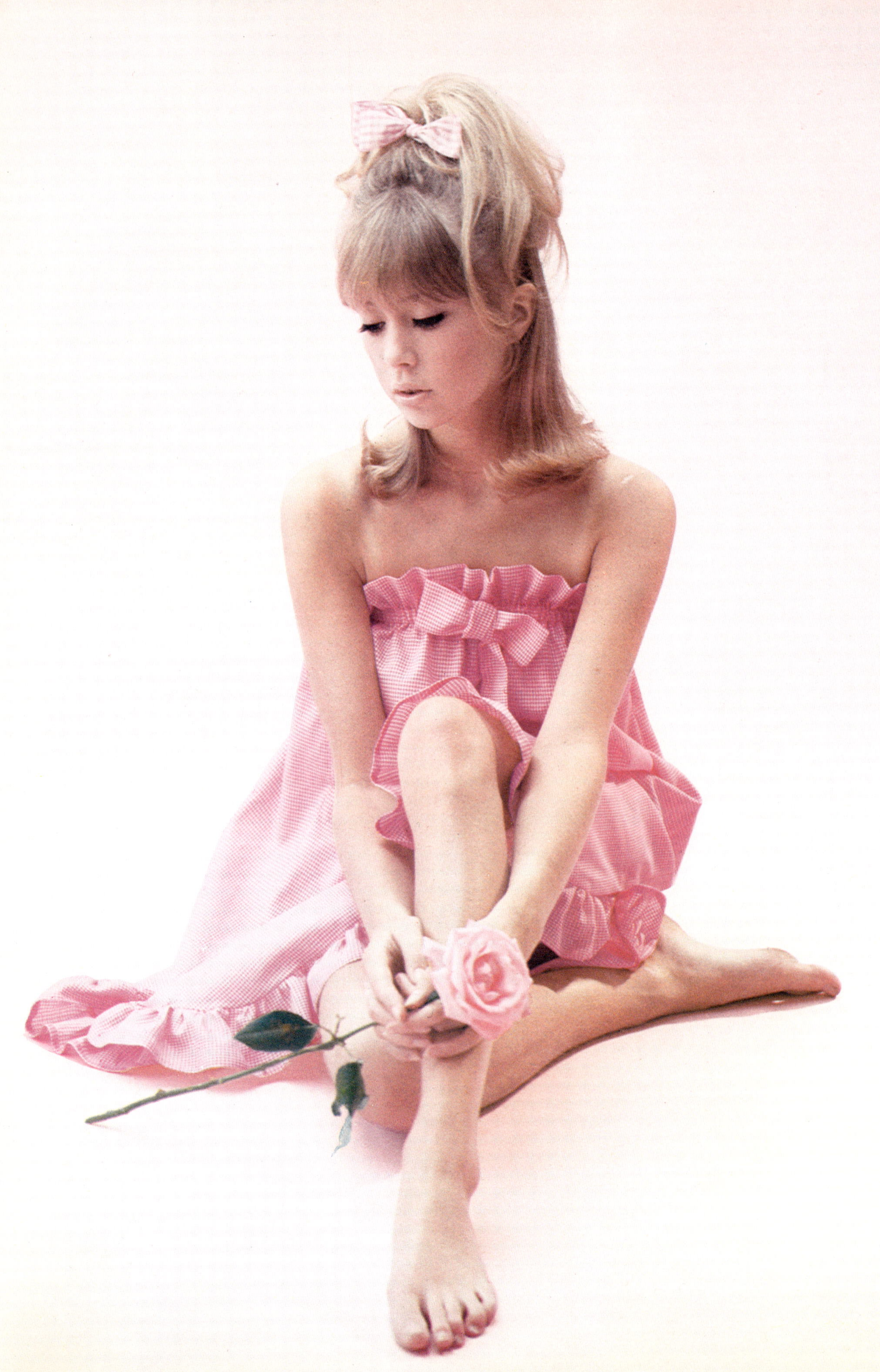

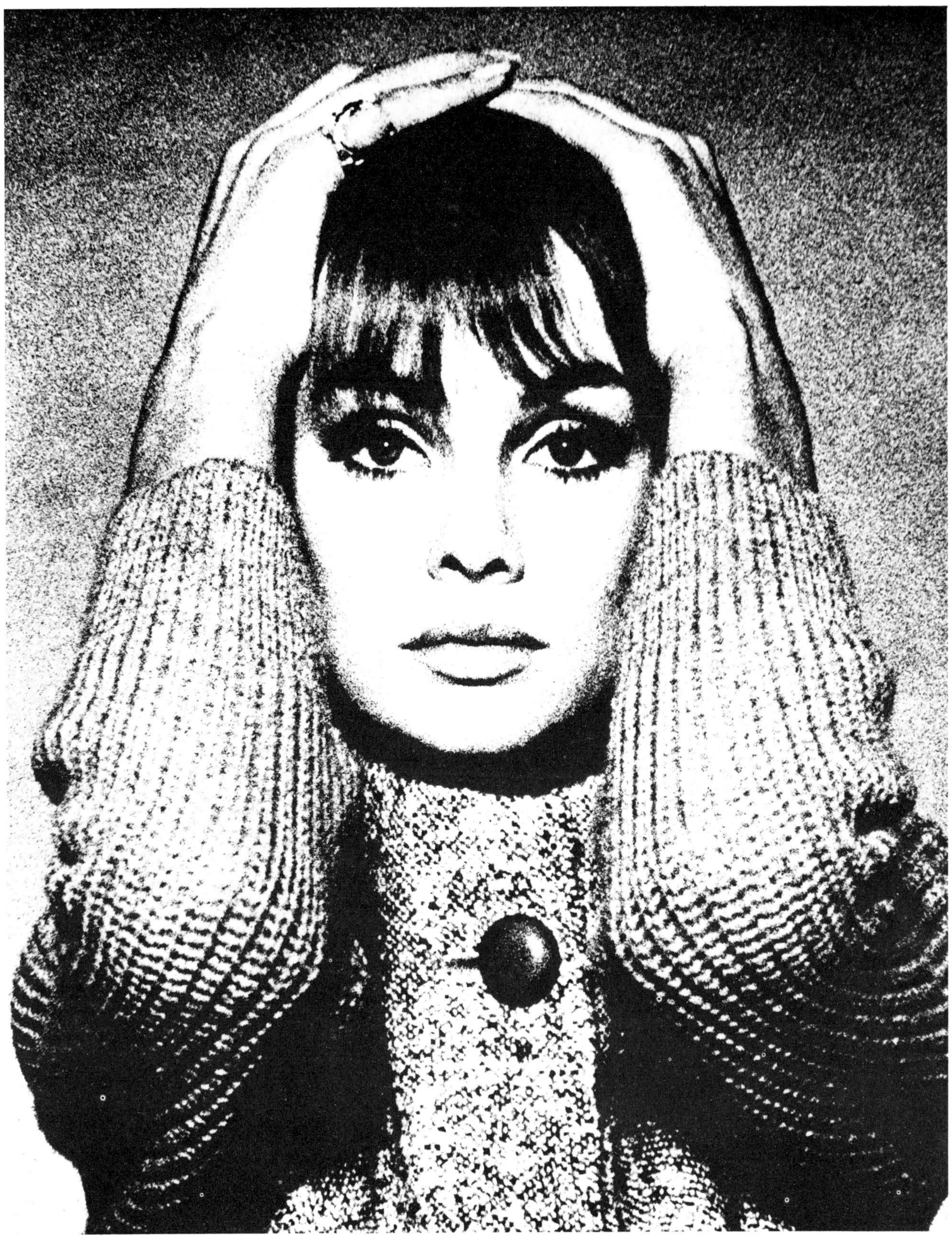

Above: Jean Shrimpton, photographed by David Bailey. Their partnership brought a major change in fashion photography and made her a household name

Opposite: Patti Boyd by David Bailey (Courtesy the John French Photo Library)

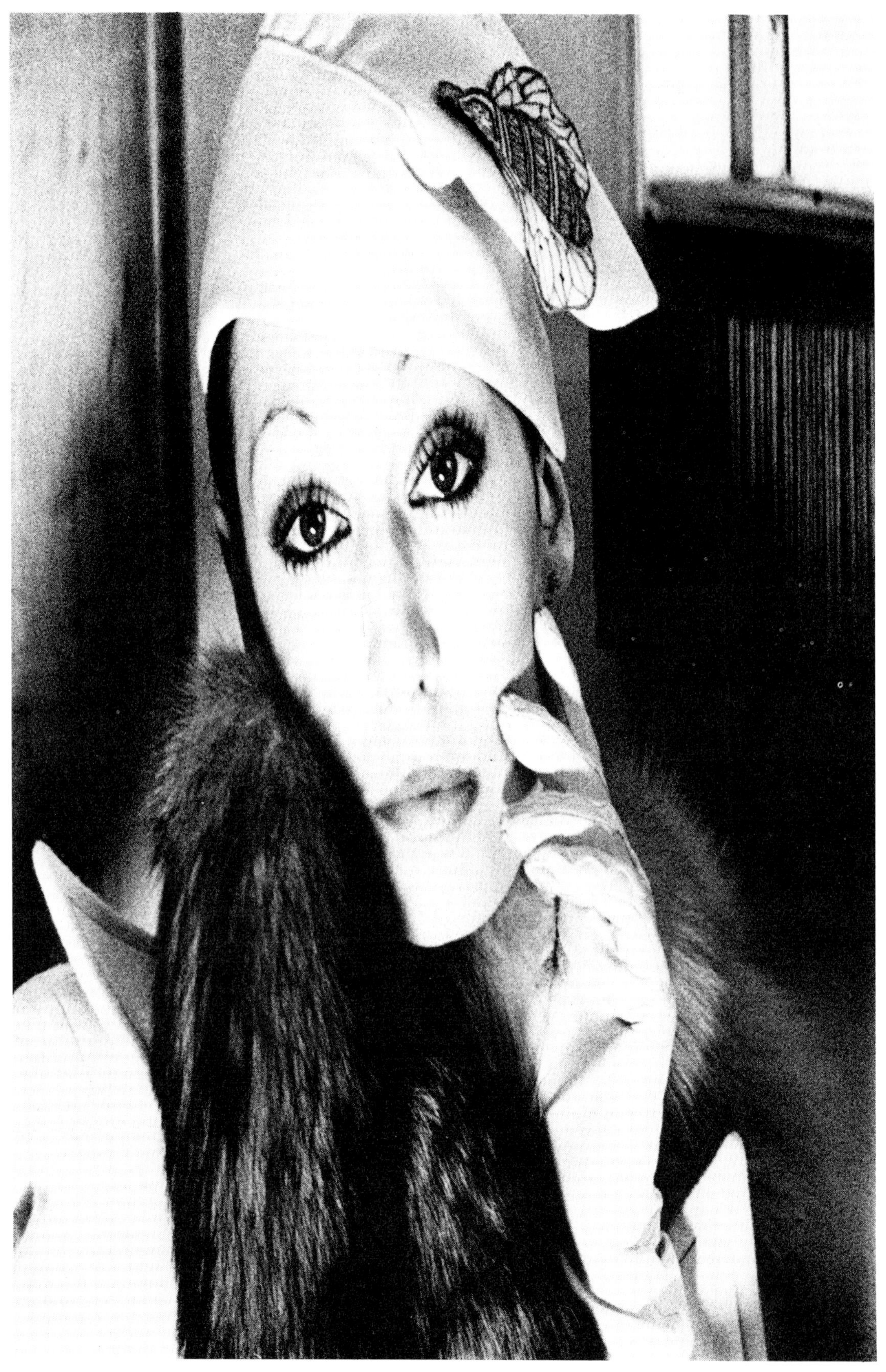

**Angelica Huston for *Vogue* –
David Bailey
By kind permission of Condé Nast
Publications**

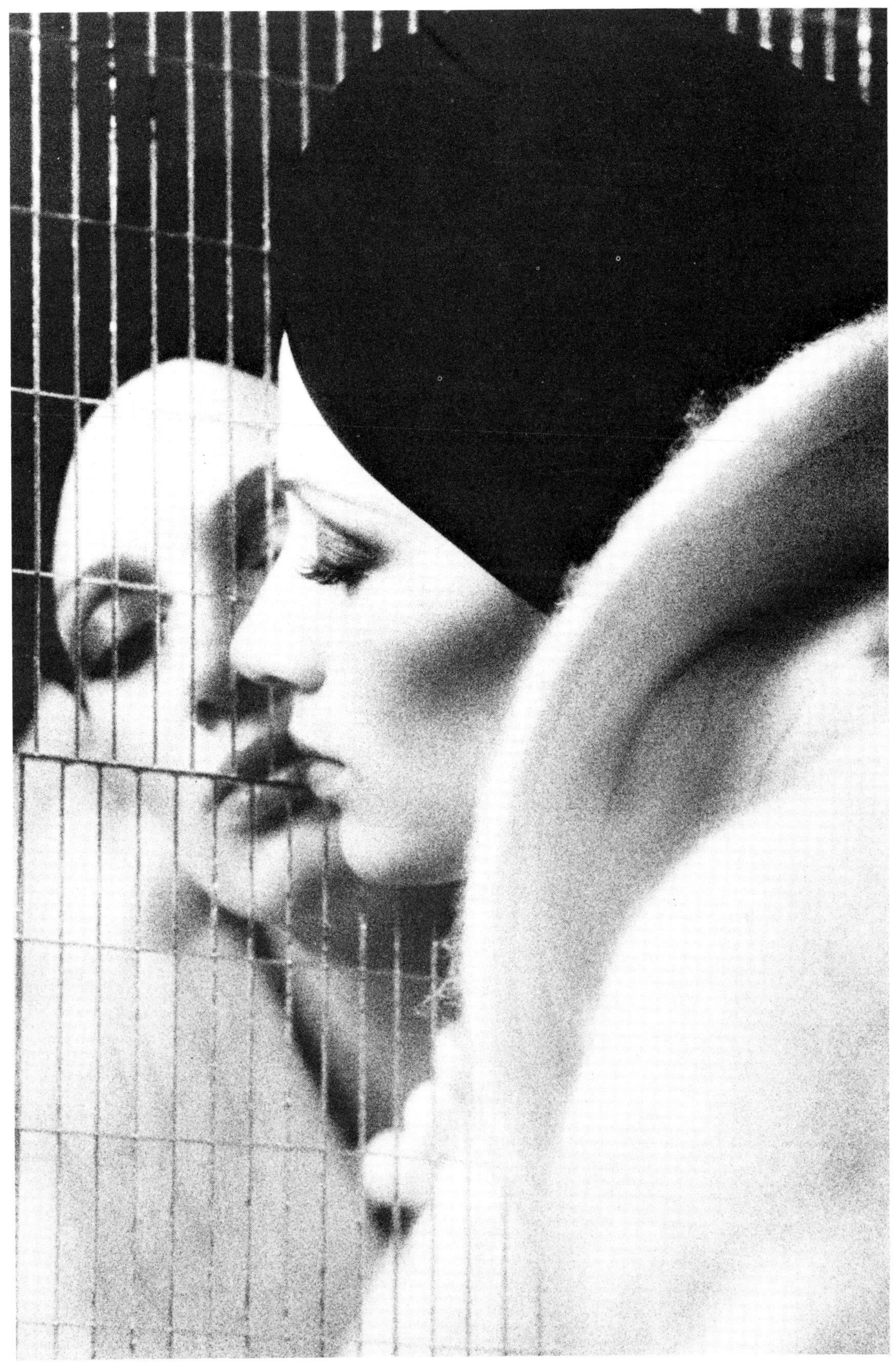

Donna Mitchell for *Vogue* –
David Bailey
By kind permission of Condé Nast
Publications

acknowledged phenomenon. Her name became as famous as her face, which appeared on practically every fashion cover in the world within twelve months. She was acclaimed as the world's greatest model by both Paris and New York. She was photogenically perfect; her body is faultless, and her proportions were unrivalled—exaggerated and feminine. One of the most adaptable of models, she could switch from sophisticate to tomboy with equal ease with her natural style and individual approach. She dared to be herself in an artificial industry. As David Bailey says: 'I was not conscious of the impact we were having, because what we were doing wasn't worked out. I just took pictures of Jean the way I liked her to look. I think the thing about Jean was that she wasn't the stiff, dummy-kind of posed shop-window mannequin. She was somebody you felt you could have touched, almost. When she first came to my studio, she sat down, perfectly naturally, thoroughly at ease. She didn't pose like some goddess against Greek pillars. Jean's look was what every girl wanted to look like. Apart from Jean Shrimpton there have only been about six models since I've been going, that were really for me: Celia Hammond, Tania Mallet, Sue Murray, Penelope Tree, Moyra Swan, and Marie Helvin.'

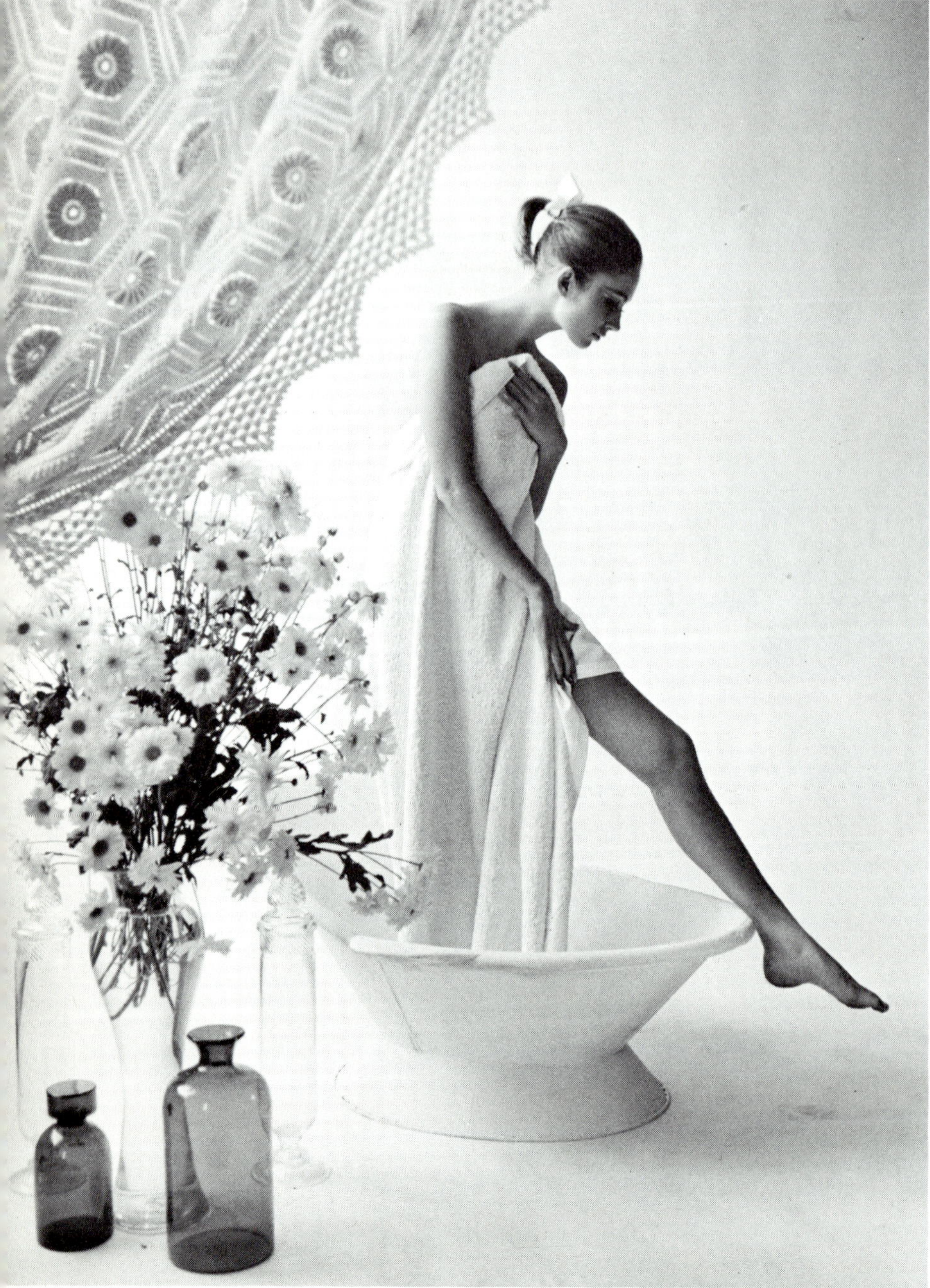

Left: Sue Murray, another of Bailey's favourite models, in a photograph by Richard Dormer

Opposite: A photograph by Richard Dormer with Twiggy in the foreground, and Patti Boyd at the back. The male model is the late Earl Knapp

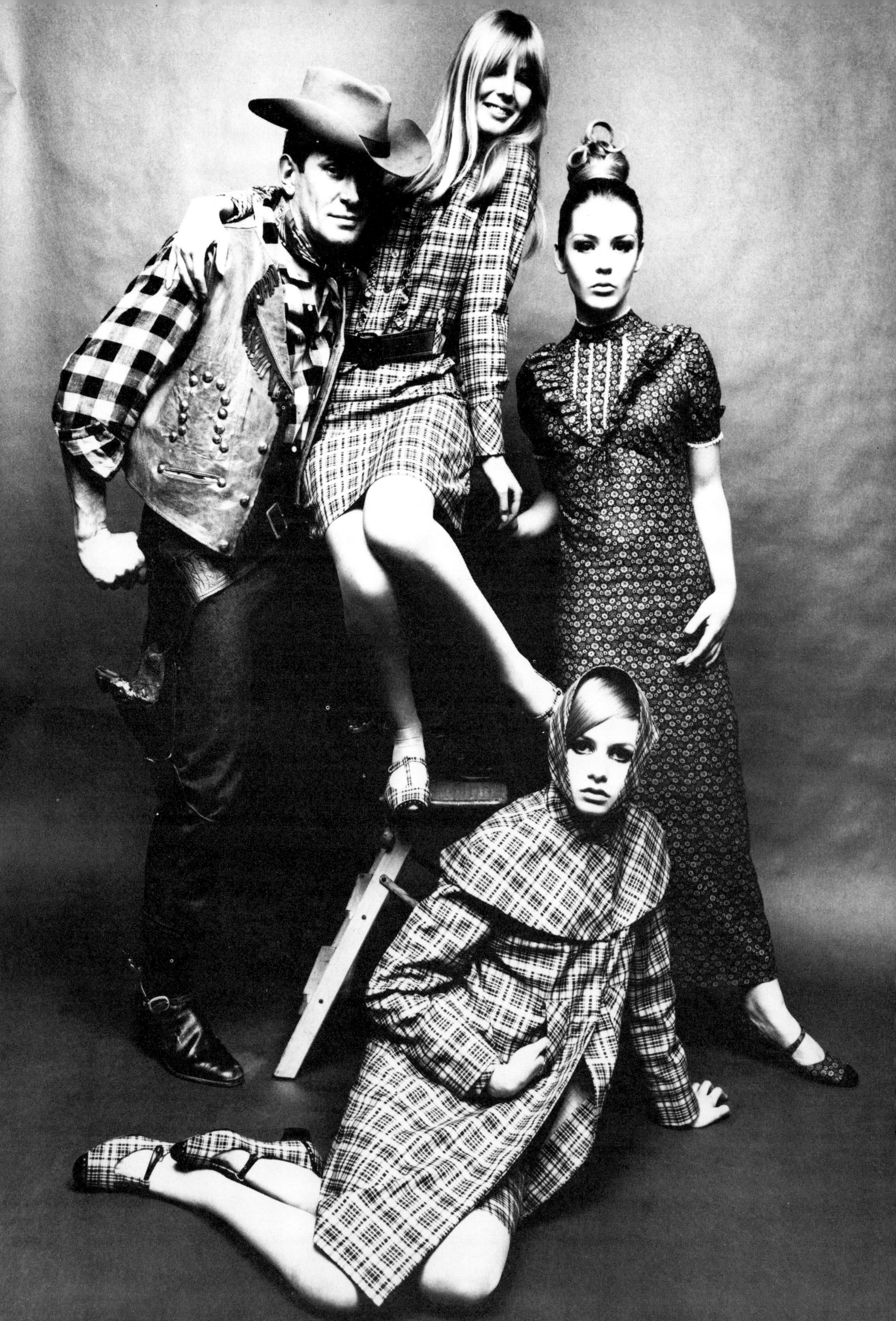

Beautiful People

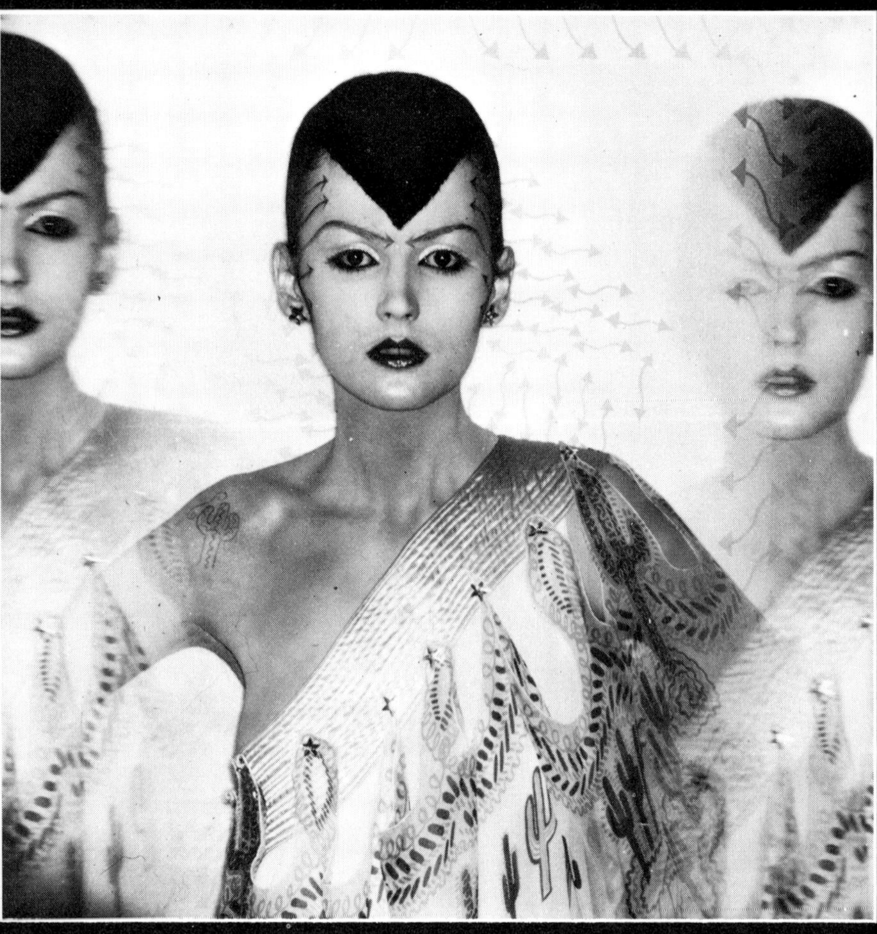

Sue Purdy in a Zandra Rhodes'
creation photographed by Barry
Lategan for *Vogue*. By kind
permission of Condé Nast
Publications

With the growing fascination for models and modelling in the sixties, came a change in the status of the model girl, independent of changes in fashion and the ideal of female beauty.

The world of glamour and travel seemed wide open to every young girl who wanted it, and dreams of unreality were fulfilled by all who ventured forth. The heyday of models and photographers was upon us, on all levels. There was no embargo, no holds barred to anyone who dared to be themselves.

Young models began painting their faces in multi-colours, as if to recreate the illusionary tones and shapes dictated by psychedelic music so prominent in the sixties. Fabric designer Zandra Rhodes created floating chiffon dresses in exquisite and original forms and colours, inspiring models to carry the imagery further, onto their faces; beauty marks of silvery half-moons and resilient stars were appliquéd onto their complexions. Bright red hair with yellow streaks harmonised with their free, freaky fantasies.

Among the great many models, the following girls have been singled out for

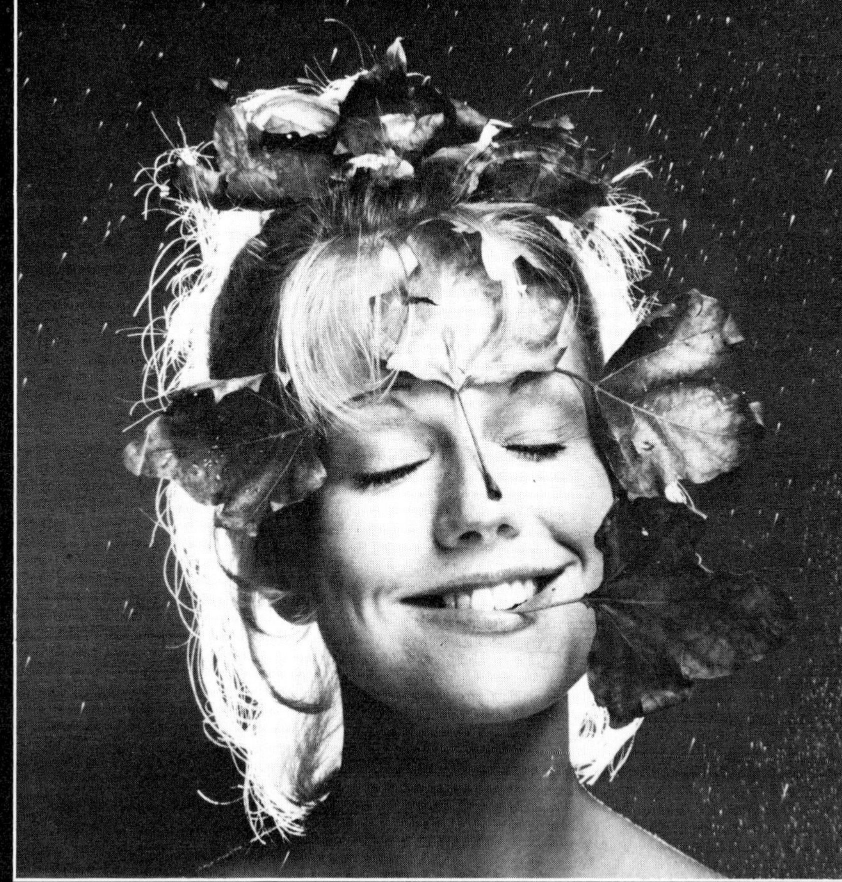

Sally-Ann Vancliffe embodies the spirit of the sixties. By courtesy of Peter Hope-Lumley

their particular individual brand of beauty which drove them on to personal achievement in their chosen profession:

Patti Boyd was more of a personality than a model and swept into the limelight when she married the Beatle, George Harrison.

Jackie Cahill was sweet looking, and one of the teenage types so popular in the fifties. One of John French's great favourites, she wore her hair with a fringe and tied in bunches in the period of gingham dresses with full skirts.

Grace Coddington was a fashion model in the true sense, rather than the heart-beat of her generation, but she changed her style all the time to keep abreast of what was going on, whereas Jean Shrimpton always kept the same sort of look. She was a very professional model. Off-duty she wore kooky clothes, and became known as 'the Cod'.

Debbie Condon was a very good American model, and also extremely professional. Although she worked for Balmain and other couturiers as a show model, she did mainly photographic work. She had a chipped tooth in the front of her mouth and had a false piece which she stuck on when advertisers and editors wanted the cute, teenage look. She was one of the first models to have painted-on freckles.

Marie Lise Gres was photographed by David Bailey on many occasions with Shrimpton. She is a French girl, but always lived in England.

Geishie; 'She was very pretty', remarks a top fashion editor, 'she was going out once with a wealthy boyfriend, and the photographic sessions I had with her were chronic. She would just sit and tell me how he tried to shoot her, or the row they'd had. Then she'd burst into tears, and she'd have to put her make-up on all over again. I could *never* get Geishie onto the white paper in the studio! But she was a very sweet girl, and a very good model—once she got cracking!'

Celia Hammond was Britain's second top model, after Jean Shrimpton, in the sixties. Brought up in Indonesia where her father was a tea-planter, and later in Australia, but educated in England, she went to the Lucie Clayton agency to learn modelling, and was discovered by Norman Parkinson. Within six months of meeting Norman Parkinson she went with him to Paris to cover the French collections for *Queen* magazine.

Vicky Hodge appeared more in the sensational press than in the glossies,

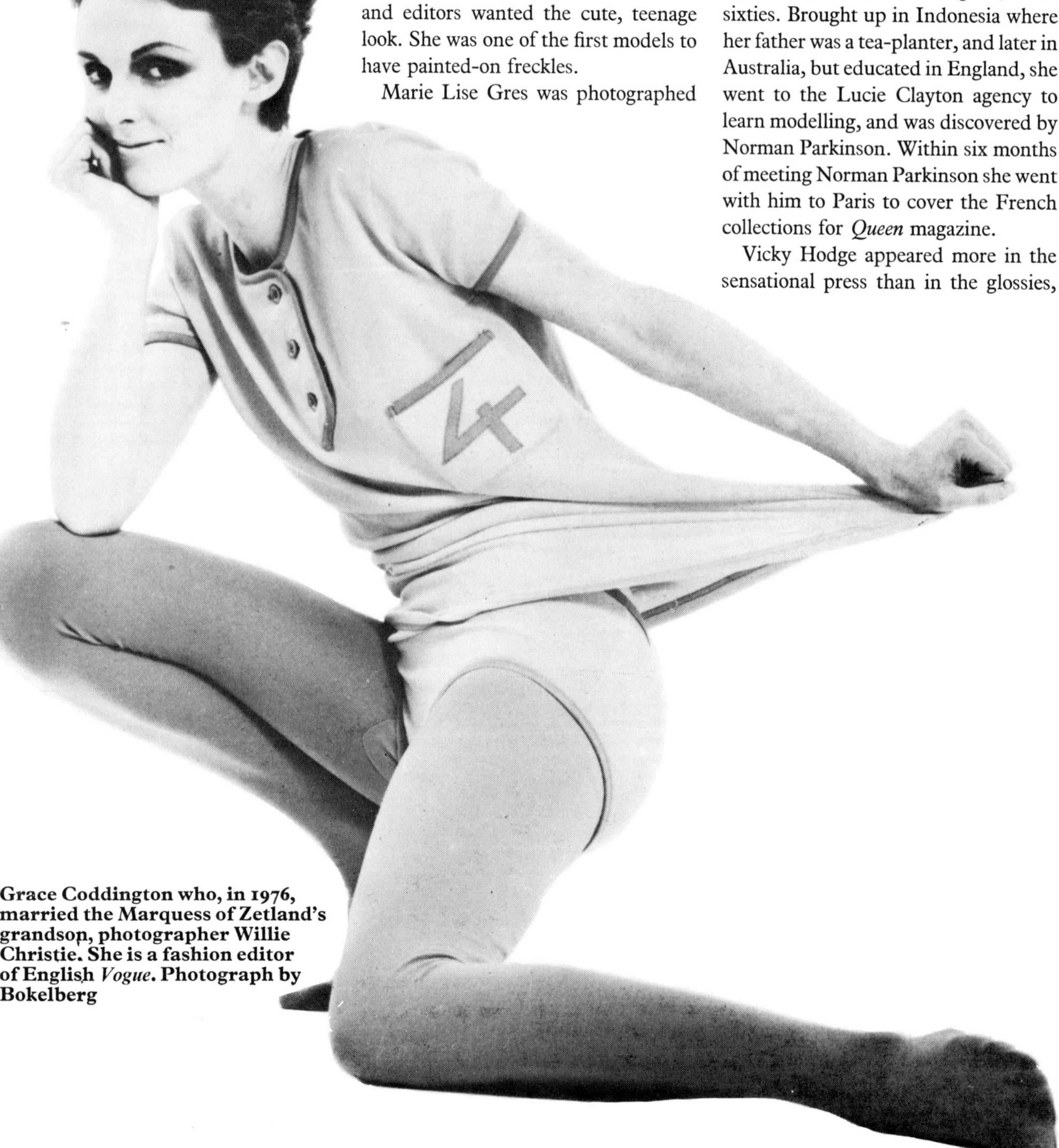

Grace Coddington who, in 1976, married the Marquess of Zetland's grandson, photographer Willie Christie. She is a fashion editor of English *Vogue*. Photograph by Bokelberg

like *Vogue*. She was purely 'London' though, and not known internationally. *The* nude model of the sixties, she comments: 'If photographers couldn't get models to take their clothes off, I and another girl were the ones. I was extremely proud of my bottom. Still am.' In the sixties, she was paid £300 a day, plus first class travelling expenses, to model swimsuits in Jamaica—a considerable amount for an English model.

Marie Helvin is now David Bailey's wife, and was one of his discoveries: 'She was the top model in Tokyo. She came here, but everybody was making her look like a Japanese doll, and I'm not really interested in Japanese dolls so I didn't take much notice. Then *Vogue* suggested I use her, so I sort of changed her looks. I've always been mad about Anna May Wong, so I tried to push her into that exotic, mysterious area.'

When it comes to photographic models, one rarely sees coloured or oriental models in advertisements: 'It's no good doing an ad for Max Factor or Revlon with a girl that the majority of people can't identify with. It's very difficult to put make-up on a black girl.

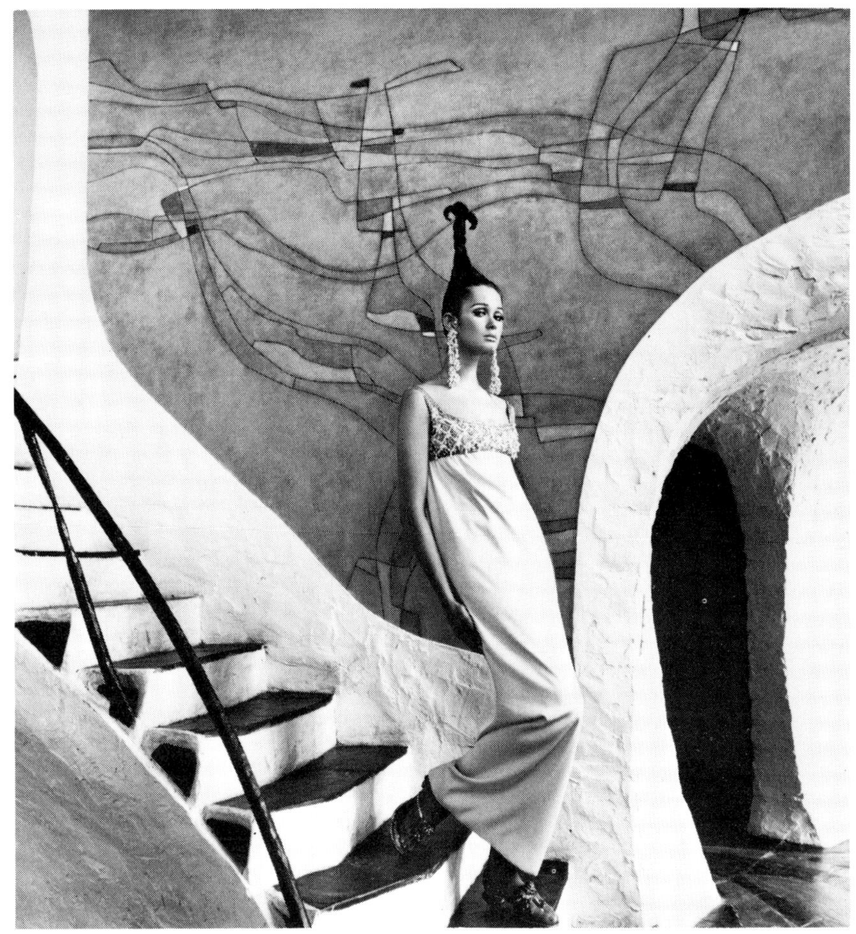

Above right: Marie Lise Gres, photographed by Henry Clarke

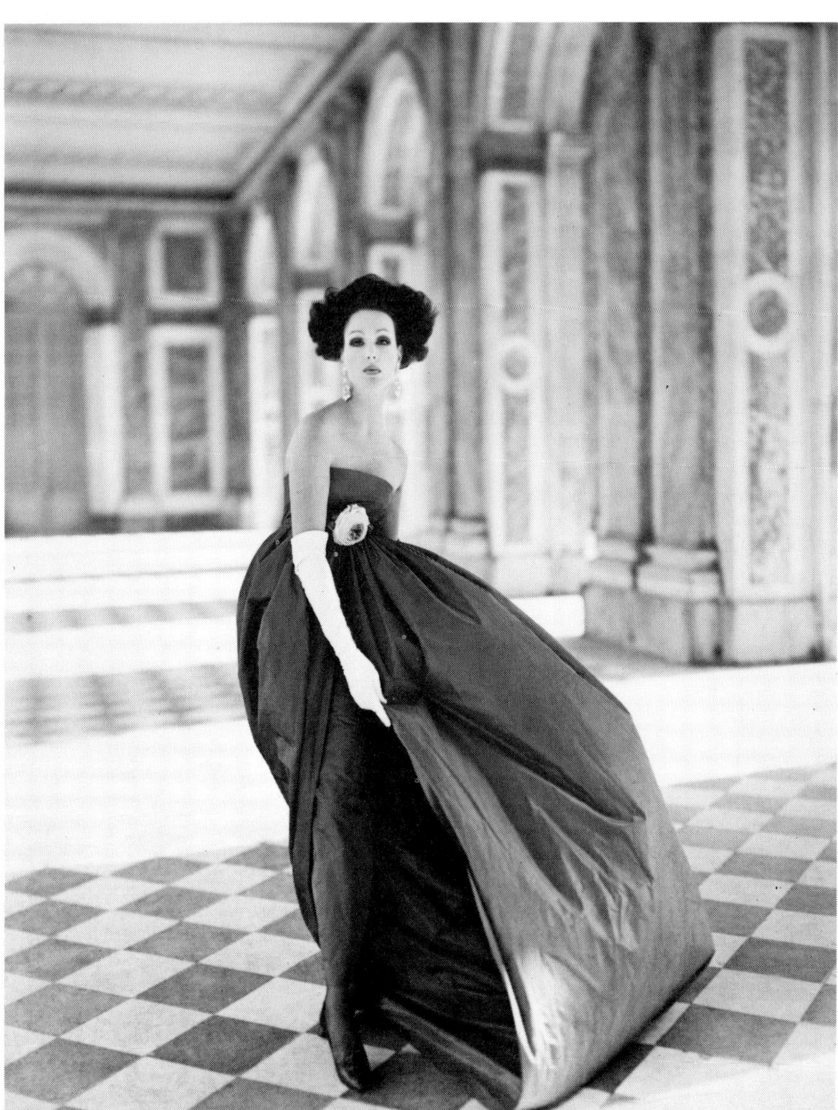

Right: Betsy Pickering, photographed in a Pierre Cardin dress by Richard Dormer

If you put make-up on made for a black girl, you're selling to a black market. In fact, I was the first to put a black girl on the cover of all *Vogues*. That was Donyale Luna. And that was the first cover of all black girls.

'It's not odd. If we're doing a fashion magazine in China, we're not going to have an English girl on the cover. People buying in China aren't going to believe they're going to look like Lauren Hutton.'

Angelica Huston modelled a great deal for *Vogue*. She has a great, cold, hard, elegant look. 'She was a personality,' says David Bailey, 'but an international one. A fantastic model. She was a great kind of original beauty.'

Maudie James who was one of the traditional English-rose types, was first photographed by Lord Snowdon in 1966, for an article called 'Fresh Faces'. She did many magazine covers, and worked for all the top photographers in London, but suddenly word was out: 'No more Maudie James'. They had found another new face to replace hers and she works consistently in Europe these days.

Jill Kennington has the most marvellous Mediterranean-blue eyes. Although not very successful in England, she made it when she went to America and then Italy. She was discovered by Sir Norman Hartnell: 'She was a natural, she arrived without any training, and became a very fine model indeed.' When she first began photographic modelling she was stiff and awkward to photograph, but although she's thirty-five now, she has been a top model for ten years. She has never been photographed with a male model, or with another girl. In her publicity material, she displays only her name—never her face.

Tania Mallet 'Of all the top photographic models, I think Tania is most like what people imagine models ought to be', says Jean Shrimpton. 'I think she is ravishing to look at. She is witty, biting, earthy, and fascinating, all rolled into one.' She has high cheek bones, soft, silky skin, and cold, slanted doe-like eyes. Leading fashion editors found her difficult to work with, but full of fun and personality. 'She did charity shows for me', recalls Sir Norman Hartnell. 'She was a lovely person and was very nice to me.'

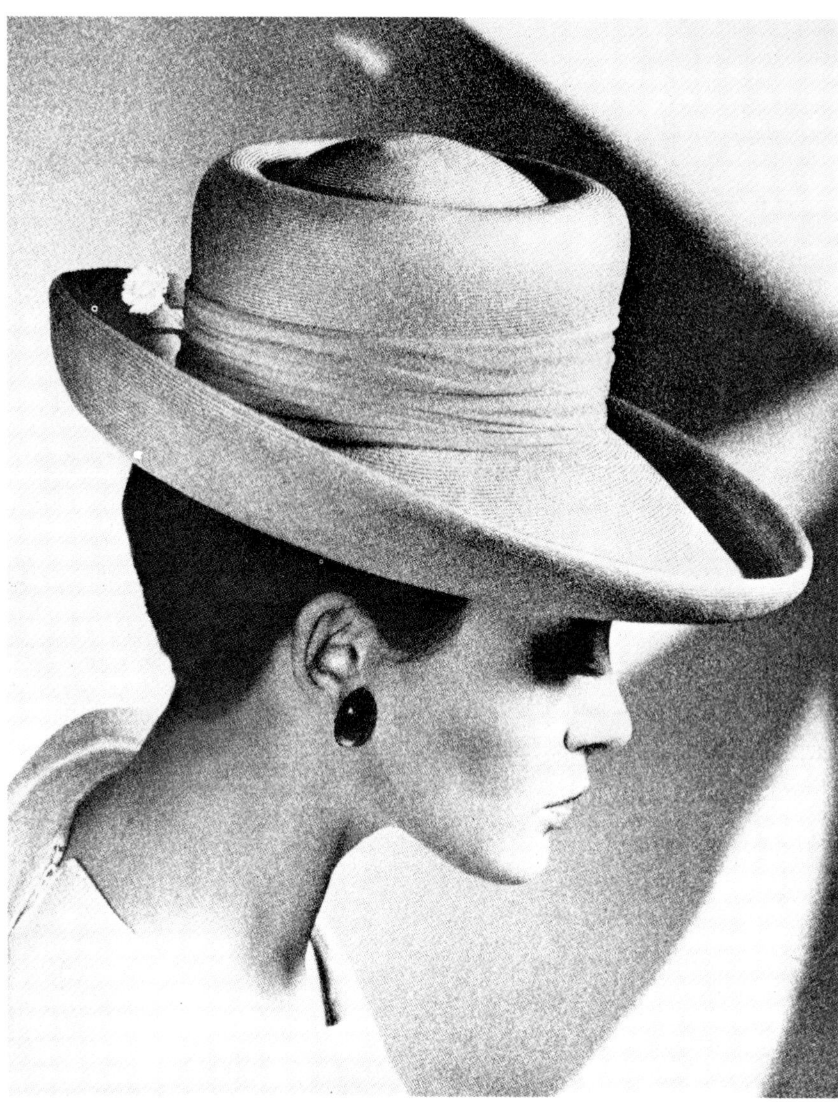

Jill Kennington, by Richard Dormer

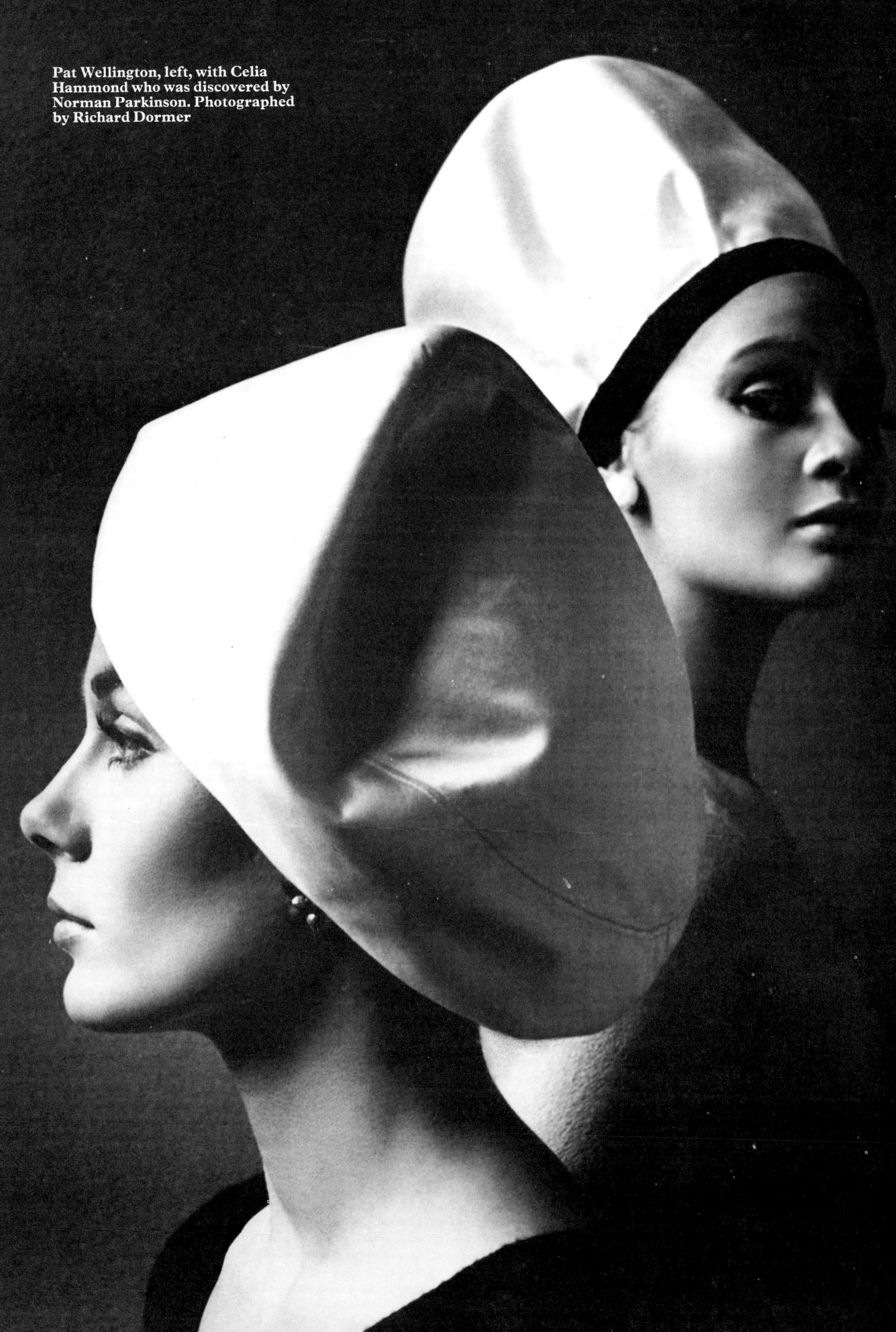

Pat Wellington, left, with Celia Hammond who was discovered by Norman Parkinson. Photographed by Richard Dormer

Sue Murray is considered by David Bailey to be a superlative model, one of the best. He was the first to photograph her, and they worked together a great deal. 'Sue was more my conscious invention, whereas Jean Shrimpton was an unconscious creation', he says. She tended to get overlooked as she seemed to be in Jean's shadow all the time.

Greta Norris was a beautiful model with sexy lips and straight blonde hair, who stemmed from Paris. She became better known than many of the *Vogue* models because she worked a lot for the more popular magazines, *Nova* and *Cosmopolitan*. She also appeared in many British Rail posters, in a bikini, inviting the public to British seaside resorts.

Sandra Paul was very good for advertising because she wouldn't offend anybody. The English-rose type, sophisticated, upper-class looking, she has corn-coloured hair and huge brown eyes, and is much in demand in Paris and New York. Her career began at Lucie Clayton's modelling school, then Norman Parkinson saw her and photographed her. Her picture appeared on the *Vogue* cover almost at once. She was photographed regularly by Brian Duffy.

Sue Purdy has been hailed as the face of the mid-seventies and her face was chosen to launch the *Vogue* book, *In Vogue—Six Decades of Fashion*. Daughter of author Tony Purdy, she spent her childhood travelling around the Far East until she was fifteen. After a spell as a secretary and a PR girl, she was 'discovered' by photographer Barry Lategan when she was nineteen. London's top beauty and hair photographer, Lategan moulded the blonde grey-eyed beauty with the expert help of make-up artist Barbara Daly. A compulsive, excitable girl, Sue has an ethereal aura about her. Now she works a lot in Germany, and is very much in demand in Japan, where she works for the largest cosmetic company, Kanebo. Her next step is to New York—where she will almost certainly reach the top.

Before he discovered Jean Shrimpton, David Bailey's work was first recognised when he photographed Paulene Stone. Ex-*Sunday Times* fashion editor, Brigid Keenan, who worked on the *Daily Express* at the time, says: 'The first thing of any note that happened to us was using David Bailey for a feature called Autumn Girl, and Bailey photographed Paulene Stone on all fours, talking to a squirrel. It's a terribly significant picture and it was the first time I'd seen a model photographed as though she was an ordinary girl. I think she was a great model.

'Terry Donovan saw the picture in the *Express*', David Bailey goes on, 'and said to me, "That's something new, baby." And so, this "new thing" I found I had, was first with Paulene Stone, not with Jean Shrimpton.' Paulene became one of London's top models, better remembered as 'Redbird', proof that the traditional coolness and chic were very much alive. Paulene was more 'London' than international in her work. She worked more for newspapers and *Woman's Own* than for glossies like *Vogue*.

Sarah Stuart was by no means a top model, but worked consistently throughout the sixties. She had a certain striking look, and an ambitious mother who helped her career, which culminated in her marriage to the Aga Khan in October 1969 at the age of twenty-nine.

Moyra Swan is currently one of Britain's top fashion photographic models. First photographed by David Bailey, they work together a great deal for *Vogue*, for whom she has done many covers. 'I like her because she is adaptable', says Bailey. 'She is everybody's idea of a model. I usually work with friends, and Moyra's a friend.'

Penelope Tree has a strange, individual look, classed in the same category as Veruschka and Donyale Luna for their fantasy, exotic image. 'Penelope Tree is the most original model there's

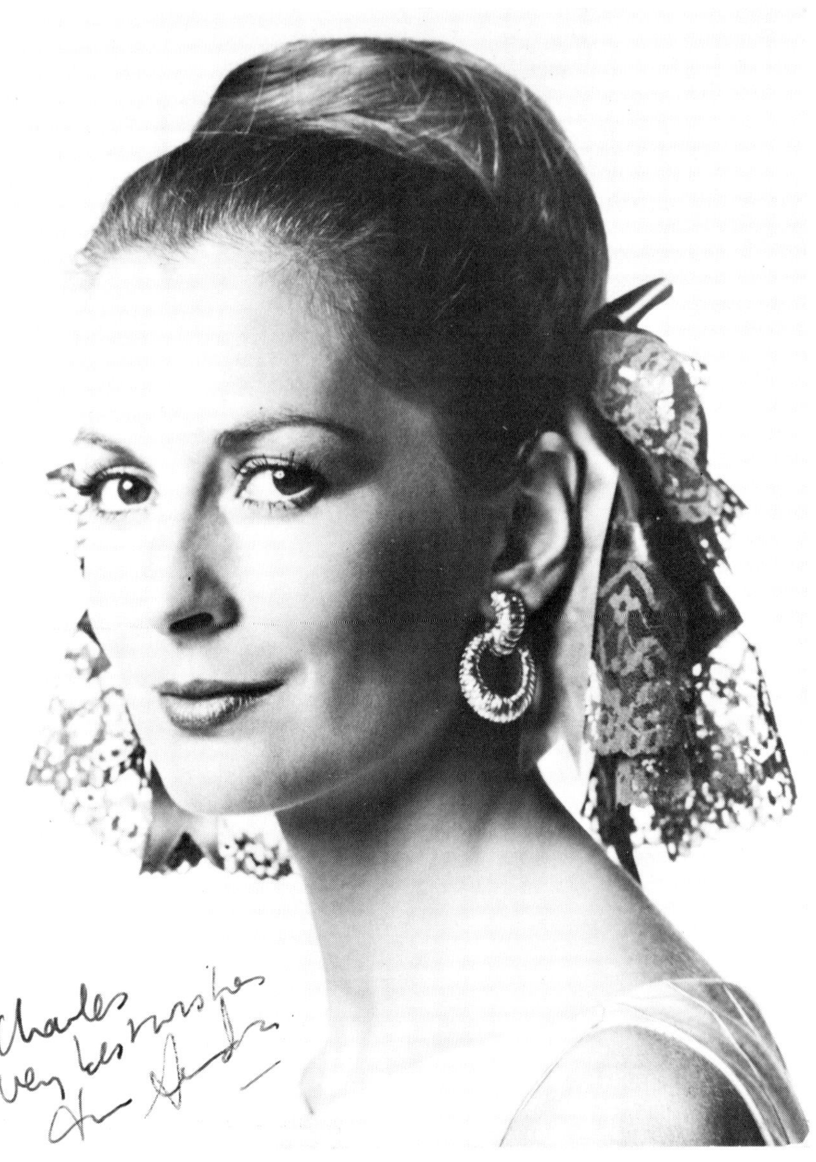

ever been', comments David Bailey, for whom she has worked consistently for many years. 'She's the most original looking girl I've ever seen.'

Jean Shrimpton's natural successor was Twiggy and, like Shrimpton, she became an international success almost overnight. She shot into prominence when girls of the sixties tried to emulate the ordinary, sweet, 'girl next door' look. Acclaimed throughout the world by the time she was seventeen, her success is justifiably attributed to the astute management of Justin de Villeneuve, who groomed and nurtured her for stardom.

Twiggy had her first, unsuccessful brush with fashion when writer Prudence Glynn went to see Lesley Hornby, as she was then known, for *Woman's Own* magazine. She and the art director were looking for a 'new face'. She

returned to tell her editor that the photographer felt that this was not the face to launch a thousand magazine covers. Later, however, photographer Barry Lategan, who was the first to photograph Twiggy in London, had a call from hairdresser Leonard with whom he had worked before with other models. Lategan had developed a reputation for hair and beauty photography, and agreed to see the girl whom Leonard said he knew through a friend of his, Justin de Villeneuve. 'I want to do a haircut on her', he added. Justin de Villeneuve had known Leonard from their old barrow-boy days, and had taken his young protégée to have her long, blonde frizzy fair hair re-styled. Leonard cut it into a short, boyish style, and sent her along to Barry Lategan's studio.

'The first thing that struck me when

she walked into the studio', Lategan recalls, 'was her friendliness. "Ullo!" she said. She was very natural and warm. On that first day, Justin said to her, "Stop biting your nails, Twigs." I said, "What did you call her?" and he replied "Twigs. Twiggy. Because she's thin." I said, "That's a terrific name. Call her that." ' He took Lategan's advice, and the name and the first photographs taken by Barry Lategan rocketed the child into an overnight phenomenon. The *Daily Express*'s then fashion editor, Deirdre McSharry, was shown the photographs, and she gave

Below: Paulene Stone, widow of film actor Laurence Harvey, photographed by John French

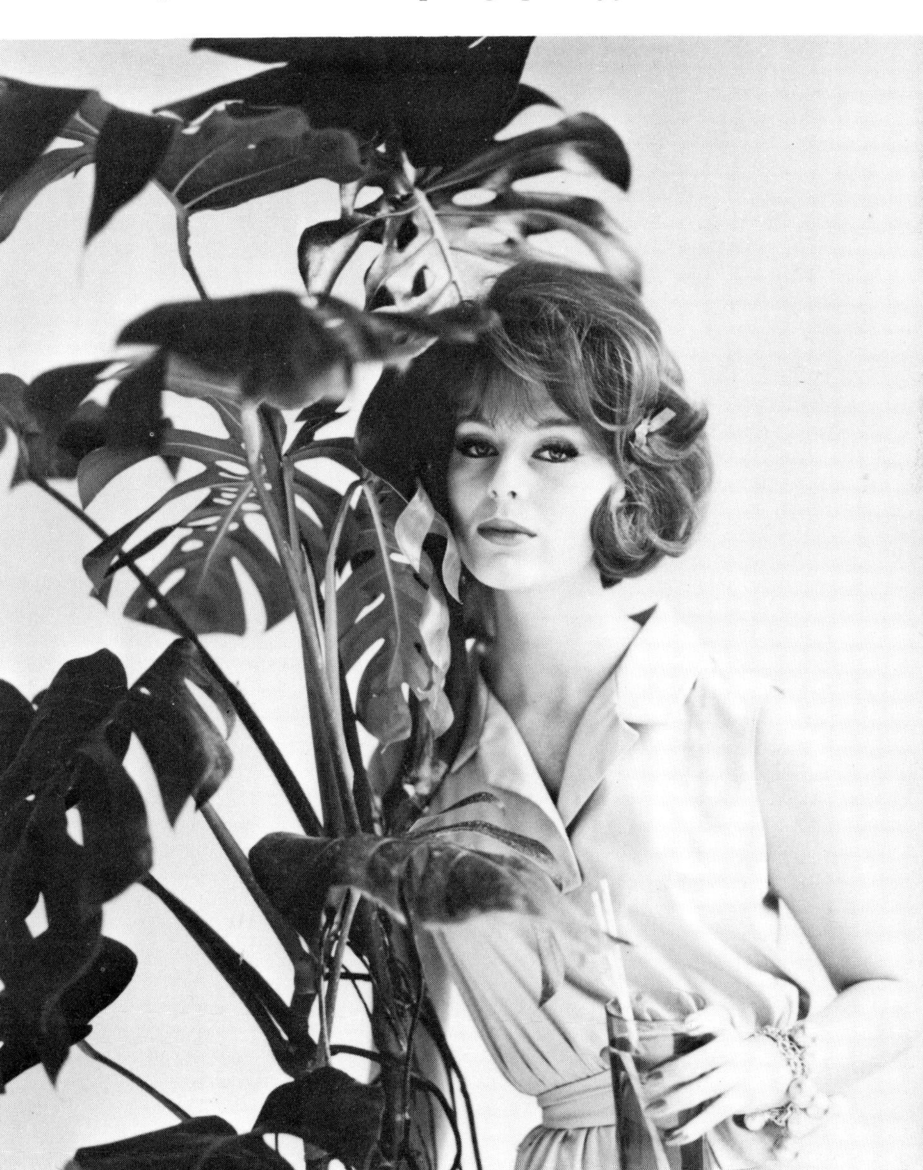

Opposite: Sandra Paul, former wife of Robin Douglas-Home, nephew of the Tory ex-prime minister

her full-page coverage headlined, 'This is the face of '66. Twiggy, the Cockney kid with the face to launch a thousand shapes and she's only sixteen.' Yet up until then she had done no modelling.

Whereas, after Jean Shrimpton, models such as Brenda Harper, Anne Larson, Imogen Woodford, and Ros Watkins, had an older, sophisticated look, Twiggy introduced the 'innocent, child-like' look to modelling and became a model cult-figure. She 'personalised' the look of a model, and other models began copying her style and gave themselves similar nicknames, such as Bluey or Smokey. While Justin de Villeneuve created the Twiggy entity, Barry Lategan created her photographically because he took the best pictures of her. 'When Twiggy sat in front of the camera, her awareness of what she was

doing was extraordinary', Lategan continued. 'Being photogenic is never a question of features alone. It's a sense of projection: and Twiggy had that.'

Although the media was instrumental in creating Twiggy, the subsequent reaction by fashionable young London photographers was to gang up and not use her. Until then models were always handled by an agency, and photographers called the tune, but Justin de Villeneuve escorted Twiggy everywhere, and took her away from studios at 5.30 when photographers wanted to work on into the evening. He started demanding terms for models which they never had before, and so a natural reaction against the two of them developed, but it had no effect on Twiggy's career whatsoever. She took London, Paris and New York by storm. The

5ft 6in desperately skinny girl with a boyish haircut, enormous innocent eyes, and natural warmth, radiated the Mini-era. Her name became a household word and jokes and gags were cracked about her flat chest.

'Twiggy was a product, whereas Jean Shrimpton was something that "happened",' comments David Bailey, ever-loyal to the model *he* created. 'Once something is established, then you can make a product of it. I compare it to the difference between the Beatles and the Dave Clark Five. The Beatles was a natural innovation whereas the Dave Clark Five was a product.'

The top cosmetics cover girls in London in the mid-seventies include Sue Purdy, and Micki Gardener, who is Australian born and has a perfect heart-shaped face. She modelled in

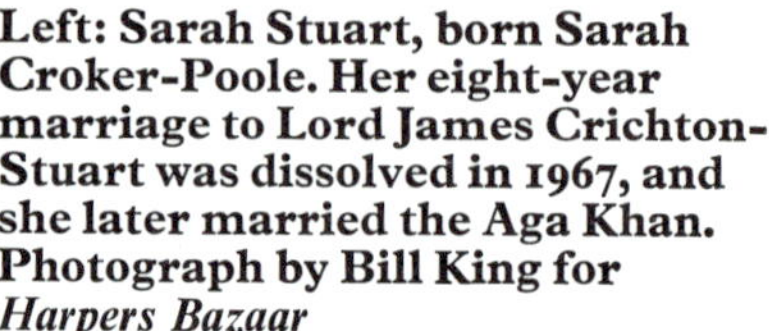

Left: Sarah Stuart, born Sarah Croker-Poole. Her eight-year marriage to Lord James Crichton-Stuart was dissolved in 1967, and she later married the Aga Khan. Photograph by Bill King for *Harpers Bazaar*

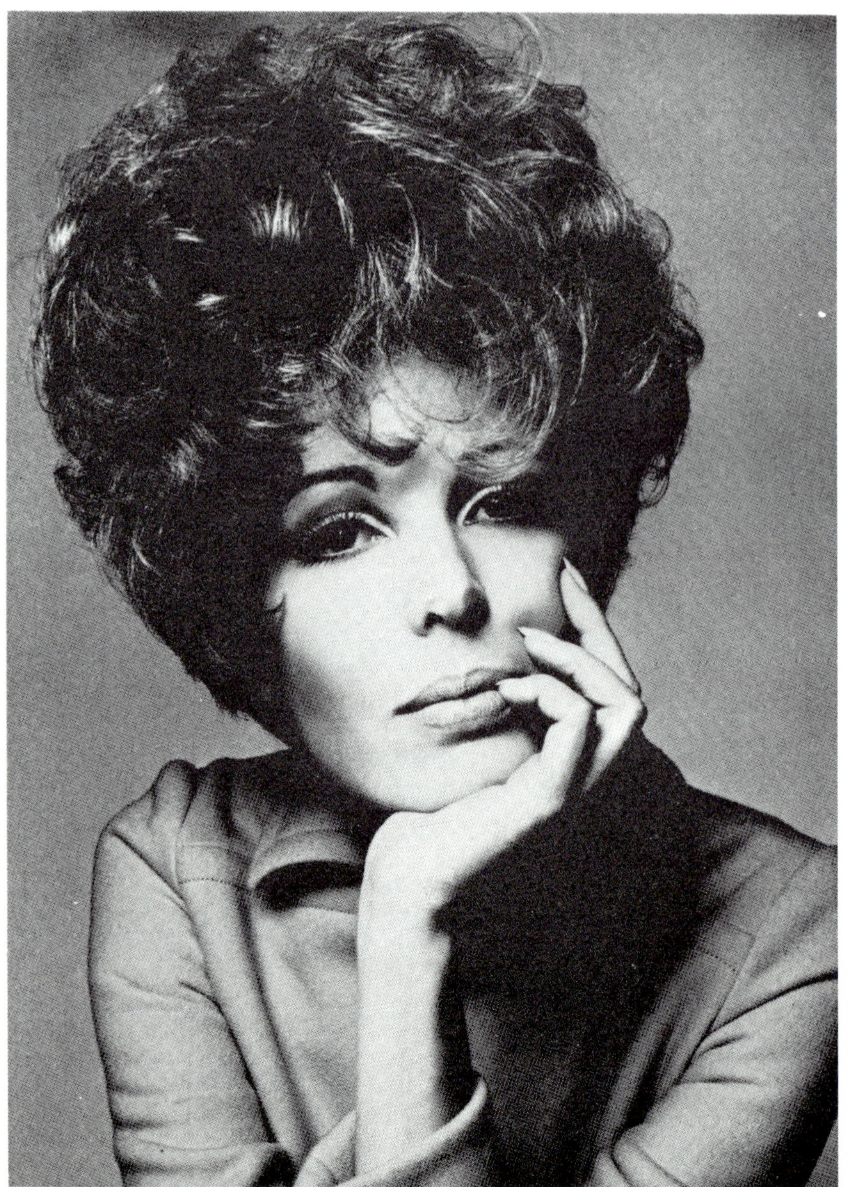

Opposite: Twiggy, the natural successor to Jean Shrimpton, whose 5ft 6in frame, huge innocent eyes and natural warmth took the world by storm when she was only sixteen. 'Created' by her mentor, Justin de Villeneuve, she was first photographed by Barry Lategan in 1966, and heralded as the face of 1966 by the *Daily Express*. **Photograph by Barry Lategan**

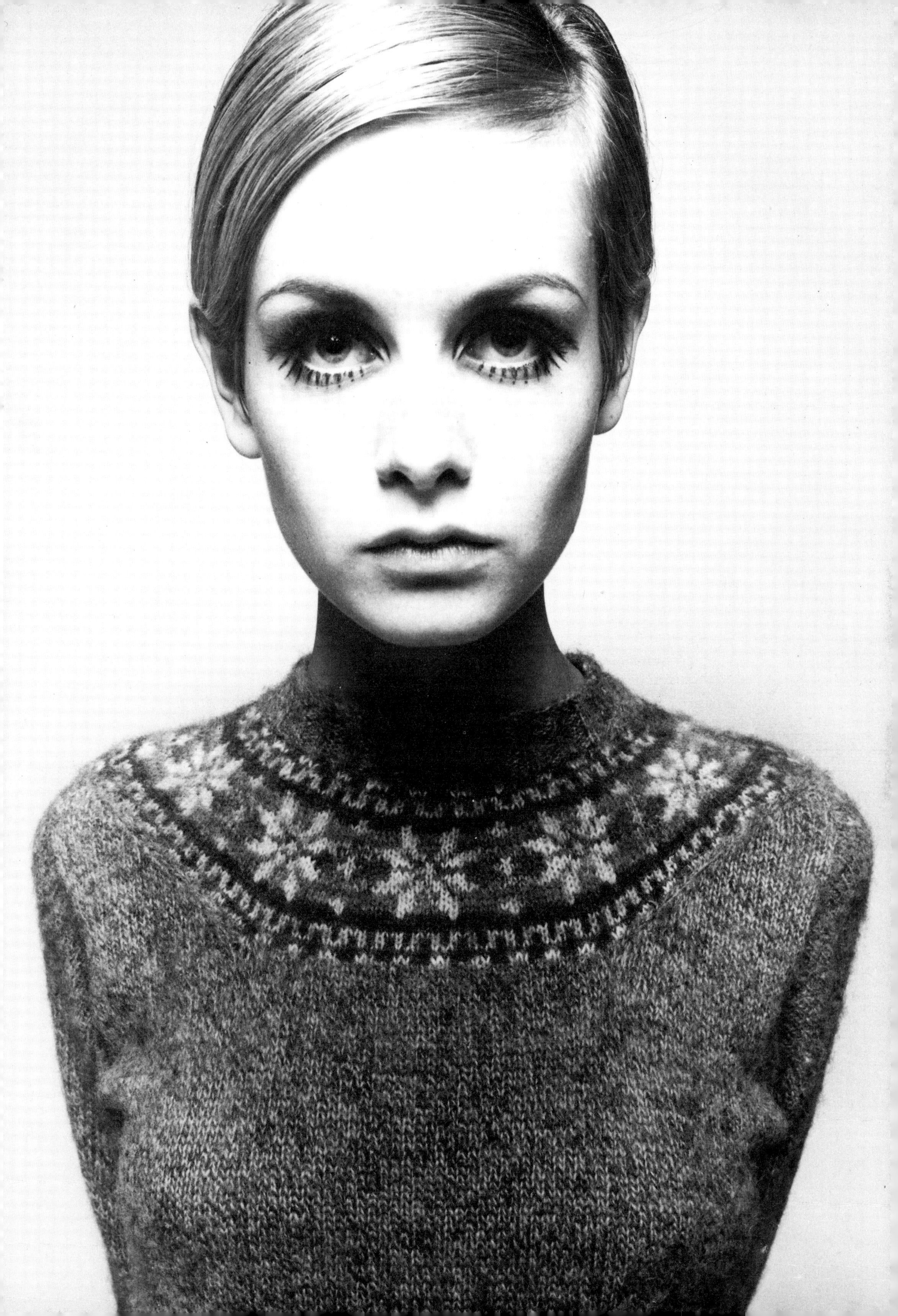

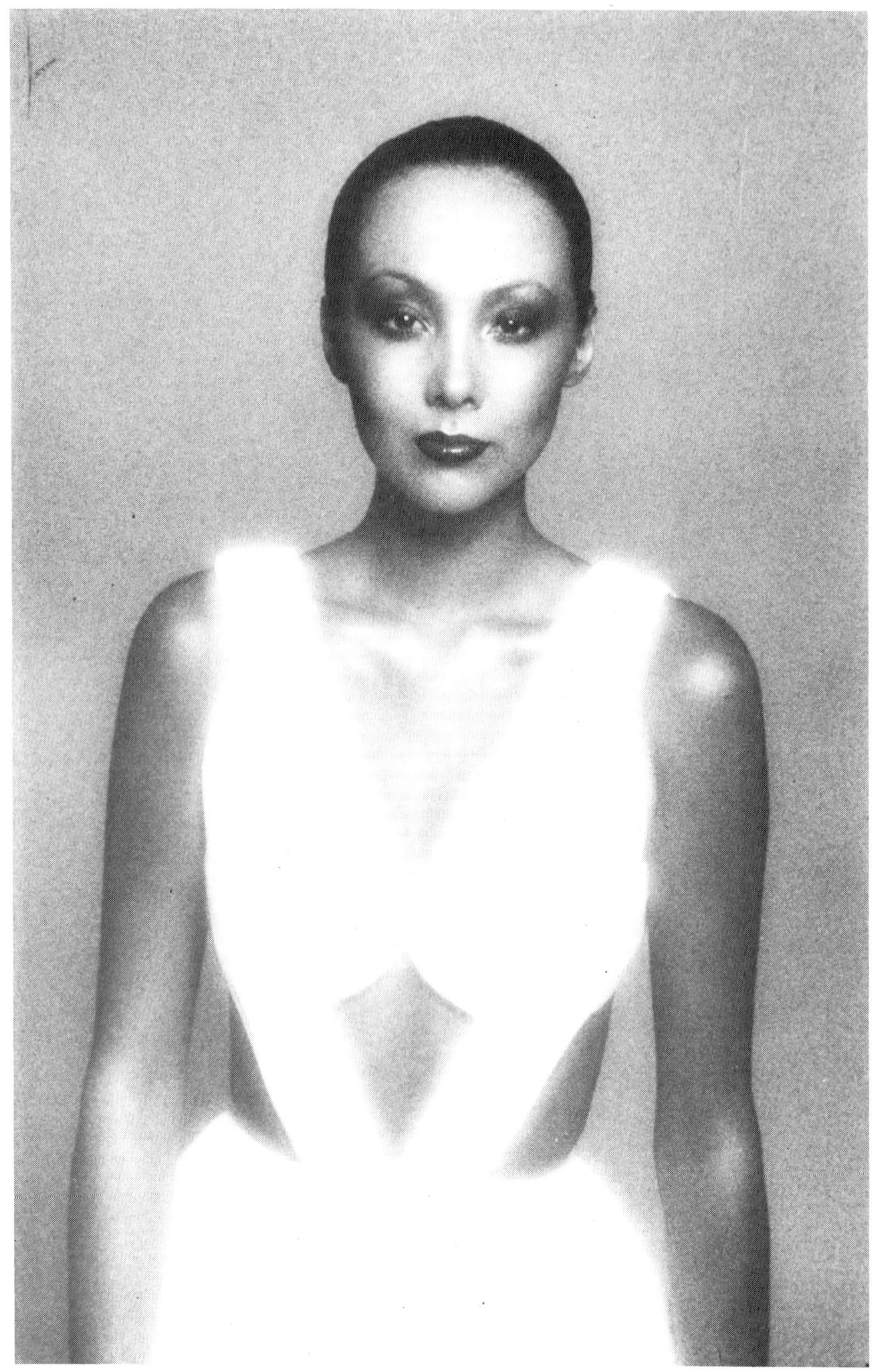

**Above: Marie Helvin, by her
husband David Bailey—*Vogue*
France**

**Opposite: Vibéké, photographed by
David Bailey—*Vogue* France**

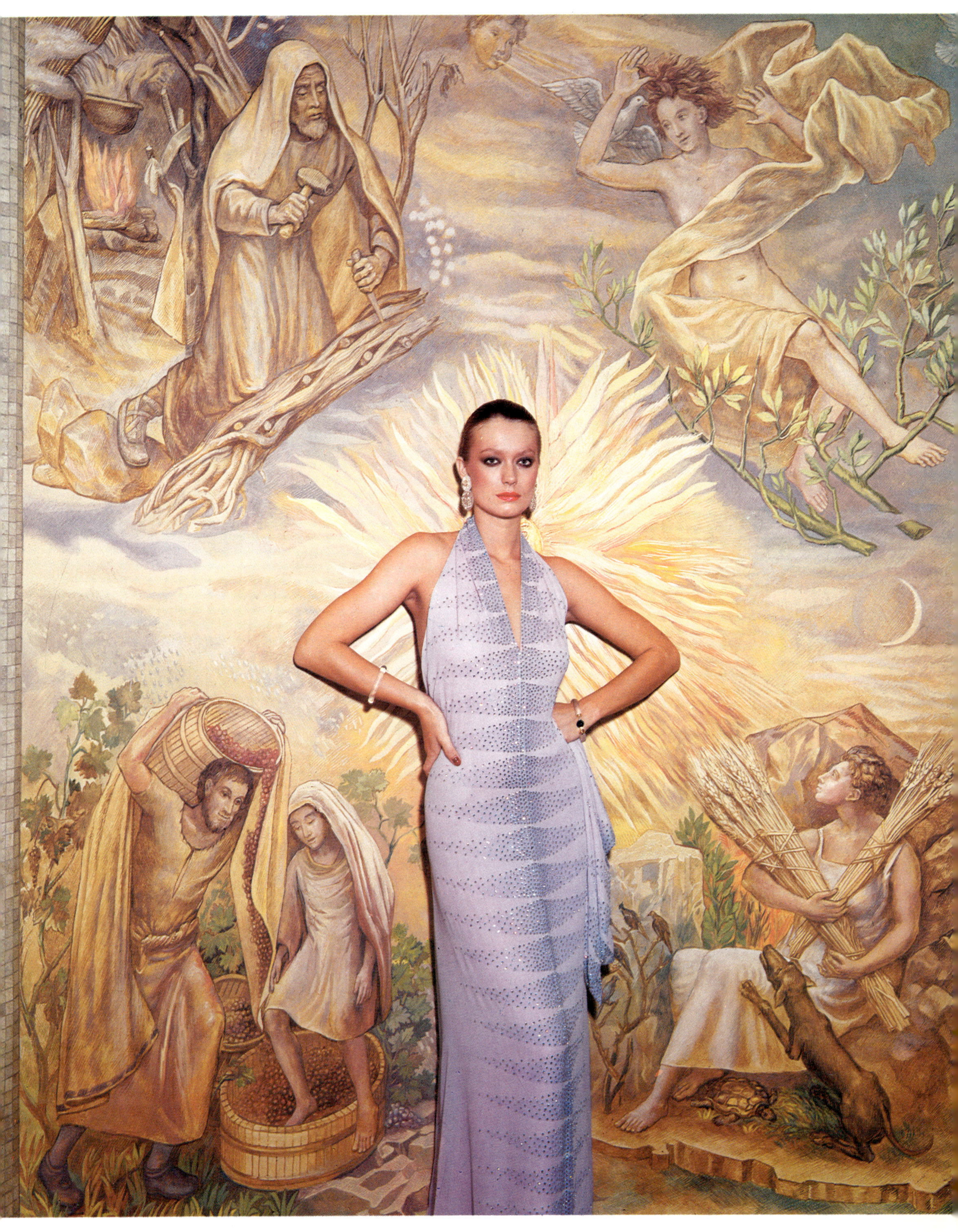

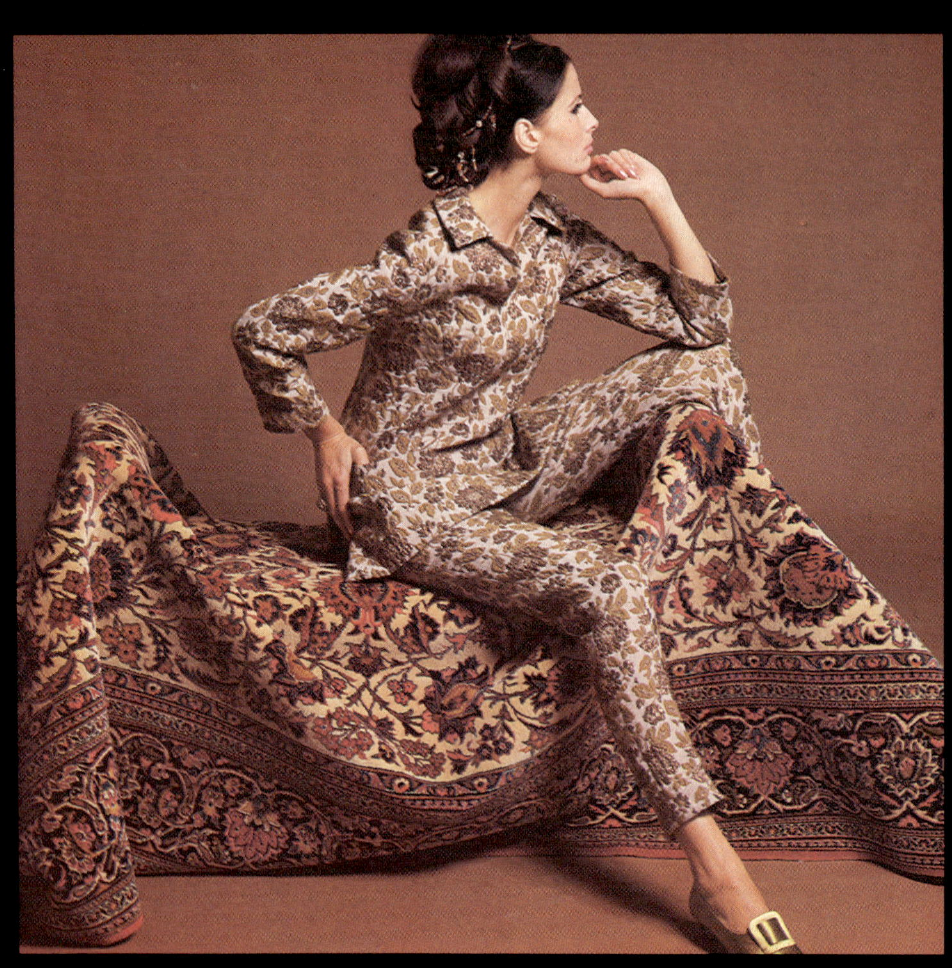

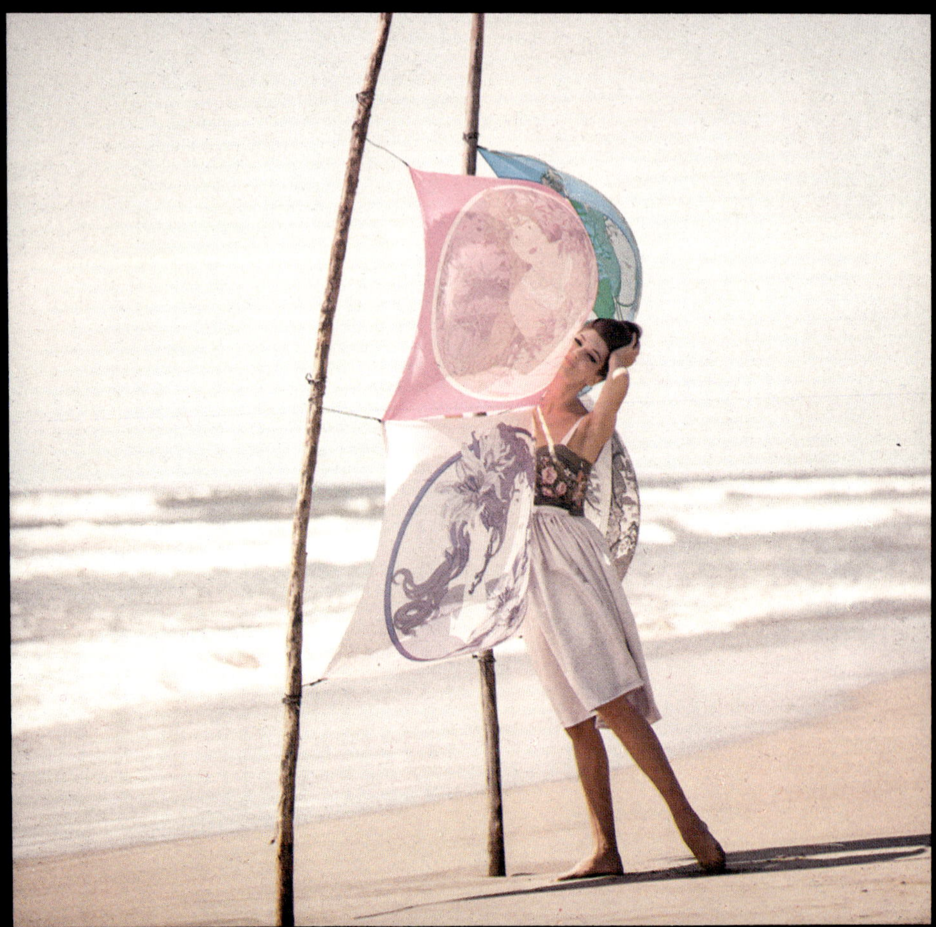

Italy for two years and now lives and works in London, specialising in hair pictures. Esther DeDeo, tall, dark and wafer-thin, was born in Pittsburgh, Pennsylvania, and was originally a mathematics teacher. She later married, lived and modelled in New York, and then moved to Australia for five years with her husband who is in advertising. Rose Marie was acclaimed Miss Teenage America at the age of seventeen. She came to London and played Adam Faith's girlfriend in *Stardust*. Cathee Dahmen, an American Indian who started work as an artist's model, made her name in New York. Then, five years ago, she came to England. She married the English actor Leonard Whiting (the young Romeo in Zefferelli's film *Romeo and Juliet*), and they have a four-year-old daugher, Sarah.

The permissive society of the sixties had introduced nudity, the pot era, boutiques, and discotheques. The world began to turn upside down and the youth trend proved financially rewarding for many. The kids were making money, some of them becoming millionaires. In 1966 anybody under twenty-five was convinced that through music, fashion, and drama they could build a new society, but their wares—pop music, trendy gear and way-out art—were exploited to the hilt. Businessmen made money out of the industry and talent of these youngsters, but many lost it in a few short years when times changed, and the seventies came along with inflation, recession—and depression. Britain was in a mess; businesses went bankrupt at a rate of thousands a month; it was as close as it could get to the 1929 collapse in America.

Model girls of the seventies have reflected these changes by becoming rather like the aloof models of the fifties, except they have a harder, tougher look about them. With a few exceptions, the sixties girls all tried for the ordinary, sweet, girl-next-door look, but the seventies girls have an almost frighteningly tough look, no doubt because of the clothes they have to show. They need to have strong looks to go with the clothes and the multi-million pound empires they advertise; to go with the tough times the seventies have brought us.

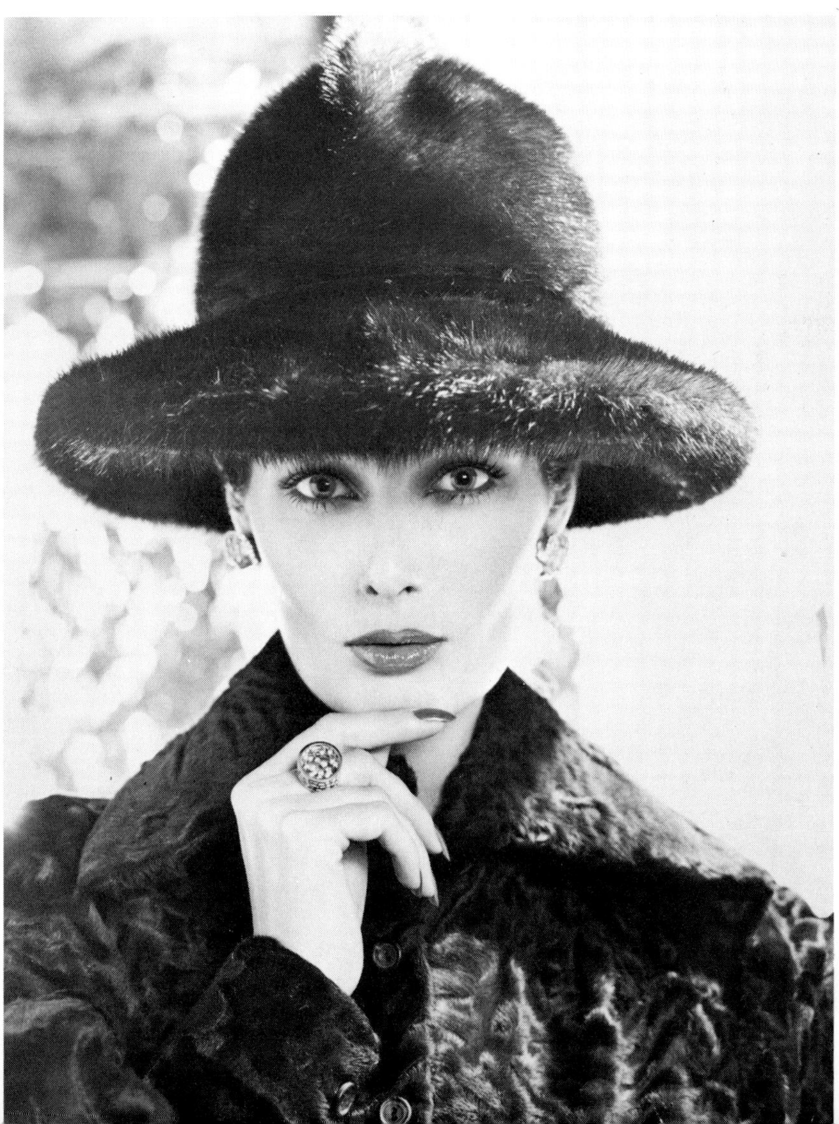

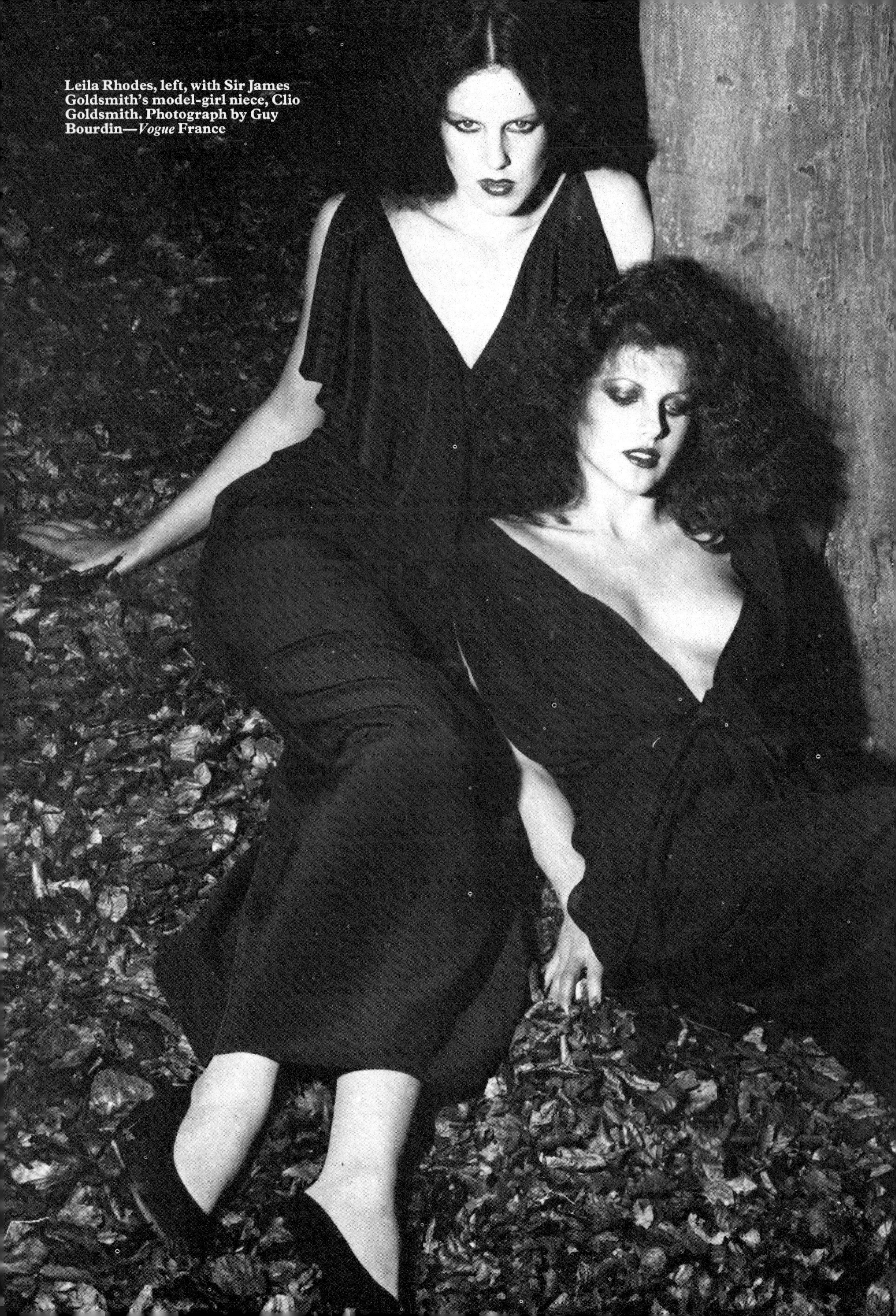

Leila Rhodes, left, with Sir James Goldsmith's model-girl niece, Clio Goldsmith. Photograph by Guy Bourdin—*Vogue* France

Models in Europe

Paris dominated the fashion scene from the mid-nineteenth century to the end of the 1930s. In the twenties and thirties, models arrived to work in Paris from Germany, Sweden, New York, London, and Russia. World War II put paid to any fashion trend-setting in the forties, and as a consequence there were few models around during that period. New York dominated the international modelling scene in the fifties with a handful of English models making the big-time and a freak swing to London as a centre of the model world occurred in the sixties, producing two of the super-models of all time, Jean Shrimpton and Twiggy.

However, the model scene in the seventies has swung back to Paris where it all began in 1852. Here, a handful of top photographers reign supreme, projecting the beauty, flair, and creativity of models who flock to the capital. Each top photographer in Paris has his own style and pet models whom he uses constantly, having the power to hire and fire as he sees fit.

Young models are encouraged to begin their careers in Paris where they can build up a portfolio of good photographs of themselves, and find employment with the many magazines who constantly search for new faces. A sixteen-year-old girl, new to the business, can command 1,500 francs a day in Paris; and although this is half of what she could get in New York, it is good money for an unknown girl fresh out of school. But that is for photographic advertisements. She is paid much less for editorials. For *Vogue* in Paris, the girls get 300 francs a day ($60). English *Vogue* in London would pay her £70 a day. For *Elle* and *Marie-Claire* in Paris, they get 400 francs a day. But although editorial photography pays them less money, it is their best shop window. For a girl starting in Paris, the magazine to go for is *Elle*; it is published weekly, and so the turnover is tremendous. Everybody buys it. The girls who achieve the covers of *Elle* or *Marie-Claire* would work for it for nothing because of the exposure they receive.

French girls rarely make good models. They are, moreover, extremely unprofessional. Surprising facts, since Paris is the Mecca of fashion. But French girls have neither the physical

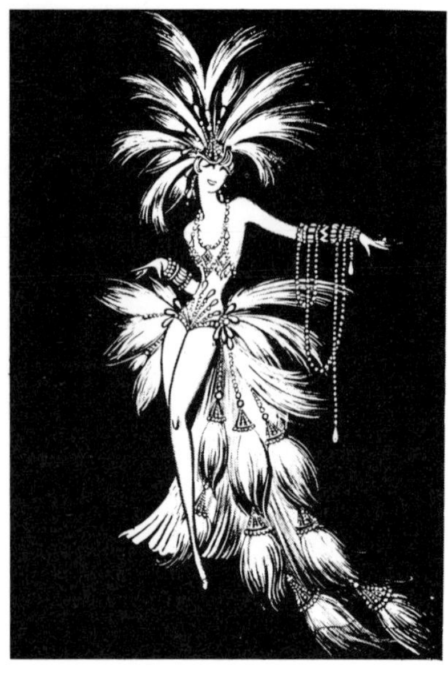

Left: A design for a showgirl at the Folies Bergères, by Alex Shanks

Below and opposite: Two studies of Simone d'Aillencourt during her assignment to India and the Far East with Henry Clarke

dimensions, nor the right temperament required for the job. Latins tend to be short in the leg and long in the torso, whereas a good model needs long legs and a short torso. The best models who tend to have these proportions are American, English, and Scandinavian. Even the spectacular show girls at the Lido and Moulin Rouge in Paris are English or American; no doubt because the astute French get them cheap!

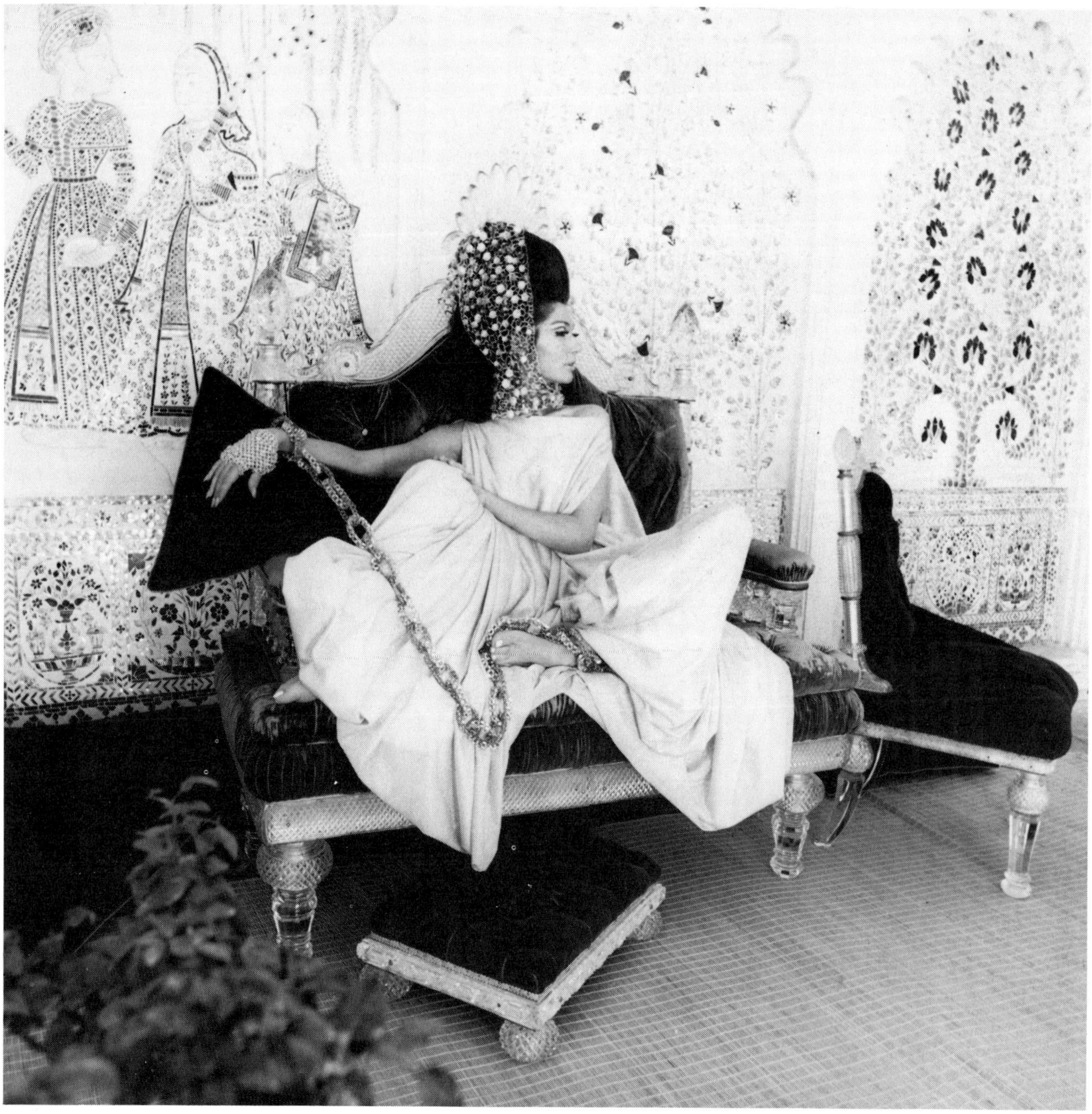

Of the top models who worked in Europe, the majority were Swedes, Danes, Germans, Americans, and British. Wilhelmina, the top model in America, however, was Dutch. She worked consistently in Europe in the sixties. Bronwen Pugh, Balmain's top model, was Welsh and Nina Ricci's head-girl, Nadine, was Russian. The girls leading the field in Europe today are Jeanette Christjansen and Vibéké Knudson who are Danish; Christiana Steidten, German; Ann Anderson, Carrie, and Gunilla Lindblad, Swedish; Suzy Dyson, English; Susan Moncur, American; and Marie Helvin, Japanese.

French girls simply do not have the right mental attitudes for modelling. If ever you hear a girl quarrelling with a client in France, she is bound to be French! The trouble lies in the fact that French girls take the job because they need the money, and they make this too obviously known to the client. Otherwise they're in it for 'kicks', and

although they like the glamour, they don't take it seriously. They certainly reduce this glamorous, fascinating and highly lucrative profession to sloppy indifference.

There are, of course, exceptions, notably the four outstanding French models of all time, Bettina, Simone d'Aillencourt, Nicole de la Margé—and the unforgettable Praline. Ironically, both Nicole and Praline were killed in motor car accidents at the peak of their careers.

Praline modelled for Lelong, and switched to Pierre Balmain when he opened his couture house in 1946. Ginette Spanier, who was Balmain's *directrice* until she became Queen Bee

of the new Nina Ricci ready-to-wear boutique in the Avenue Georges V, in 1976, remembers that Praline was a gay, marvellous, luscious, funny, divine girl.

'Praline was superb', Ginette Spanier enthuses. 'Sometimes when she was showing at rehearsal and a collection of little working girls had crept downstairs to see her, she would open her mink coat and reveal herself stark naked. She did so much to keep the firm gay and spontaneous and happy.

'She was always nipping off somewhere, to do a show in Antibes for instance, which obviously infuriated Balmain, because it would be in the middle of our collection! On one occasion I had to go to Orly airport to plead with her to return. The scene between us was terrifying. I think the people all around thought I was pleading with her to leave my husband alone.'

Praline led a film star's existence in Paris and even went on the stage in a theatre show; she was the symbol of the Parisienne mannequin. She was killed in a car crash on her way back to Paris from Deauville at the peak of her career—and had a funeral like royalty.

In Paris, just after the war, there were no photographic models as such, the models did shows as well as photography. The mannequins at the famous couture houses were known to customers by their names, and a couple of Dior models married rich men—one of them the owner of *Paris Match*. Victoire, who was another Dior model, was clever enough to find a shop in the Place Victoire and promptly rented it, naming it after herself.

One of the few French models to achieve international stardom as a model in the fifties was Simone d'Aillencourt, who, born in France, went to London at the age of twenty-one to learn English. She married the French film maker José Bénazéraf, had two children, and nowadays, having retired from modelling, runs one of the top model agencies in Paris, Models International in fashionable Avenue Victor Hugo.

When Simone arrived in London, she was asked so frequently by strangers whether she was a model that she decided to try her hand at it. She read newspaper advertisements for model agents, and went along to see Lucie

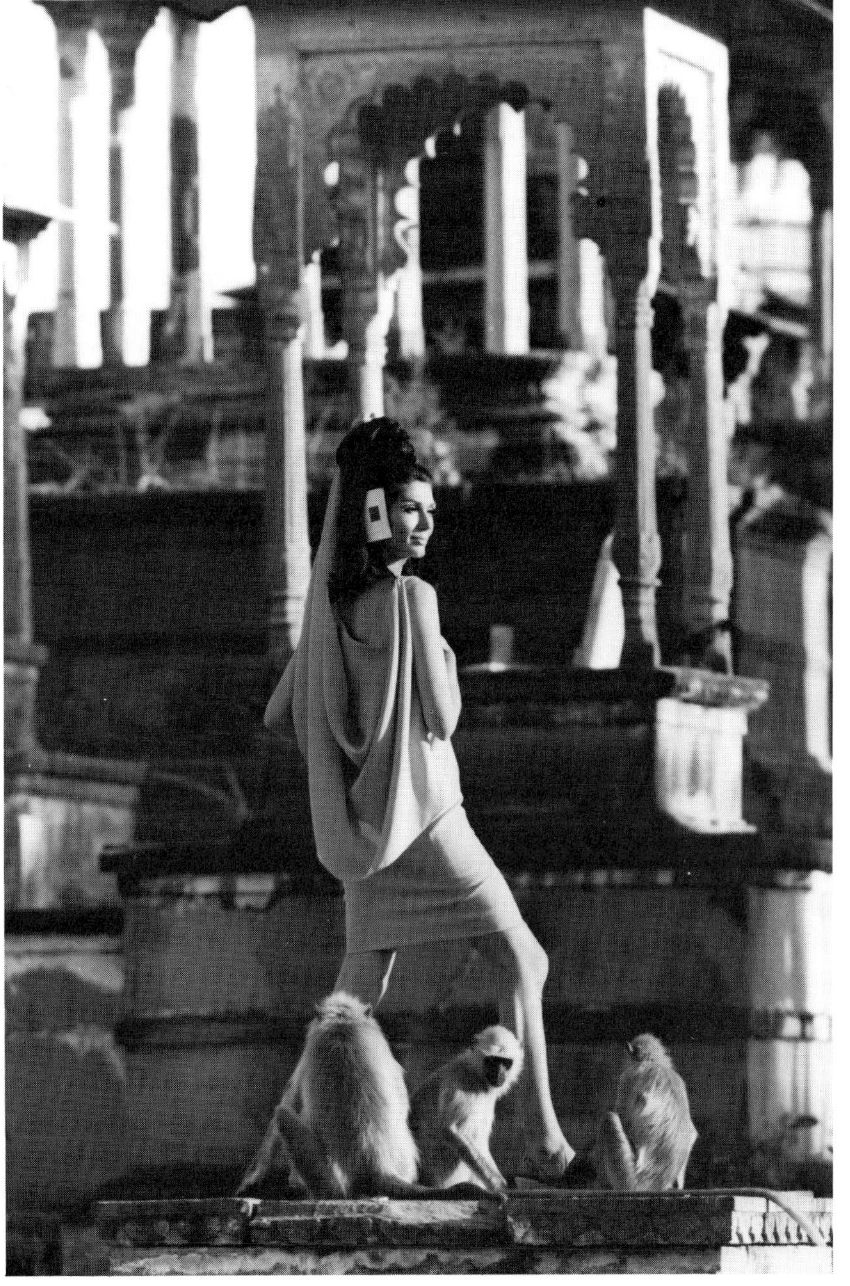

Clayton. She told them that she had had no experience and when they suggested she join their model school for tuition, she declined, explaining that she had come for work, not for schooling. They persuaded her to join one of their courses, but after two days she felt she didn't need tuition and told them so.

However, they realised that she had potential and sent her along to do a collection in Edinburgh, telling her they would pass her off as a famous French model, newly arrived in London, having shown the Dior collections.

Simone returned from Edinburgh and called on the famous fashion houses in London. She showed Hardy Amies' collection and, whilst there, met the fashion editor of English *Vogue* who asked to see her at the end of the show. 'Although I told her that I'd had no photographic modelling experience, she asked me to the studio the next day, and there I met the *Vogue* photographers, Americans Henry Clarke and Don Silverstein. So I started working for *Vogue* immediately, later being photographed by Norman Parkinson.' She

continued to work in London, and when a French editor saw her photographs in English *Harpers Bazaar*, he telephoned her, not knowing she was French, to invite her to Paris.

She returned to Paris to do the collections for photographer Tom Kublin for English *Harpers Bazaar*, but William Klein, who was photographing the collections for *Vogue*, wanted her as well. He had already booked a handful of well known American models, but now he wanted Simone instead. 'When do you finish working with Kublin, each day?' he wanted to know. 'Not until midnight', she replied. And so he persuaded her to join him at his studio after midnight, to work until five in the mornings, for *Vogue*.

She decided to work in Paris permanently, and was employed by every major photographer and magazine. The great American model agent, Eileen Ford, saw her and began sending her letters encouraging her to go to New York. 'You'll love New York and New York will love you', she wrote. Simone took some time to decide, as she was

rather frightened of the prospect of going to New York, but finally went and began by working for *Harpers Bazaar*.

Diana Vreeland, who was the fashion editor for *Harpers Bazaar*, employed Simone for eight months. She was a great entrepeneur, discovering many models and photographers, always helping them in their careers, developing and guiding their talents.

Henry Clarke was one of the top photographers working in Paris and London in the fifties who worked with Simone: 'She started in London, and was brought over by an editor we had at *Vogue* called Pat Cunningham. Simone had a kind of homely chic about her. I used her then, in a small way, in the fifties, and she went on from there. Bit by bit, bit by bit, she worked on herself. It was magic what this girl did to herself. Her legs were straight, but somehow when you photographed her, they looked like Dietrich's legs. I don't know how she did it, but she had studied carefully how to arrange those legs, how to stand; and if she sat, how to place them. Her face, without make-up; zero. But when she had the full thing on, the shading, the make-up, the hair, the eyelashes, she was dazzling. These girls in the fifties did their homework. They worked out everything they had to know for their trade. In other words in order to be as beautiful as they could be.'

Nicole de la Margé was one of the best French photographic models, although her name was never known to the public. David Bailey claims that there were only two really great models as far as he is concerned: Nicole de la Margé and Jean Shrimpton. He found Nicole to be a natural model, but can't define why she was so rare. 'Nicole just didn't have a face', Bailey says, 'but she was an unbelievable artist. You'd say, "Go away and come back looking like Audrey Hepburn", and she'd come back as Audrey Hepburn.'

Left: Simone d'Aillencourt, photographed in the bubble on the Seine by Melvin Sokolsky

Opposite: Nicole de la Margé, one of the great French models of the sixties, photographed by Henry Clarke

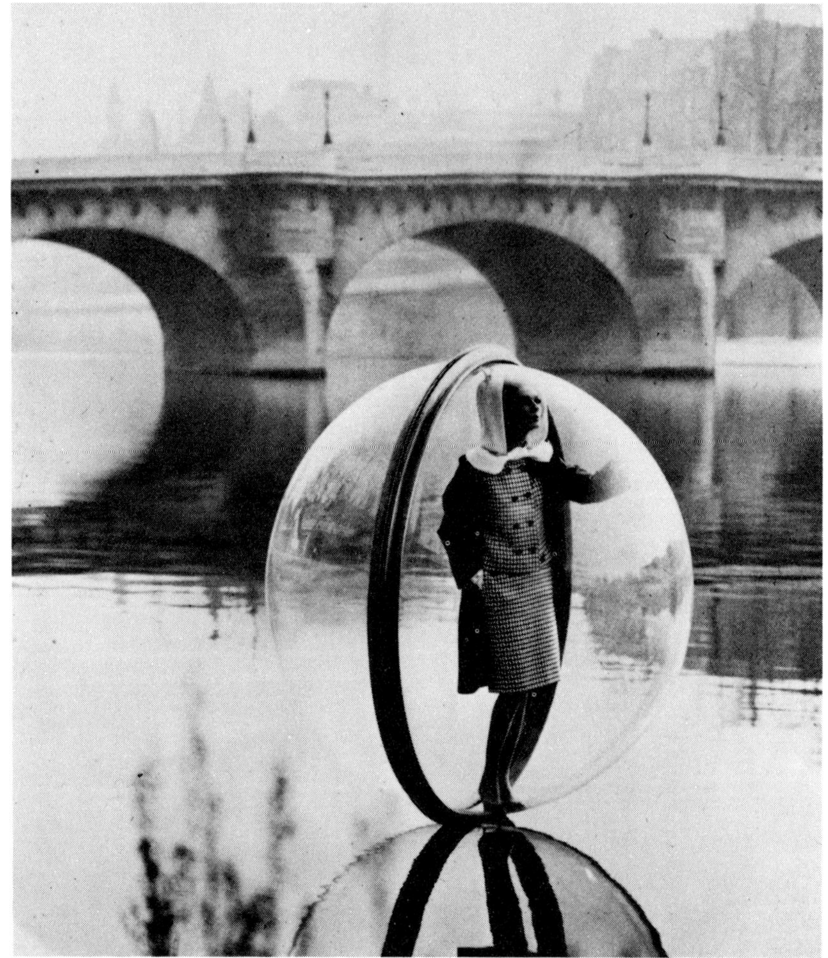

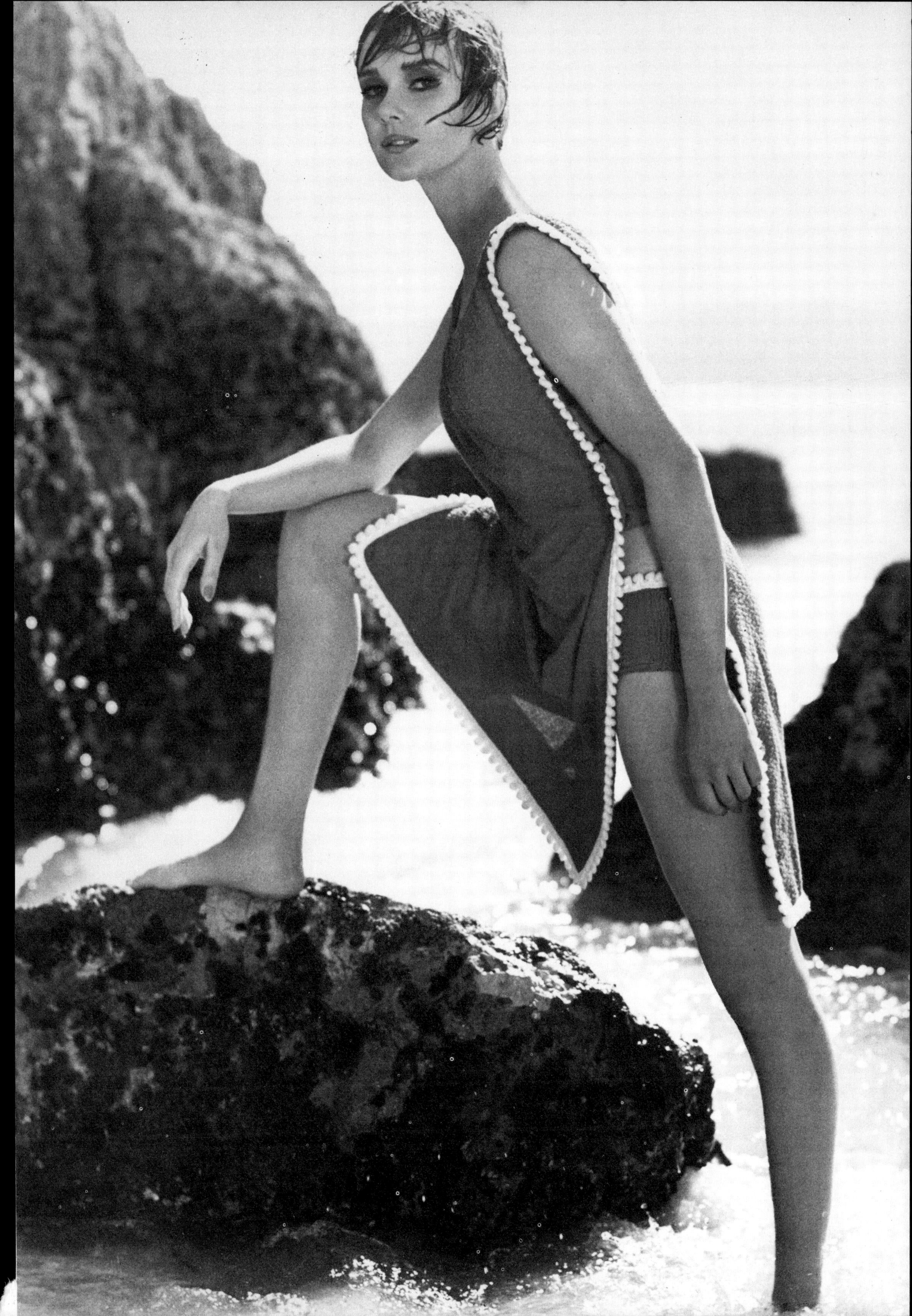

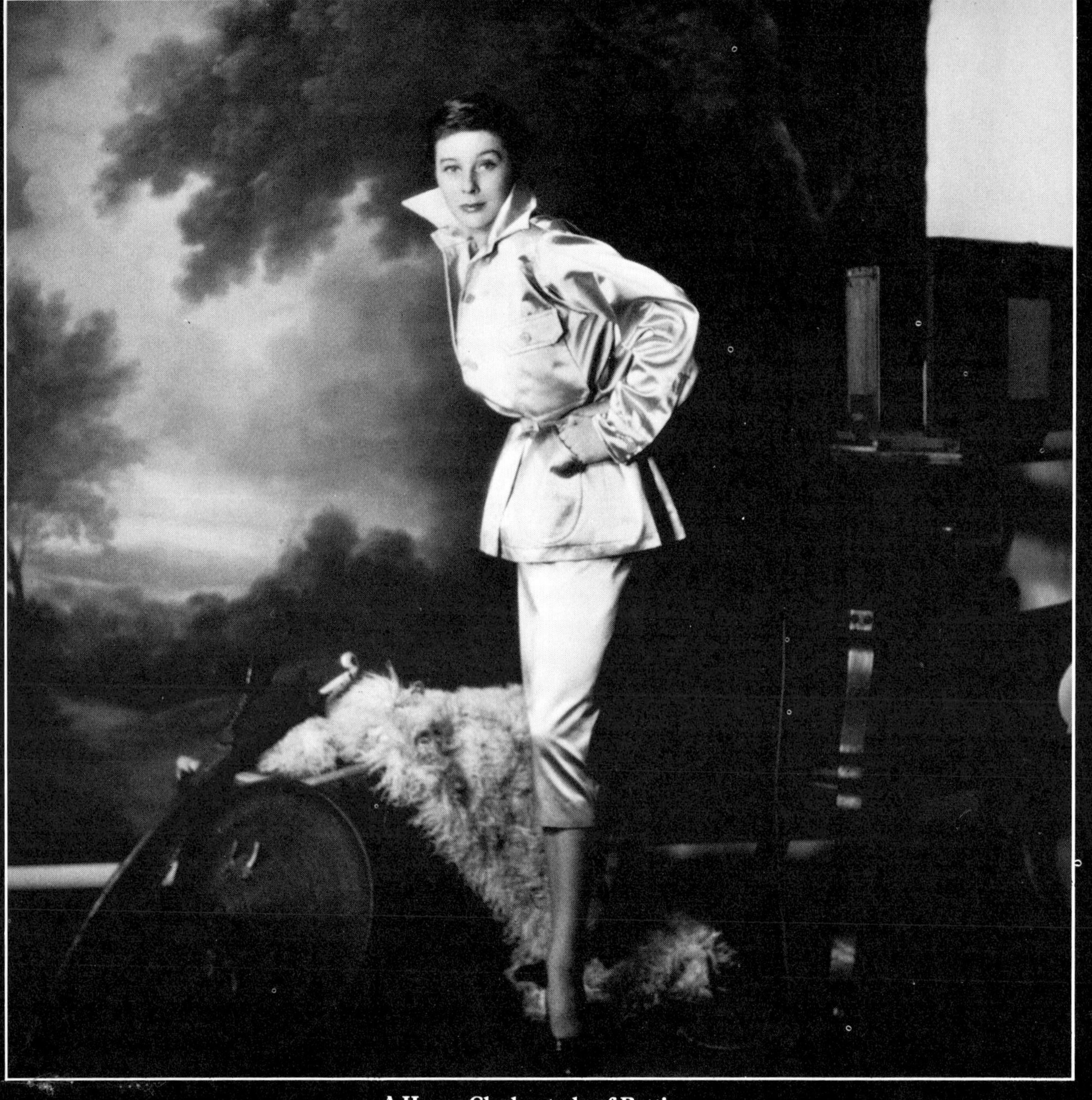

A Henry Clarke study of Bettina,
one of the most famous French
models of all time

Nicole de la Margé began her career with *Jardin des Modes* in Paris and then moved over to *Elle*, where she personified everything the magazine represented—fashionable, wearable clothes that were elegant. She was, in fact, a very very plain little thing with an ordinary face. 'I met her one day in a shop in Paris during the collections', recalls Brigid Keenan, former fashion editor of *The Sunday Times*, 'and I just walked straight past this plain little girl. She caught me by the elbow and said, "Hey, aren't you going to say good-morning?" I looked her full in the face and I didn't recognise her because she hadn't got her make-up on!'

Henry Clarke, too, found her superb, a marvellous model, although she was small. 'She made everything out of nothing', Clarke says. 'Without make-up, she was like a white paper-bag. You could hardly see her eyes, but when she finished putting on those lashes and painting that mouth and shading her features, she was superb! Absolutely first-class!'

She was a brilliant make-up artist. She could make her face look like anything she wanted. When she tired of being the *Elle* girl, she went to London at the beginning of 1968. She arrived at the time when models weren't very professional, and she would teach everybody at a modelling session. She insisted on having a full-length mirror so that she could see herself as the camera saw her, and that started a great vogue at the end of the sixties. Every model who thought she was anything had to have a full-length mirror, but only Nicole knew how to use it.

She used to boss the fashion editors around, telling them how to accessorise the clothes. She knew exactly how she should be lit because she knew the structure of her face so well, and told the photographers how to do it. Working with Nicole was easy; she did the picture for everyone concerned. She was purely a fashion model, and rarely appeared in advertisements.

She was killed in a car crash in the early seventies.

Fashion photographers found great difficulty in taking pictures of the house models in couture houses in Paris because the girls were invariably un-photogenic and lacked a still quality. They could certainly walk and show clothes superbly, but, as they lacked the stillness and camera technique required of this demanding craft, photographers took along with them their own free-lance models to be photographed wearing the collections.

The exception was Bettina, who could do both. She was a great show model as well as a photographic model. Her success, however, was confined to Paris and London, for American clothes simply did not suit her style.

Bettina, who was a railwayman's

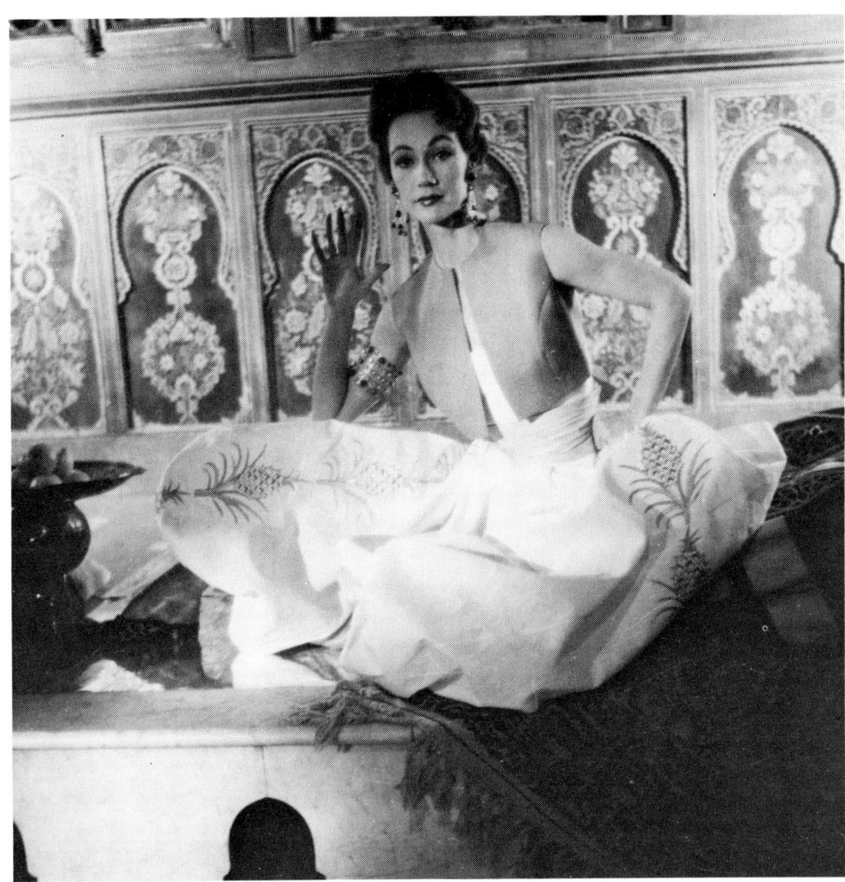

Film producer Anatol Litvak's wife Sophie, photographed in a Givenchy dress by Henry Clarke

daughter from Brittany, was Jacques Fath's top model. Her image was so popularised by the magazine world that she had great influence on a certain type of woman. She was a great inspiration to Jacques Fath, and he, in turn, introduced her to the Café society, which moved between Paris and Acapulco, between Rome and Sardinia. Mixing in these surroundings, it was little wonder that she found herself in the circles frequented by Prince Aly Khan, a dare-devil horseman, motorist, and aviator, who had married Lord Churston's

daughter, Joan, in 1936 (one of her sisters, Lydia, married the Duke of Bedford). He fell madly in love with Bettina, who gave up her eleven year modelling career the day she met and fell in love with him. Their much publicised relationship was brought to an abrupt end when he was killed in a car crash five years later.

Other well known models in Paris were English-born Jean Dawnay who, in 1947, became one of Paris' top models, working for Dior. She married Prince George Galitzine, and retired from modelling. Valerie Thurlow worked for Balmain, together with American model Debbie Condon, who climbed the pinnacle of success working for Balmain, Balenciaga, Cardin, and Dior. The popular model, Sophie, married American film producer Anatole Litvak, and Eliette Mouret married the jet-set international conductor Herbert von Karajan.

Nina Dyer, another well known English model, married the German steel manufacturer, Baron Heini Thyssen. Later, when their marriage ended,

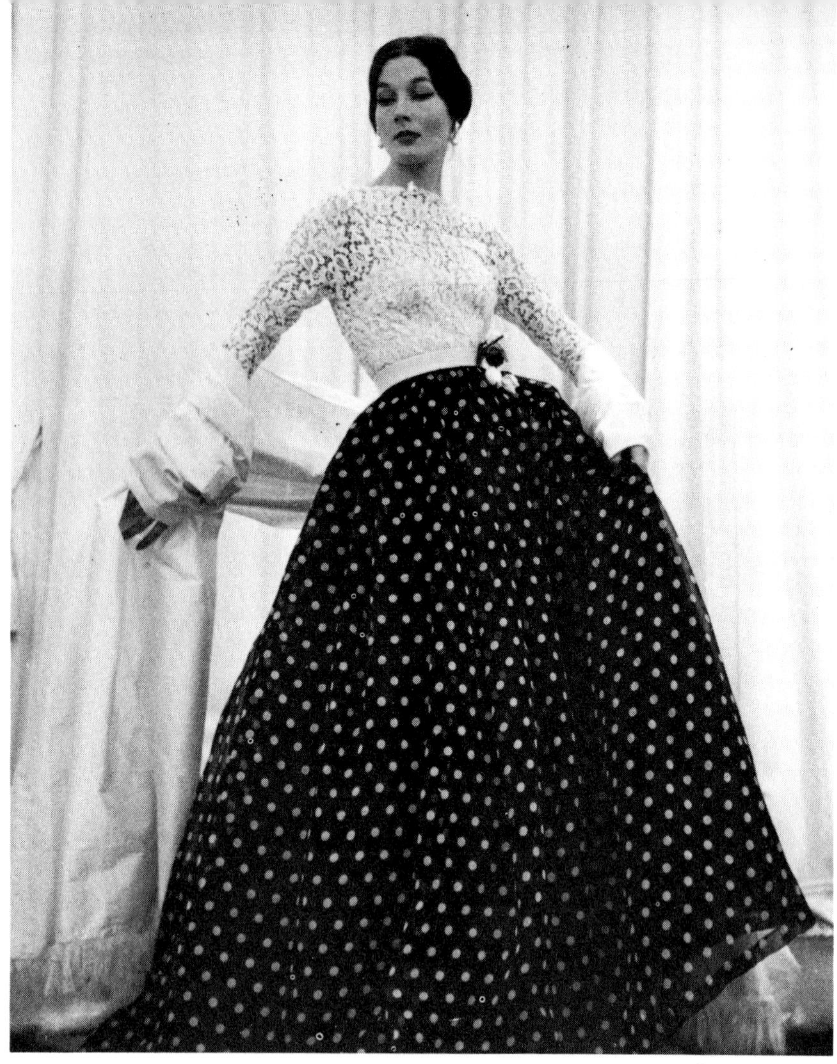

he chose another top British model as a wife—Fiona Campbell-Walter. Nina remarried, and became Princess Sadruddin Khan, Prince Aly's sister-in-law. She adored animals and was to be seen accompanied by a pair of black leopards sporting diamond-encrusted collars, specially designed by Cartier. She had a tragic end, committing suicide.

Of the British girls to make their mark as models in Paris, Bronwen Pugh was one of the most successful of all. The daughter of an English judge, she had been an elecution teacher, and gave up a career as television announcer in London when her first marriage ended. She went over to Paris to become Balmain's top model and won acclaim from the press. She retired from modelling when she married Lord Astor of the Cliveden set and, when he died, went to run a home near Godalming in Surrey, where she helps tend the needy.

'Very tall and incredibly slim, she walked with long, easy strides, her arms motionless against her sides', is how Pierre Balmain describes the extraordinary Bronwen Pugh. 'In her big, light-coloured eyes there was a complete absence of expression and ignorance of what was happening around her. She had a habit of slightly disarranging her hair as she entered the salon, giving herself a nonchalant air that is a sign of supreme English elegance.'

Photographer Richard Dormer first met her when she was at Balmain's. Although he agrees that she was a superlative model, he found her difficult to photograph. 'She wasn't really a photographic model', Dormer says. 'Her angular bones, emphasised look and exaggerated walk and stance, although highly effective for showing the exquisite clothes, were unsuited to the camera's lens.'

Eugenia Shepherd, high-priestess of fashion for the *New York Herald–Tribune* recalled her return to the Paris collections after she had first seen Bronwen. 'Balmain still has that husky Welsh mannequin, Bronwen Pugh', she reported, 'who drags a coat down a runway as if she had just killed it and were taking it home to her mate.'

Sue Blair, the blonde, 5ft 8in American model, worked for the Nina Ricci couture house in the fifties, in the days when there were fourteen or eighteen models at most of the fashion houses. Today there are four, and very few couture houses. The majority have gone over to *prêt-à-porter* (ready to wear). When Sue Blair joined Nina Ricci's, she was the fourteenth girl whom the resident designer, François Crahay, used as a model for his designs. These days Crahay is the designer at Lanvin. American girls were more sought after in Paris than the European girls because they were more professional and kept their appointments, whereas the French girls were lax. The Americans move beautifully because they tend to be less inhibited than their continental cousins. Models either have that vital inner sense of chic, or don't—like star quality it is indefinable and cannot be taught.

The photographers whose work is in such demand in Paris, and who the models prefer to work for, are few. For *Vogue*, there is Guy Bourdin, a Frenchman, who is perhaps one of the finest fashion photographers in the world at present. Helmut Newton stems from Germany; Hans Feurer from Switzerland; Sarah Moon from Britain (she was once a model herself); and Henry Clarke, the daddy of the photographers in Paris, is American. One of the outsiders who works consistently for French *Vogue* is Barbieri, the top Italian photographer who is based in Milan.

As far as models go, Italy is fairly typical of other major European countries, Germany, Spain, Denmark, and Sweden, for there are no top, international models resident in these countries. The top girls have to be imported from Paris. There is a strange irony in this, for although the best girls come from Paris, they originated in these very countries (with the exception of Italy and Spain), and left for Paris where they learned and apply their craft. They return home to work, often appearing with the leading European fashion photographers who operate from Paris, except for Barbieri whose studio is in Milan. The next step in the European models' professional progress is New York. London, too, has a crying shortage of top models and the British photographers and glossies rely tremendously on the top models from

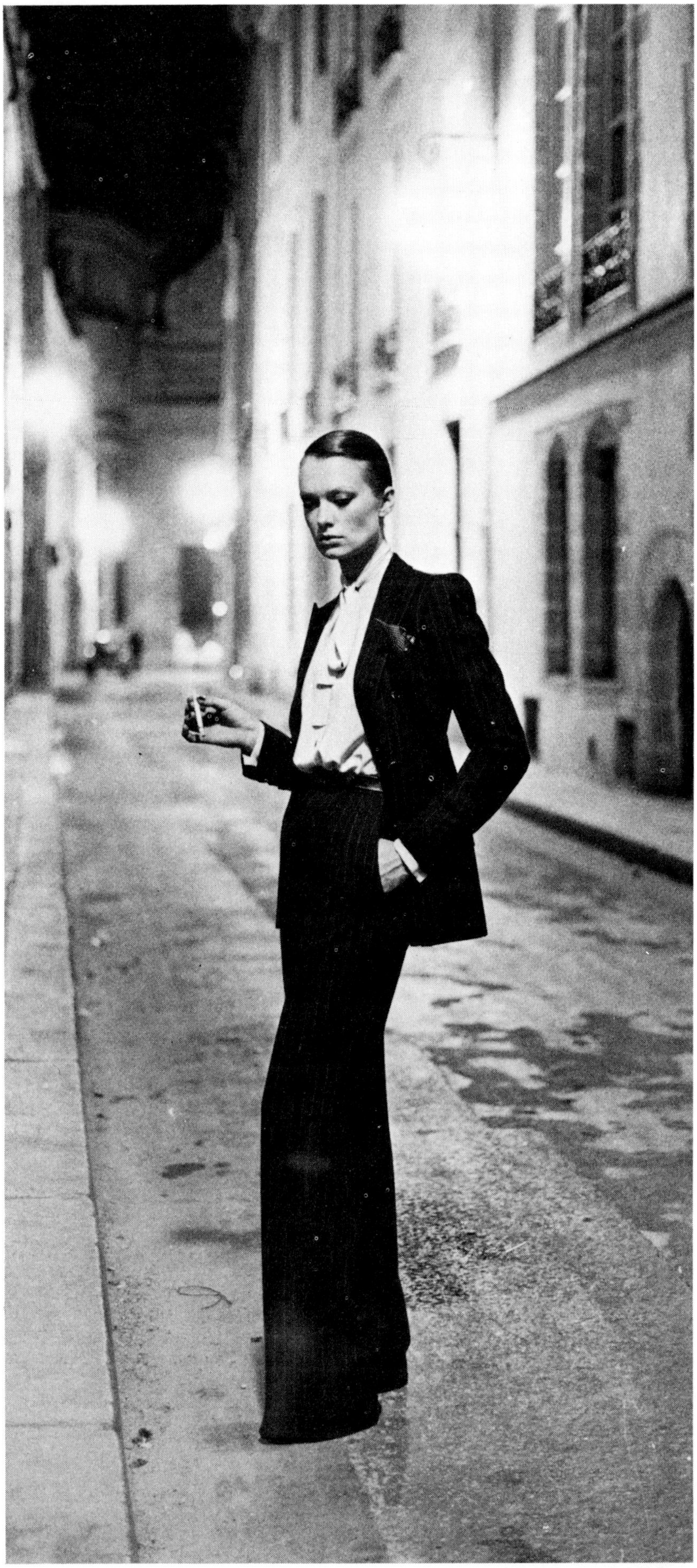

Opposite: The aristocratic-looking
Bronwen Pugh who took Paris by
storm in the fifties

Left: Vibéké, photographed in Paris
by Helmut Newton—*Vogue* France

Below: Sirpa Lane, by Helmut
Newton—*Vogue* France

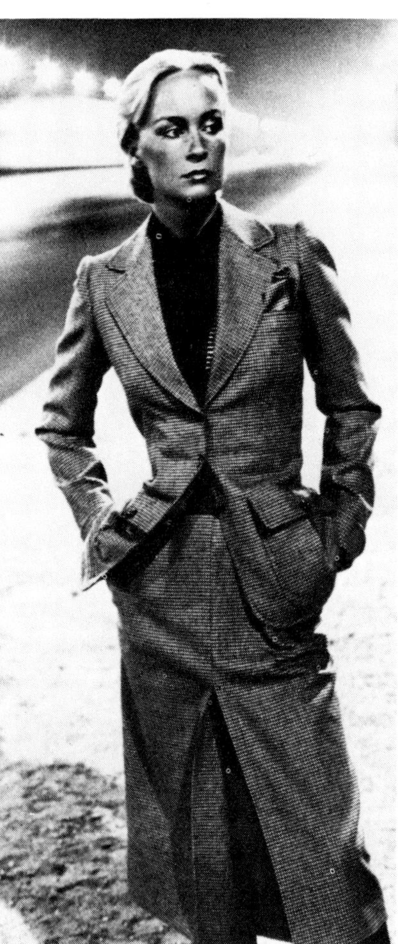

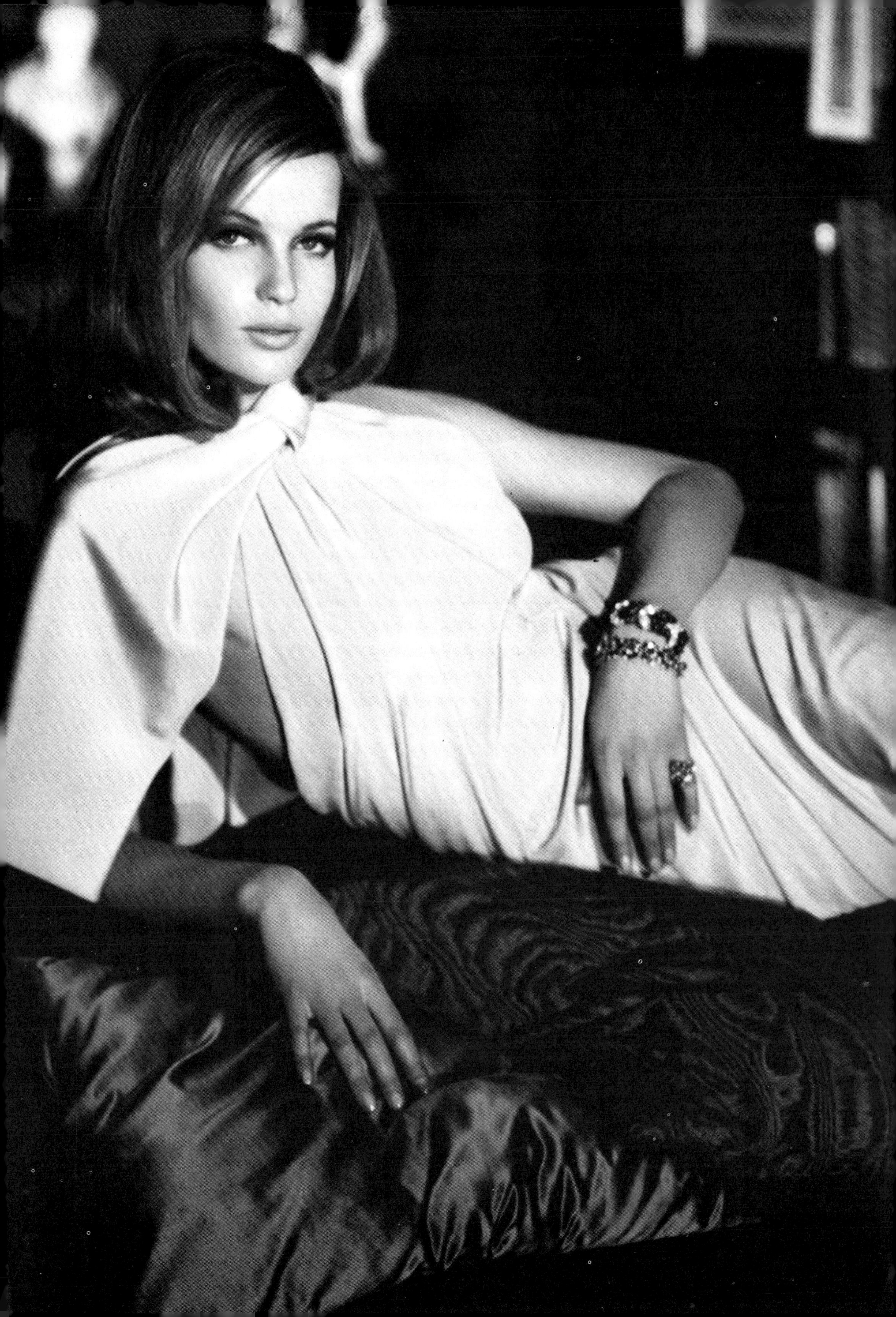

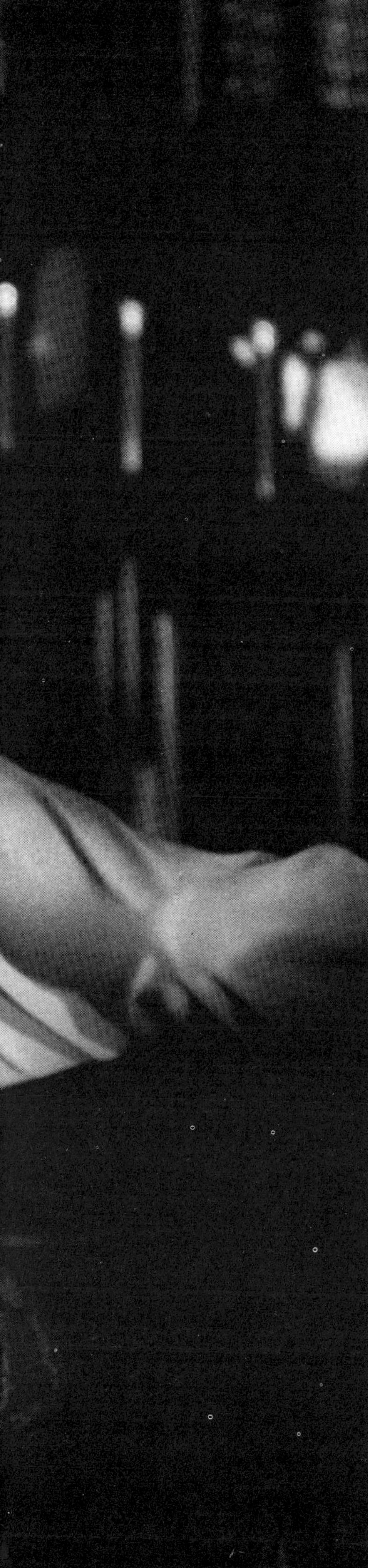

Left: The German-born Baronness Vera von Lehndorff, who modelled under the name of Veruschka, in a photograph by Henry Clarke

Below: Movie-star Marisa Berenson, taken in her modelling days by Henry Clarke

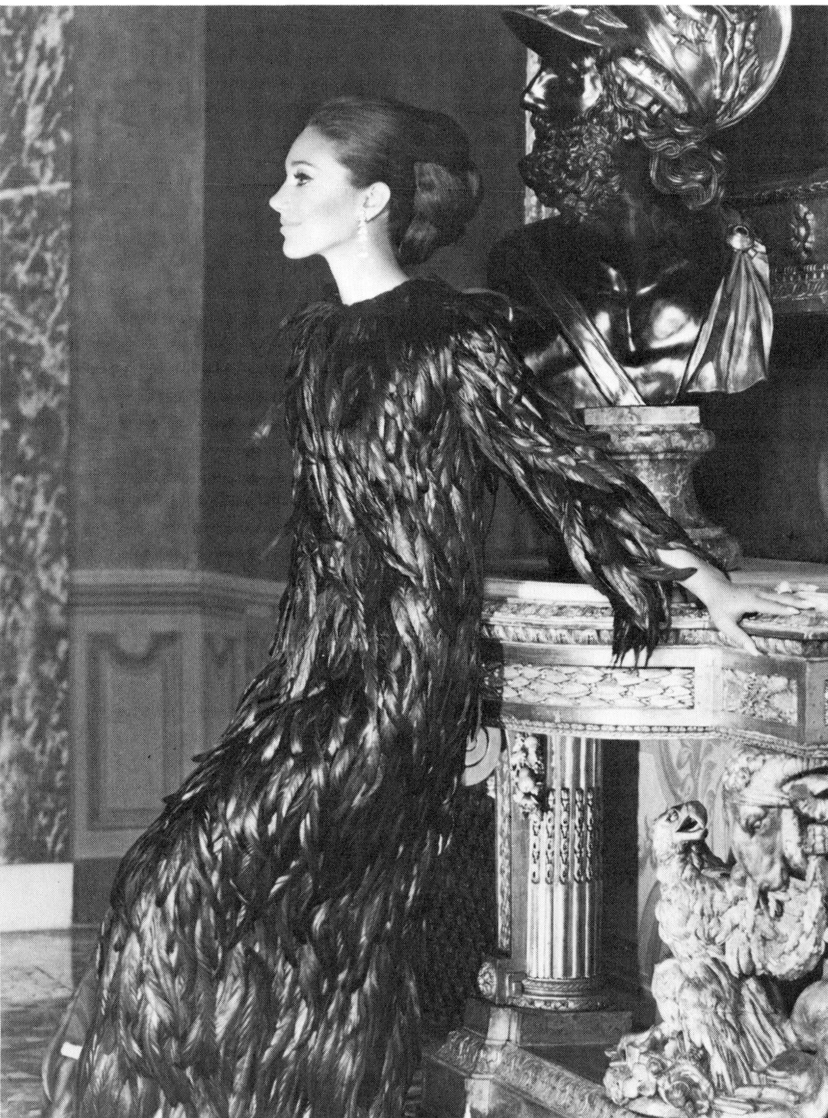

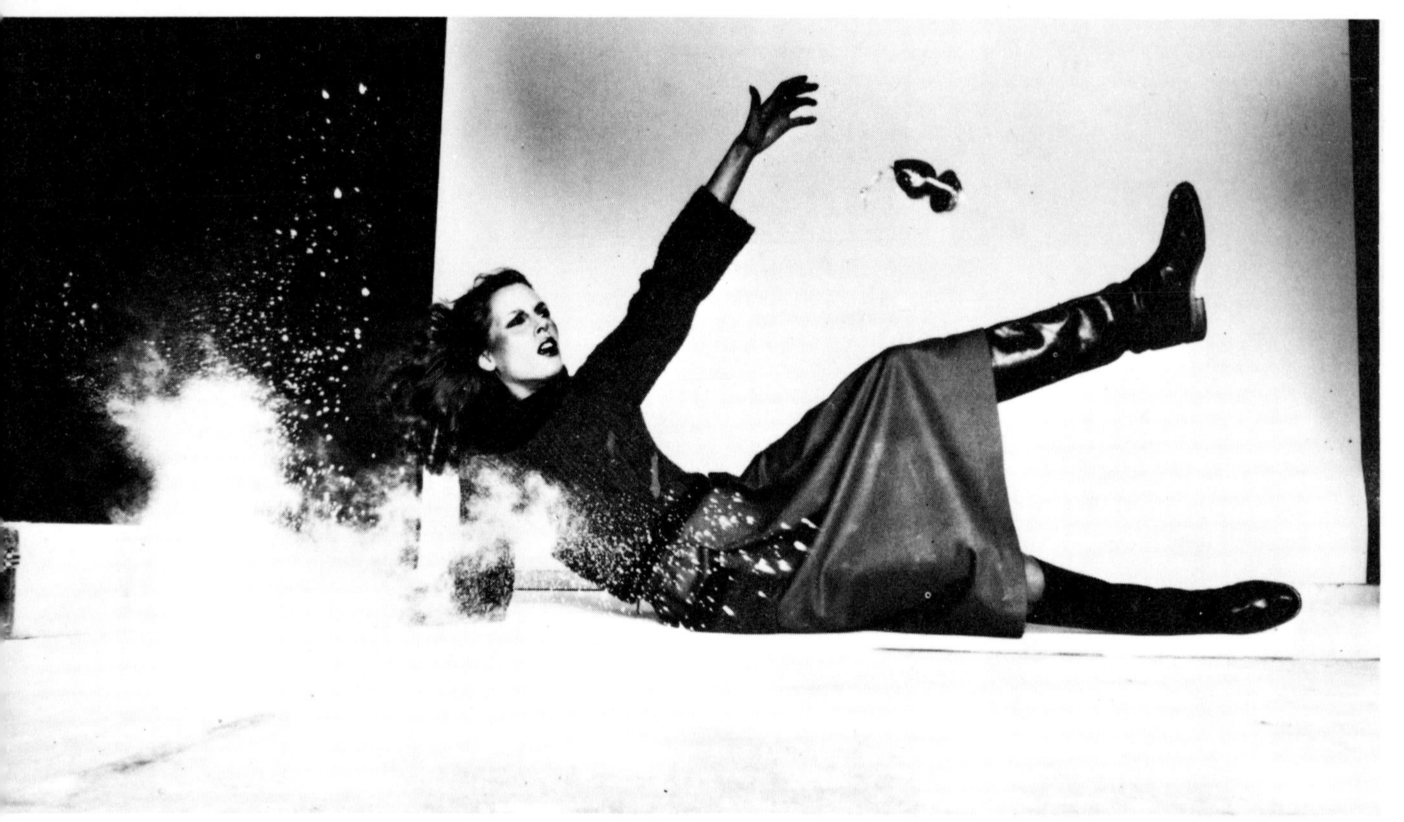

Above: Christiana Steidten, photographed by Barbieri

Paris or New York, waiting in anticipation for models of international repute to pass through London on other assignments, as they can be rather expensive to import for one specific job. Besides, fees paid in London are so low that models aren't particularly attracted to the capital, unless there is the opportunity of working with photographers of the calibre of David Bailey and Barry Lategan.

Many of the best models now working in Europe come from the Scandinavian countries. Of the top models, the undisputed choice by leading photographers, fashion editors, agents, and other models is Vibéké. Ann Anderson, Susan Moncur, and Christiana Steidten are close runners-up, with Jeanette Christjansen the highest earning and most seasoned of the five.

Simone, owner of the top Paris agency Models International, says: 'Vibéké Knudson, who is on my books, is the top girl in Europe today. She's a fantastic model, absolutely great. She is always full of life, and bubbles over.'

'She's got personality', endorses Dayle Haddon, who appears with Vibéké in the new French movie, *Madame Claude*. 'It simply oozes out of her. It doesn't have anything to do with the way she looks, she's just terrific.'

While Barbieri remarks: 'I had to book Vibéké, Ann Anderson, and Susan Moncur three months in advance to make sure I got them, I usually have to book them *six months* ahead, though, to photograph them for the collections. I work with Jeanette Christjansen too, who is extremely good.' Jeanette is so simple and beautiful and looks good in anything. I use her whenever I can.'

'Christiana Steidten is the other one I like', said Barbieri of the German model whom he photographed for French *Vogue* in the Seychelles. 'We have a wonderful rapport together. She is most professional. She gives a lot, and, like a chameleon, she changes her expression all the time. She doesn't just stand there posing for a picture, she *contributes* to it. She tells the photographer what *she* thinks she should do, and does not only what *he* wants her to do.

'The Swede Ann Anderson is one of the best now. She is fantastic because she is always fresh, spontaneous and versatile. She has a face that can appear anywhere; it fits in any magazine, *Vogue*, as well as *Elle* and *Marie-Claire*.

'The American model, Susan Moncur, is superb', Barbieri continues. 'She is acting in movies now. She's a faceless girl though. You would never recognise

Opposite: Vibéké, the top model in Europe in the seventies, photographed by Barbieri. Courtesy *Vogue*/France

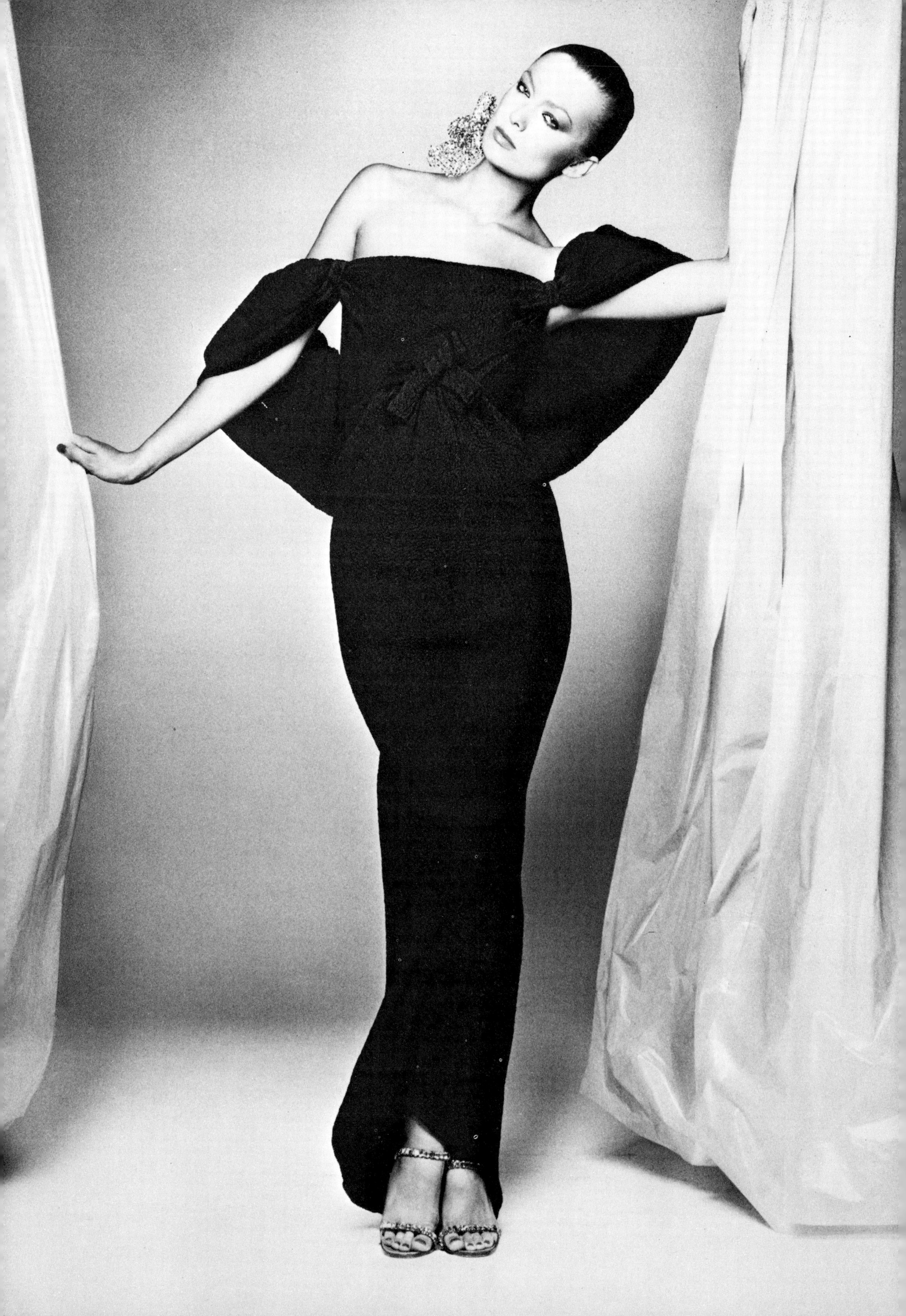

her in the street. She doesn't have a look of her own, but she changes her look every time. She is the look of the latest fashion, no matter what it is.'

Barbieri did the publicity photographs for the new Yves Saint Laurent perfume, using the Danish model Ing-Marie Lamy as his model. He found her to have one of the most fabulous faces he had ever seen.

Jeanette Christjansen, of the cool blonde hair and blue eyes, is one of the highest paid models in Paris at present. She is married to John Casablancas, head of the Elite Model Agency in Paris.

Canadian-born Dayle Haddon began her career as a ballet dancer, and modelled in her spare time to pay for her lessons. She was discovered by New York agent Eileen Ford and began modelling seriously in America before appearing in movies.

Photographed in Paris by Guy Bourdin, who persuaded her to sit for him when he saw pictures of her, she has appeared on the covers of *Vogue* regularly, and is currently appearing in the new French movie being made in Paris, *Madame Claude.*

'I'm enjoying filming *Madame Claude.* She was the most famous Madame who ever lived. She supplied the women for kings and politicians. The movie's about a political scandal in which her girls were involved. I'm playing one of the girls that she takes in, transforms, and then leaves.

'The only reason I took to modelling was to pay for my dancing lessons, otherwise I would never have gone on to become a model. It was just a series of coincidences. You see, I don't look like a model. I'm too small [5ft 6½in], and I've got a lot of other things against me, that's why it took so long in getting going.

'I've only really worked with Guy Bourdin for French *Vogue.* He had another girl booked, and when she didn't come, I got the job. Then I worked with Snowdon. He photographed me with all the fashion designers for *Vogue.*' Almost the entire issue, including the cover, was devoted to Dayle.

The only top model in Italy these days is Dalila di Lazarro, Carlo Ponti's protégée.

When other models are needed for photographic modelling work in Italy, girls have to be brought in from Paris, London, or New York. Gian Paulo Barbieri is the finest fashion photographer Italy has produced. His work appears regularly in Italian *Vogue,* and he makes periodic trips to Paris for French *Vogue.* Some of his best work appeared in French *Vogue,* taken in the Seychelles. He tends to be both realistic and critical of the model and fashion scene in Italy: 'The last top model in Italy was Isa Stoppi. She works as fashion editor for Italian *Vogue* these days. She came from Italian peasant stock, had blonde hair, enormous blue eyes, and was extremely beautiful. I think she was more beautiful in real life than in pictures. Although Isa was the last star model of Italy, she didn't have the mentality to make a lasting model. The Italians and the French do not make good models. They don't have the mentality. When they are beautiful, they cannot change their looks; and they don't want to. Models should be like chameleons. If you want a gypsy, they should become a gypsy. You put a rose and a mantilla in their hair, and— voila! But not the Italians. They always look like Italians. There are many beautiful women in Italy, but they don't want to work. They don't want to be independent. They are happy to find a rich man and marry him and never have to worry about work. The models are arrogant about working. If they go to an audition, they want the job right away. After five minutes, they give up and say, "Why should I sit there when I can find myself a rich man?"'

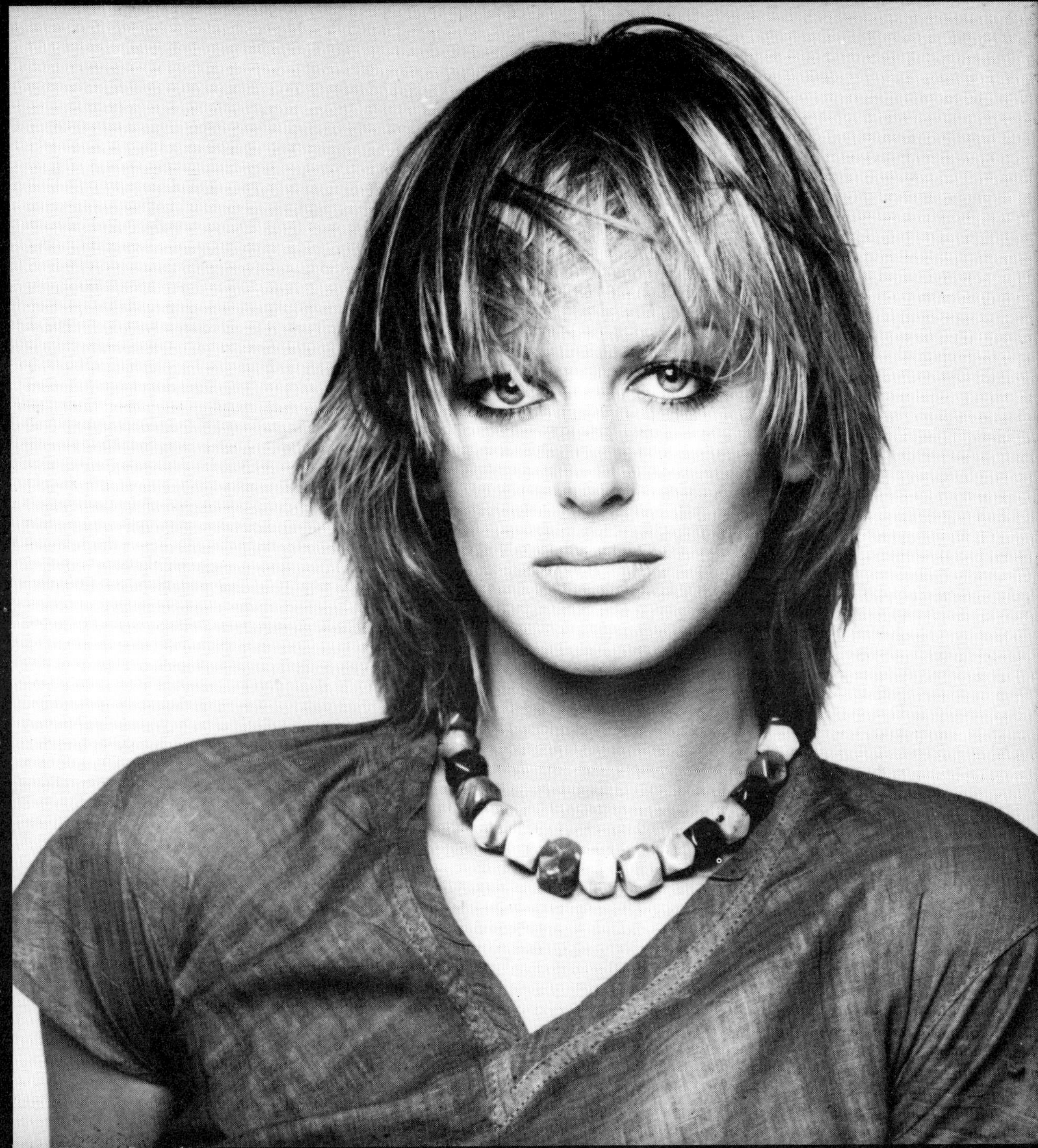

Dalila di Lazarro, photographed
by Francesco Scavullo. Courtesy
Vogue USA

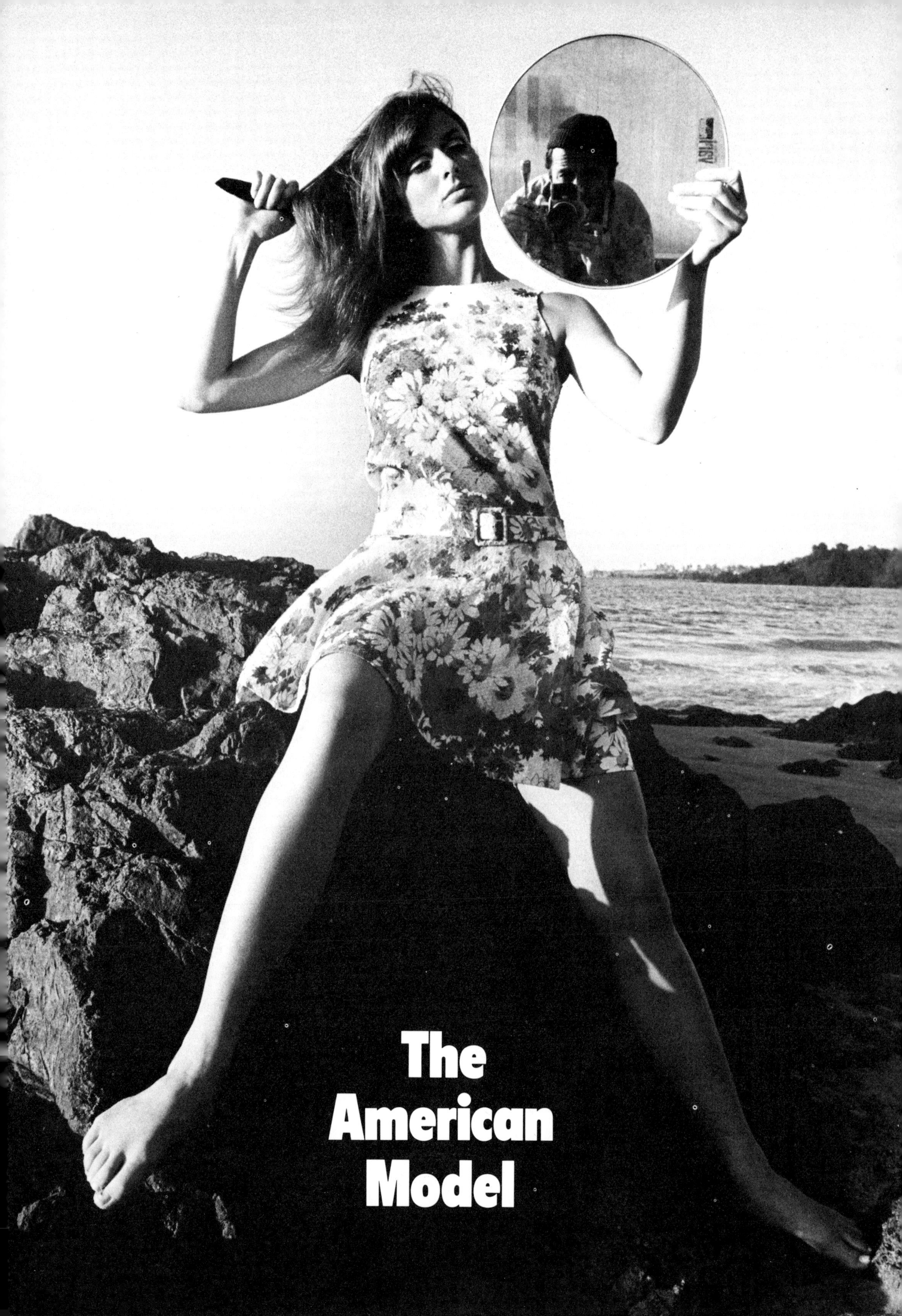

The American Model

Cover girls are the stars of today with glittering appeal and movie-star contracts provided by internationally known cosmetic manufacturers. Gone is the coat-hanger label that models once had. These days they reflect not only the fashions, but the times in which we live; their private lives and escorts being reported in the gossip columns more than ever before. However, models in New York in the fifties led more sedate lives. Their names were seldom known to the public, and readers were, moreover, interested in the clothes they modelled rather than the lives they led. The first American model whose name became widely known to the public was Suzy Parker, whose brilliant modelling career developed into movie stardom.

Suzy Parker was taught her modelling craft by her older sister, Dorian Leigh, one of the top models in America immediately after the war, until she retired to run the first model agency in Paris, in the fifties. Horst launched Dorian Leigh's dazzling career when he photographed her for *Time* magazine as the new, modern young lady of the forties. Although it was received as a revolutionary photograph, she was merely leaning on an umbrella; an innovation for those days, after the studied, stiff poses of previous decades.

Suzy Parker is without doubt one of the most famous and professional models of all time—one whose name has become a household word. Photographer Henry Clarke remembers doing a feature for American *Glamour* magazine when Horst was photographing the American collections for *Vogue*, in Paris. At the end of the collection, Horst took some pictures of the outstandingly beautiful young girl, and showed them to Clarke. 'It was a colour picture, and she was in a bright blue Jacques Fath evening gown, with all that marvellous, red-golden hair of hers cascading down, framing her perfectly lovely face. Everybody swooned. I don't think she could have been seventeen, but she had a photogenic face. All her angles were good. Like Garbo, whose face was totally mobile, Suzy didn't have to worry, because she could move and was always glorious. It was the mobility of the face that both of them had. You really had to work hard to make Suzy unattractive. She could not take a lot of make-up.' Clarke once tried eyelashes on her, but although her eyes were never really big, they appeared heavy-lidded, and with false eyelashes they seemed to look closed. She wore the minimum of make-up. A small amount of lipstick, a little eyeliner, and that was all. She didn't have to bother about shading, because she had exquisitely high cheek bones.

Suzy Parker had a tremendous sense of humour. 'We really had to fight to take the photographs', Clarke says, 'because we were always in stitches laughing, and she could never sit still!'

But although it amused Clarke, it irritated Horst, who was the first to photograph her for *Vogue* in New York. 'We had endless rows because she was always jabbering and joking. Her lack of concentration infuriated me so much once that I walked out of the studio and refused to photograph her. Then I took her to Europe to do the collections, but although we were friends, there were always complications and rows. Then Richard Avedon came along and snatched her up', and Avedon and Suzy Parker's names became inexorably linked through their work.

Horst recalls being interviewed for an article in *Esquire* about Suzy Parker. They had interviewed Avedon as well, and when the article was published, their views about her were entirely opposite. Horst said that he wished that she could have done for him what she had done in the movies: 'In the movies she sits still. When I photograph her, she is all over the place.' Suzy was annoyed with him for this remark, and refused to speak to him for many years afterwards.

Before going into movies, Suzy Parker became the first Revlon girl, succeeded later by Evelyn Kuhn and Lauren Hutton. She lived in Paris for two years and while there she married a Frenchman, Pierre Lascelles, by whom she had a daughter; but the marriage proved to be unhappy and they divorced. At the time her marriage was floundering, her father was killed in a motor accident in the United States. She was driving him and, as they crossed a railway line, the signals jammed and an oncoming train hit their car. Her father, who was seated beside her, was killed. Suzy was taken to hospital, operated on, and still has the scars on her face.

Agnetta Darren, taken by Francesco Scavullo who can be seen in the mirror

Another great model of the sixties, Wilhelmina, remembers doing a booking with Suzy towards the end of Suzy's modelling career.

'I had heard so much about her, and she had heard so much about me from Dorian, that we were both rather nervous of the competition! That was after the automobile accident when her father was killed and I distinctly remember that the booking had to be constantly retaken because it was out of focus as she never stopped jumping about.

'Suzy Parker was my idol. She was the woman I wanted to look like.'

Today, Suzy Parker is happily married to Bradford Dillman and living in Santa Barbara. They have three children of their own and she is totally domesticated, bakes her own bread, does her own gardening, and takes the children to choir practice. She was a close personal friend of Coco Chanel, and has kept all her Chanel clothes as souvenirs of the past—even though they no longer fit her. Suzy spent most of her modelling career in New York or Paris and rarely worked in London. She gave up her modelling for a successful film career, but was unsuited to the majority of the movie roles she played because she was cast in dramatic, thriller parts, whereas her forté lay more in the light comedienne roles of the Carole Lombard type. Her voice was too light for dramatic roles. Nevertheless, she is perhaps one of the most successful models to have 'made good' after giving up modelling.

Dorian Leigh, Suzy Parker's elder sister, appeared on cover after cover in New York, working mainly for *Harpers Bazaar*, photographed by Richard Avedon. On the occasions that she worked for *Vogue*, she was often photographed by Cecil Beaton who visited New York while on contract to Condé Nast.

Dorian Leigh was small, but she had perfect proportions. For a small woman she had the right length of leg, rather like Marlene Dietrich who isn't tall, but has long legs which give the impression of height. Dorian had a fantastic personality and was enormous fun.

Sunny Harnett was one of the greats of modelling in the fifties. These days she selects the models for Clairol's international advertisement campaigns. She began as a showroom model, working with Mainboucher, but, although she was shy and gawky at that time, she was sweet and attractive. Every dress she modelled had style and elegance. If it wasn't in fashion already, it was as soon as the public saw it on Sunny. She walked in off the street to photographer Scavullo's studio, and he booked her for an advertisement. He did the picture and sent her along to the Eileen Ford model agency. She was first photographed for *Vogue* by Horst, and got regular jobs thereafter.

Like Dorian Leigh, Sunny Harnett worked mainly for *Harpers Bazaar*, and was photographed a good deal by Richard Avedon. She was a willowy, elegant blonde with a wonderful big mouth and clever, twinkling eyes and high cheek bones; she was like a superb gazelle. The models in New York shop-window displays were modelled on her likeness, as well as another top model of that time, Anne Saint Marie. Both models were tall and divine looking. They were adorable, amusing, and highly professional.

Anne Saint Marie was regarded as a great American model. Extraordinarily beautiful, she was the model other models wanted to look like, and many copied her style and looks. 'She was a girl that I really created', says photographer Henry Clarke. 'We went through a week of extensive testing of make-up

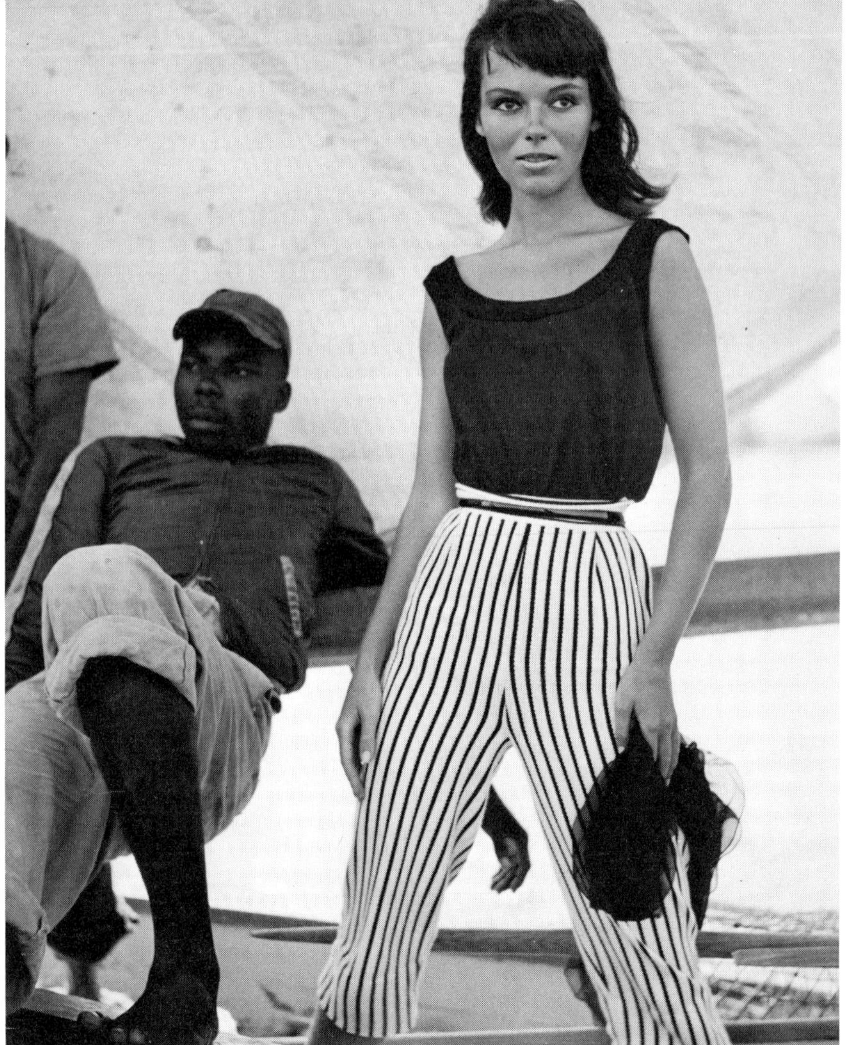

Left: Sandy Brown was a little waif, not forbidding, very sexy, wind-blown hair. *Bazaar* **disliked her picture, taken by Scavullo in 1957, with a negro lounging around, and her manning the boat**

Opposite: Sunny Harnett, one of the all-time greats of modelling in America in the fifties. Photographed in 1971 by Francesco Scavullo

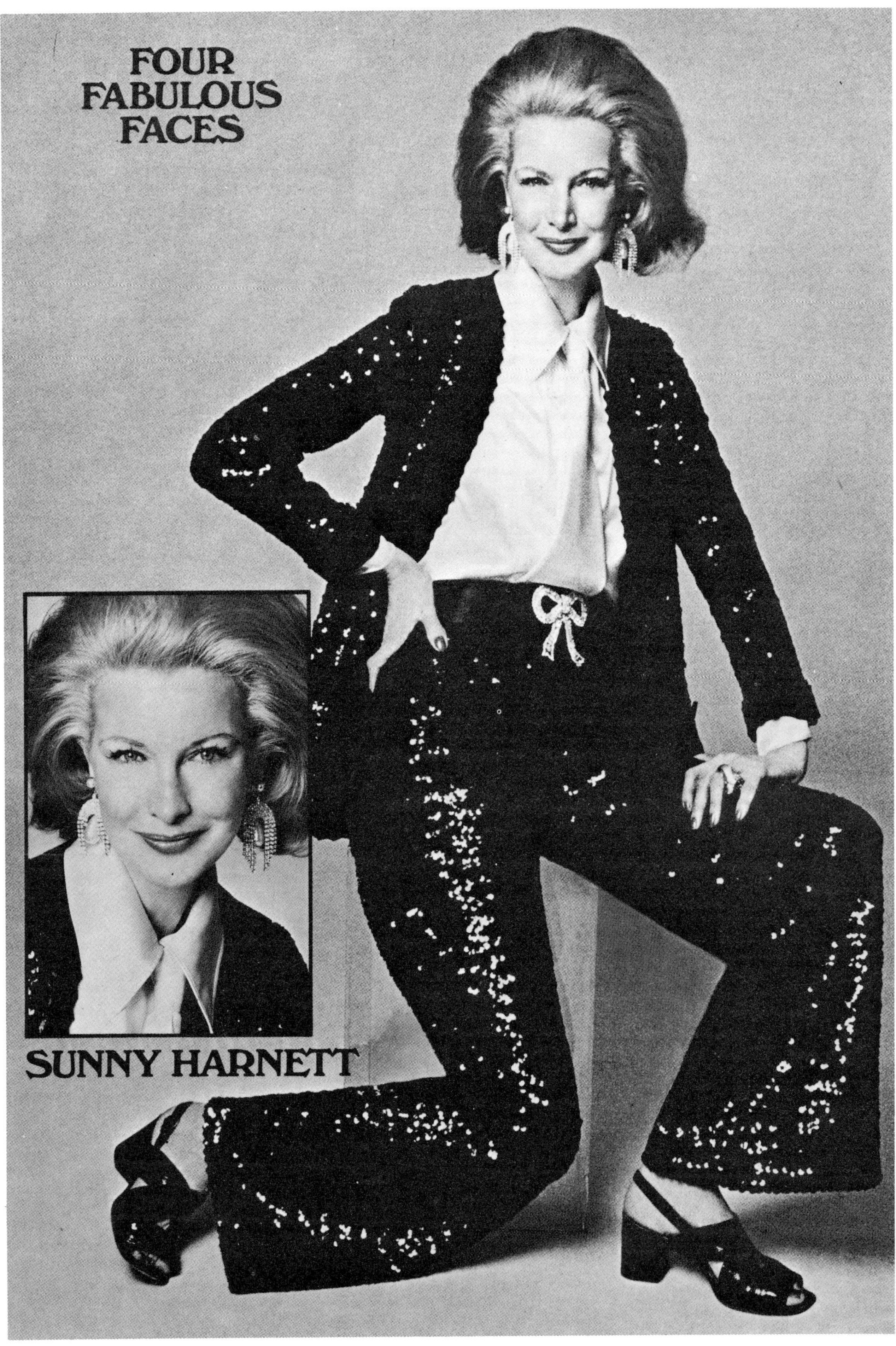
FOUR
FABULOUS
FACES

SUNNY HARNETT

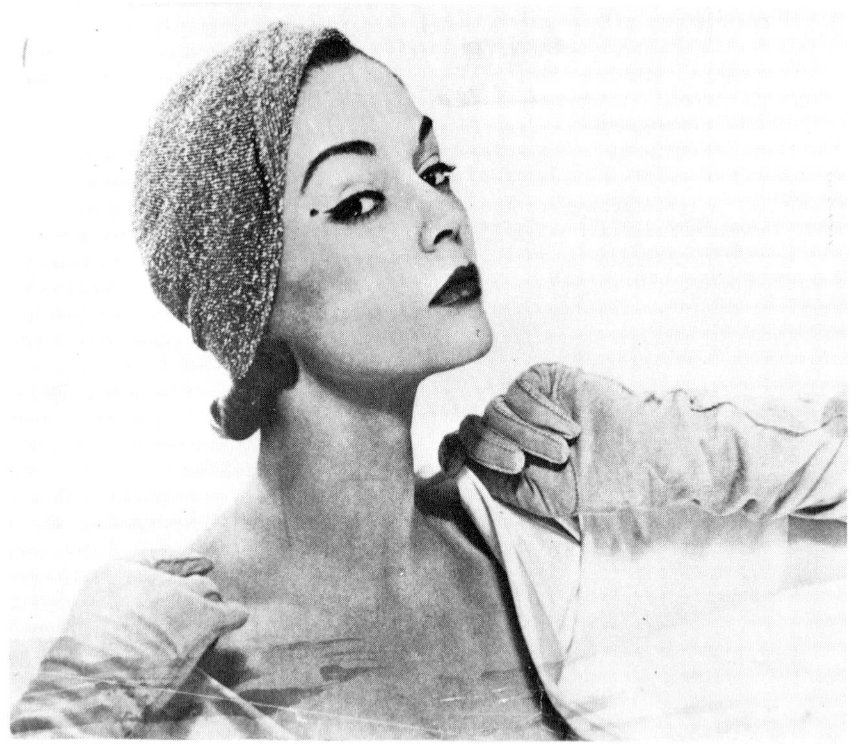

and wigs in New York before I did a collection with her in Paris, and when she came out, she really changed the model-look of that time.'

Dovima was another top model in the fifties. Horst was the first to photograph her, and then Richard Avedon took her over. 'A crazy nut', is how Horst affectionately describes the Irish-blooded model. Dovima is an anagram of her real name, Dorothy Victoria Moran. She worked a great deal for *Harpers Bazaar*, and appeared in films, notably as the model in *Funny Face* with Audrey Hepburn and Fred Astaire, who, in a scene with Kay Thompson in the bookshop in Hepburn's charge, turns the place upside down. Horst recalls a story when Richard Avedon took her to Egypt to photograph a new collection. When they returned, she was asked what she thought of *Africa*. 'Africa?' she asked, 'What are you talking about? I

Above left: The leading American model, Jean Patchett

Left: A study of Dovima, taken in New York in 1952 by the great photographer Horst

Opposite: Dorian Leigh wearing Mrs Vernon Castle's dress, photographed by Cecil Beaton

Below: Anne Saint Marie, photographed by Henry Clarke

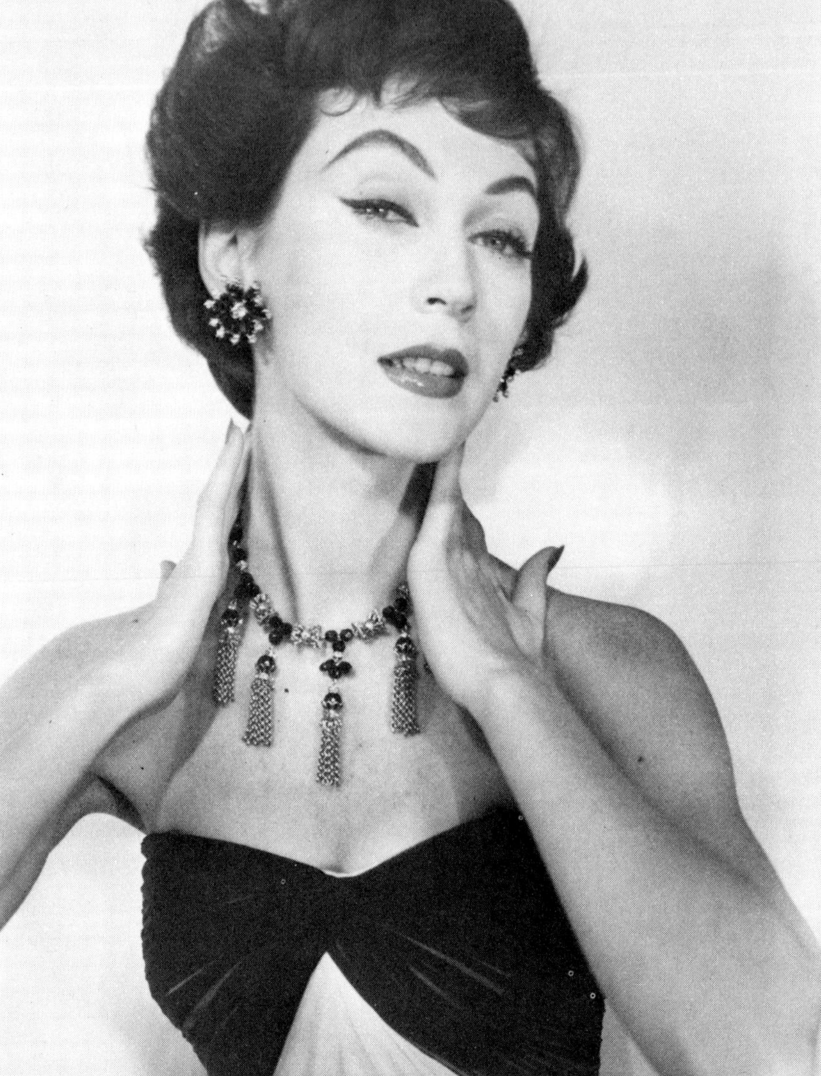

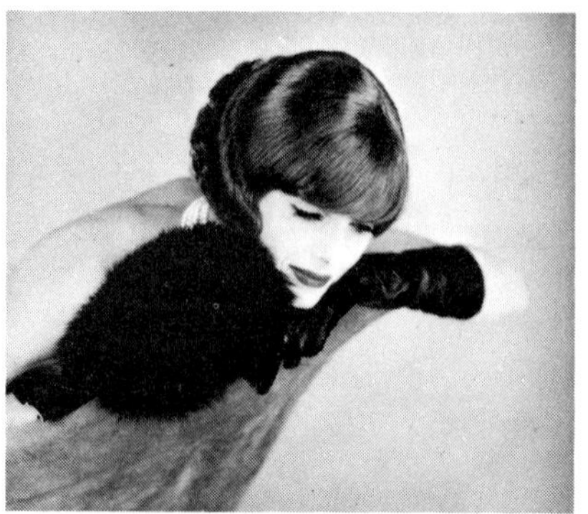

was in *Egypt*.' 'No, no', came the reply, 'you were in Africa.' 'Oh, my God', she exclaimed, aghast, 'If I had known it was *Africa*, I would have charged double!'

Jean Patchett has remained one of the most distinguished models of all time with dozens of covers to her credit. Well known for the famous beauty spot above her right eye, she had it removed recently, as it had become too conspicuous. Her two most famous *Vogue* covers are the black and white one wearing a hat and veil and an enigmatic look in her eye, taken by Irving Penn; and the other, showing only an eye and her mouth, taken by Erwin Blumenfeld. It is this last picture that graces the Bloomingdale carrier bags in New York.

Born in Preston, Maryland, Patchett —nicknamed 'Pancho'—went to Goucher College for two years, but found it too hard to carry on. In 1948, a friend suggested she try modelling in New York, but her parents wouldn't approve. However, she had an aunt living in New York who agreed to give her a bed, and she persuaded her father to hand her her next year's school fees of $600 to go there. She joined an agency, but did little or nothing after three months.

'Pancho's' money was running out, and so she went to see Eileen Ford. Although Ford's is the largest and most powerful model agency in the world today, it was only beginning in 1948.

'My impression of Eileen was a woman of about sixty, in a big plush office, and very stern', Jean Patchett recalls. 'But she turned out to be none of that. I walked into this tiny, grubby office. There were six telephones on a card table behind which sat Eileen Ford. She turned around, and I found she was only about three years older than I was. The first thing she said to me was, "You're as big as a horse. You'll have to lose weight."' Although Jean is 5ft 9in she weighed 127lb, however, she lost weight, as instructed. She joined the agency on 10 April 1948, and by the end of May had earned enough money to repay her father the $600. She did her first *Vogue* cover that September, and the *Glamour* cover in October. She began working within the first week of joining Fords, and never stopped for the next twelve years.

'I really discovered Jean Patchett', recalls photographer Francesco Scavullo. 'She walked into my studio, and I thought, "This face is incredible and she has a good body, too." I told her that she could be a great model. I took her pictures and sent her to Eileen Ford. After that, Irving Penn photographed her; she was fabulous. I only regret that at the time I was working for "young" magazines, and she was working for the sophisticated ones like *Vogue*, so I was unable to work with her.'

In 1949 she went to Paris with Irving Penn for American *Vogue* for the French collections, where Henry Clarke, who was working in Paris, desperately wanted to photograph her for *Album du Figaro*. However, *Figaro* couldn't afford to pay her fee, and although Clarke agreed to pay the balance, he found he couldn't afford it either. He was determined to work with her, and caught up with her in New York where they had a successful photographic session. 'It was a face of that period', Clarke says. 'She had a doe-eyed look about her. Her best work was with Irving Penn because of the still-life quality he likes. Jean's was a graphic face; like a poster. As the clothes those days had graphic outlines and shapes, she was the perfect model for them. She was a really healthy American, with a marvellous body and long legs.' However, she was wise enough not to over-expose herself, believing that the more you are seen, the less you are wanted.

'When you're in demand, and they can't get you, they want you all the more. I worked hard all the same, and enjoyed the travelling to Peru, Mexico, Spain, Paris, London, Nassau, Cuba, but I saw very little of the United States!'

Although she worked for all the top

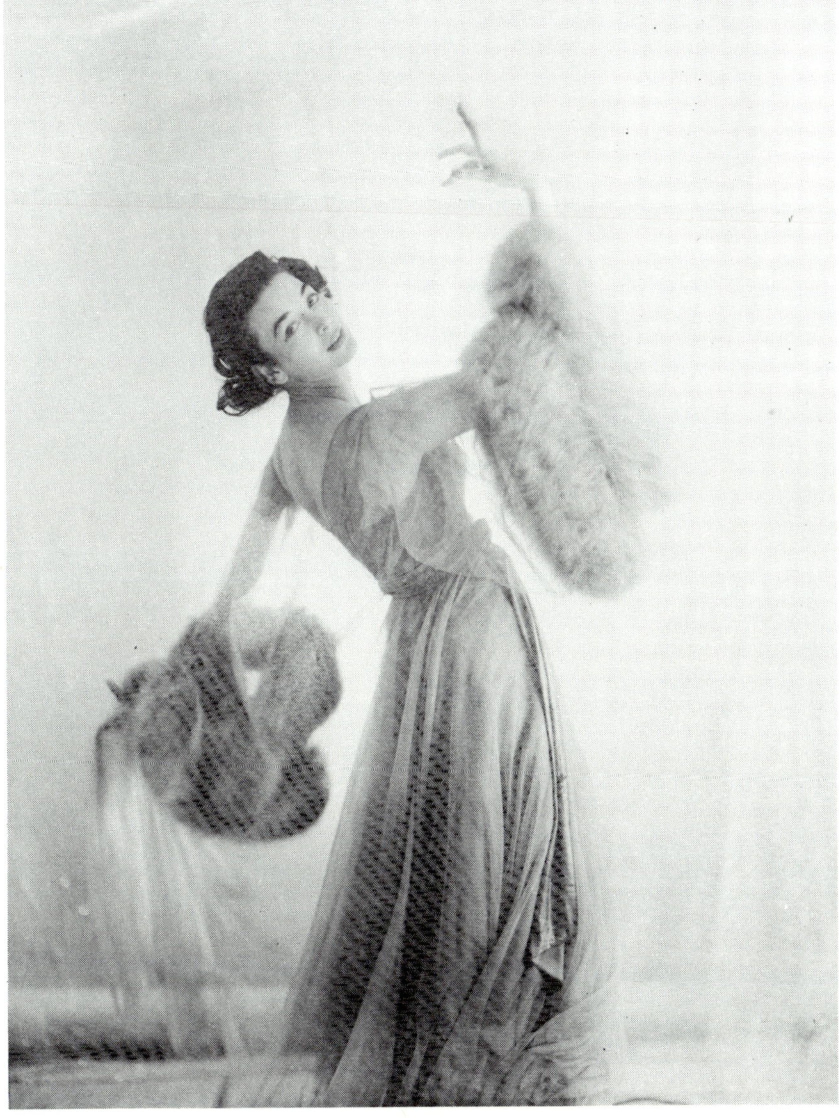

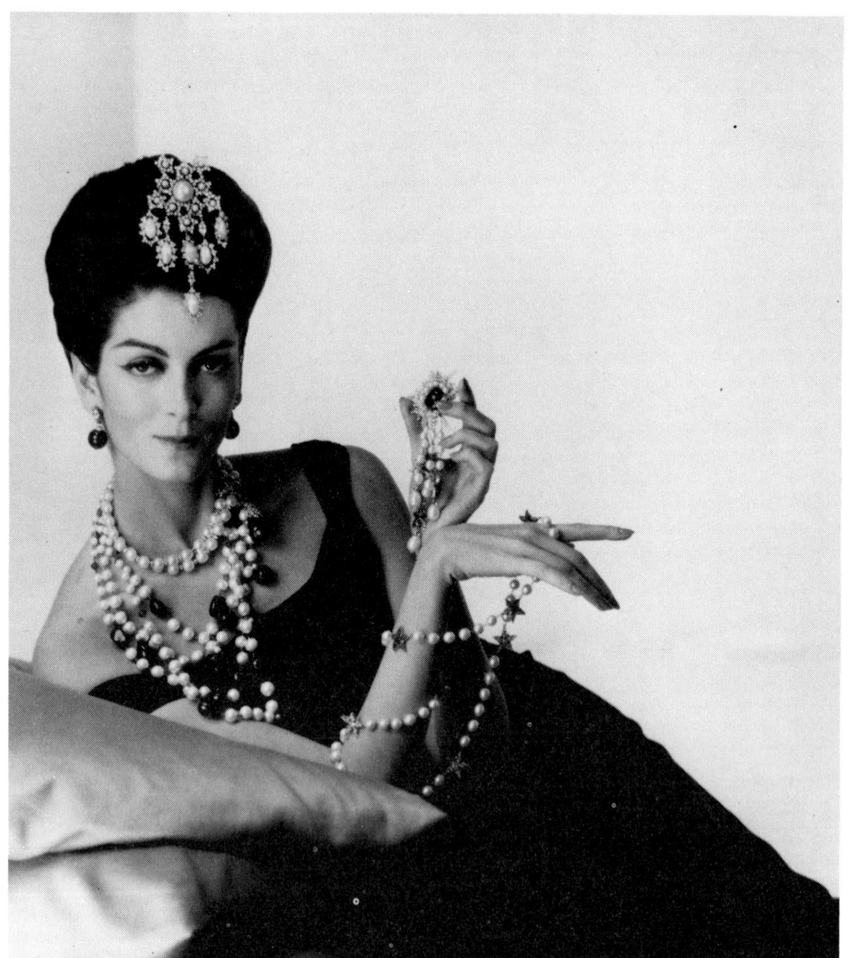

Opposite: Wilhelmina,
photographed in Jaipur, India, in
1967 by Henry Clarke

Overleaf, left-hand page. Above:
The famous advertisement in
which Marlene Dietrich appeared
for BOAC. (Courtesy British
Airways) Below: Christiana
Steidten photographed in the
Seychelles by Barbieri—*Vogue*
France

Overleaf, right-hand page. Above:
Susan Moncur by Barbieri. Below
left: Vibéké, photographed for
Vogue France in December 1976 by
Barbieri. Below right: Ing-Marie
Lamy photographed for Yves
St Laurent's *Rive Gauche* by
Barbieri

photographers, her favourite was always Irving Penn: 'When Penn took the *Vogue* cover, it was in black and white. My lips were black. I remember using eyebrow pencil on my lips.

'The Blumenfeld picture was for a hair-do. He took it in black and white, and they painted in the eye and the mouth during the processing stage.'

Although Jean Patchett became one of Penn's favourites, she somehow did not 'click' with Richard Avedon. 'I looked entirely different when I was photographed by him', she admits, and so they rarely worked together. 'Penn and I had a great rapport', she continues. 'I'd get into an outfit and stand on the white paper in the studio, and he would tell me a story. When we did the picture with the veil on, there was a box in front of me, and he said, "Now, you're going out to dinner, and just as you're leaving, you see this lovely box tied with red ribbon on the hall table. There's a mirror there and when you open the box, try the hat on in front of the mirror."

'Another time he would say, "You're at the Caravelle having lunch with somebody, and you're wearing this lovely suit. Show me how you feel."

'Or it's at the opera, and I'm looking for this lovely man I'm madly in love with. It's intermission, and I can't find him. Suddenly, I see him in the distance and I'm trying to catch his eye over everybody's heads. Another time I would have to pretend to be on the street looking for a taxi cab, or at Cartier's looking at a jewel.

'At one sitting, we would easily take five hundred pictures for one outfit.

'He called it chasing a bluebird.'

The other great models of the day were Lisa Fonsagrieves, perhaps even a greater model than Dorian Leigh, Jinks Falkenburg, Mary Jane Russell, Evelyn Trip, the O'Connor Twins, Georgia Hamilton, Linda Harper, Nell Ambrose, and Carmen.

Lisa Fonsagrieves was a model with a most distinguished career going back to the thirties. Born in Sweden, her first marriage was to a photographer, Fonsagrieves, who worked for *Harpers Bazaar*, and her second to another

photographer, Irving Penn, who worked largely for *Vogue*. Horst found her sweet and adorable, and Scavullo ,who was Horst's assistant at *Vogue* during those days, considered her the first high-fashion model he had met. 'She came into the studio, and I simply fell in love with her', added Scavullo. 'She was the most beautiful woman I had ever seen. She had a marvellous profile and moved like a dream. She is certainly one of the great models of all time.'

Carmen was the only top model that would do nudes and could still work as a high fashion model. Normally that did not exist. At that time no top model ever did nudes or lingerie unless they had the Kayser account, for their 'Girl on the Pedestal' campaign. The advertising psychology was that every man puts his girl on a pedestal—in Kayser lingerie. But the girls had to be top models to get the account since it was very prestigious.

Of the younger set, the girls who worked continually included Jackie Michelle, Sandy Brown, Anne Murray, Pat Gehagen, Carol Macausen and Dolores Hawkins who led the teenage field.

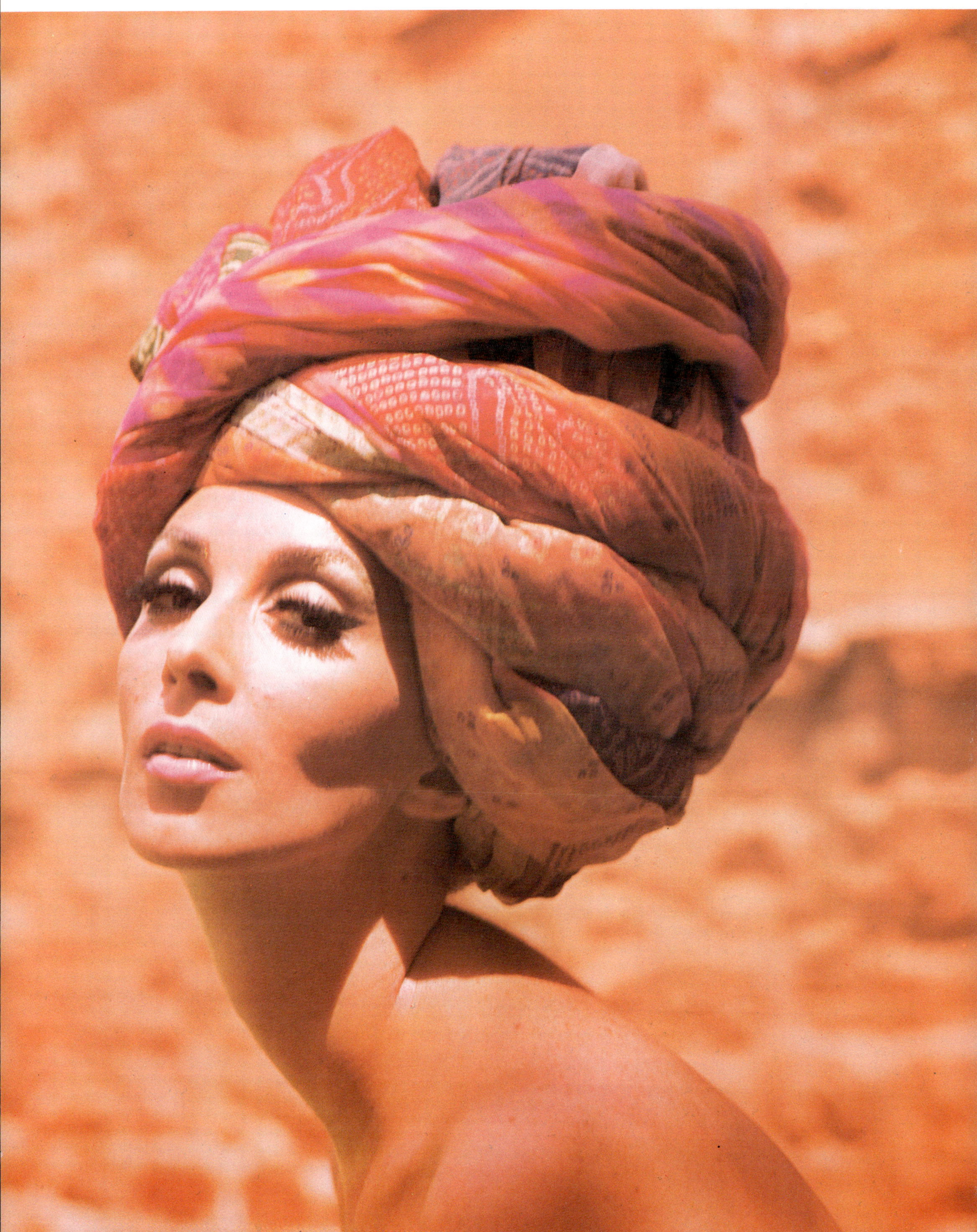

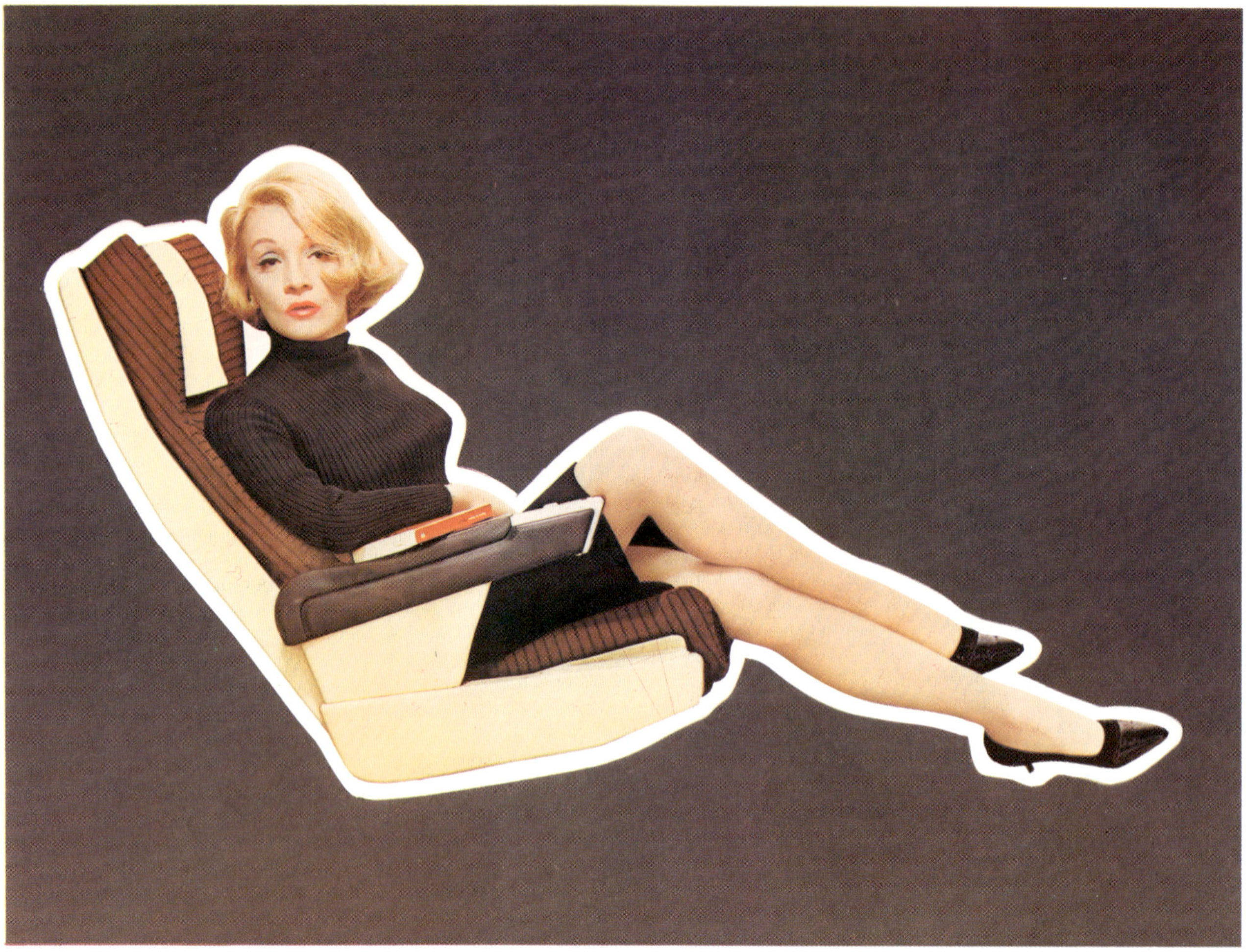

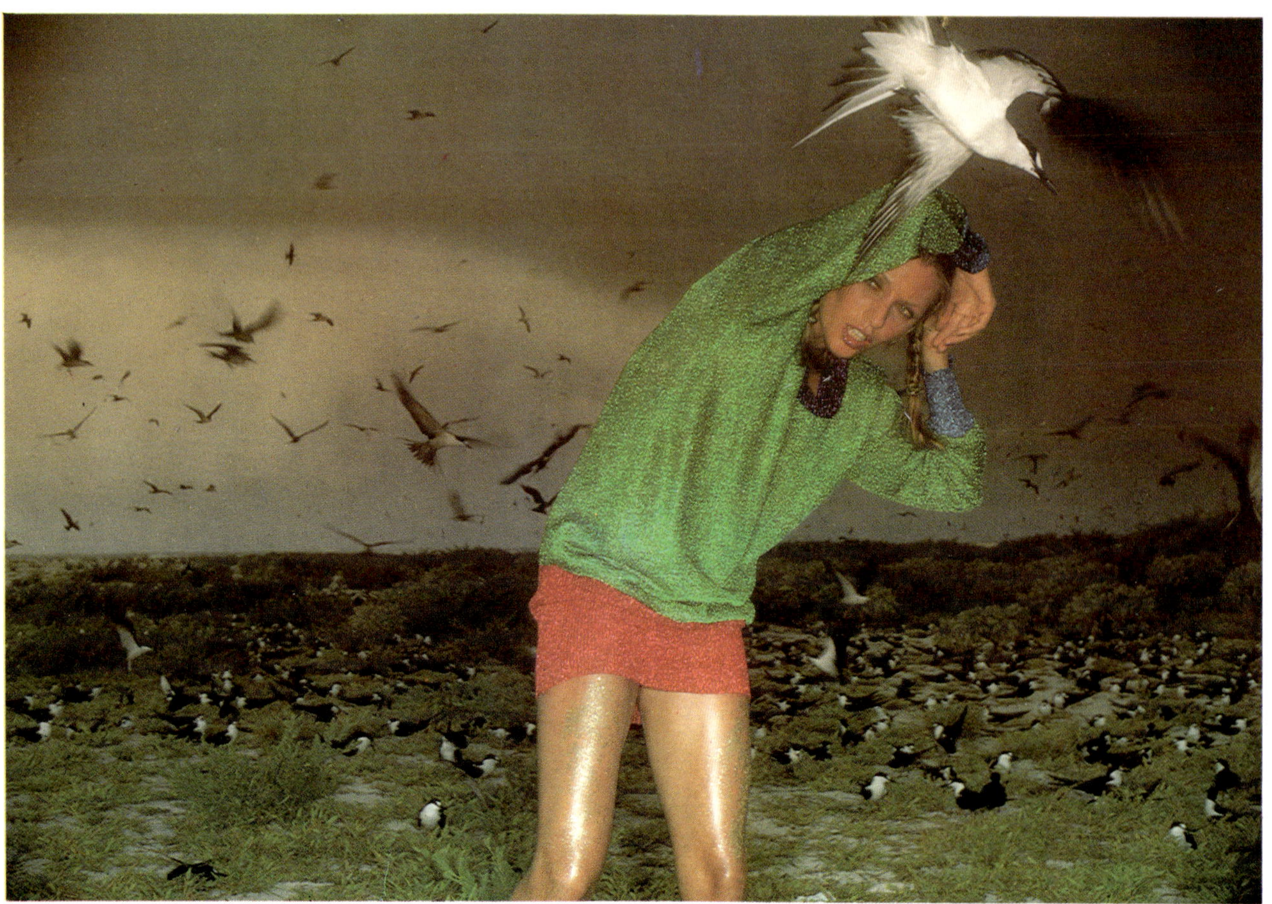

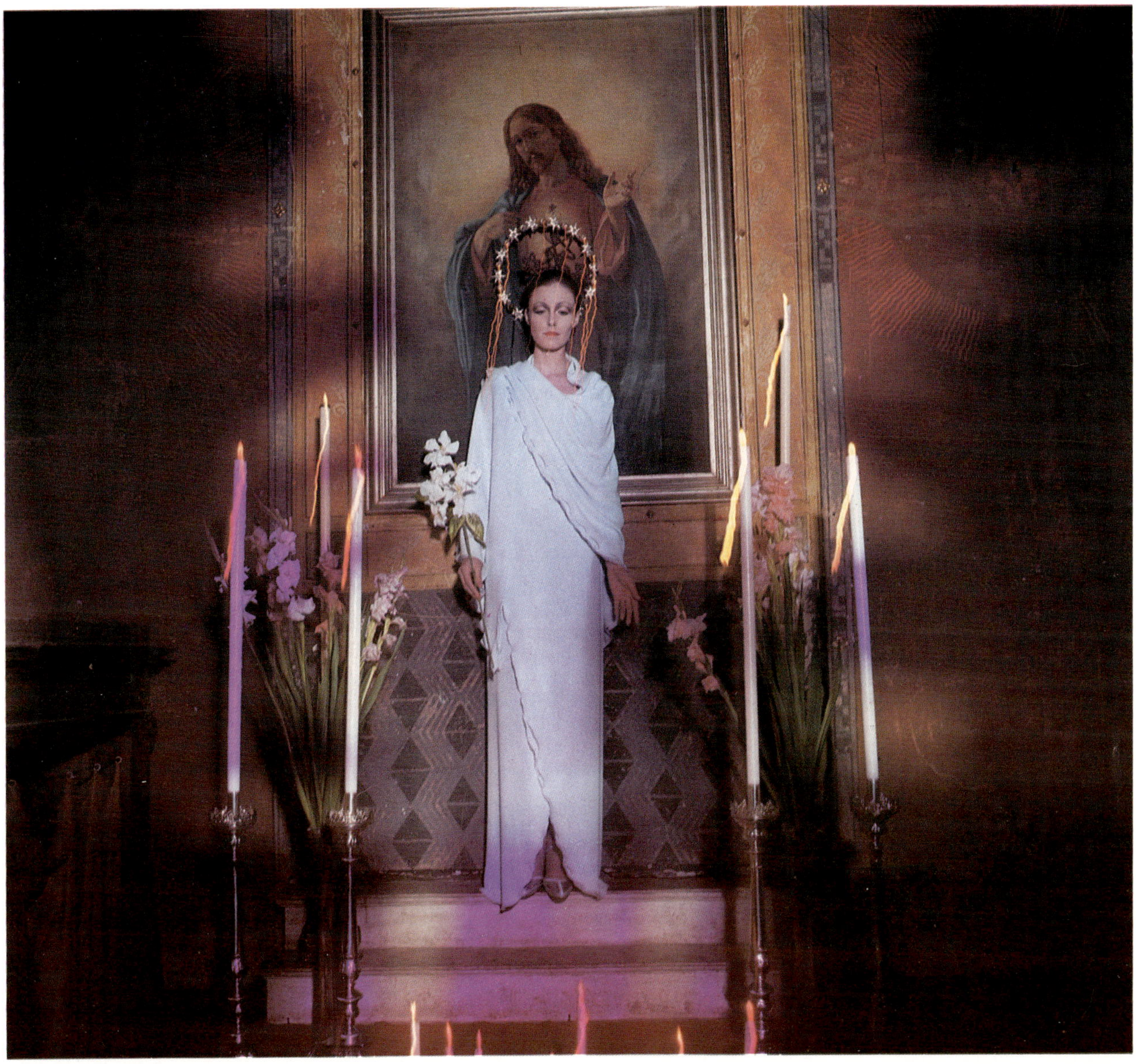

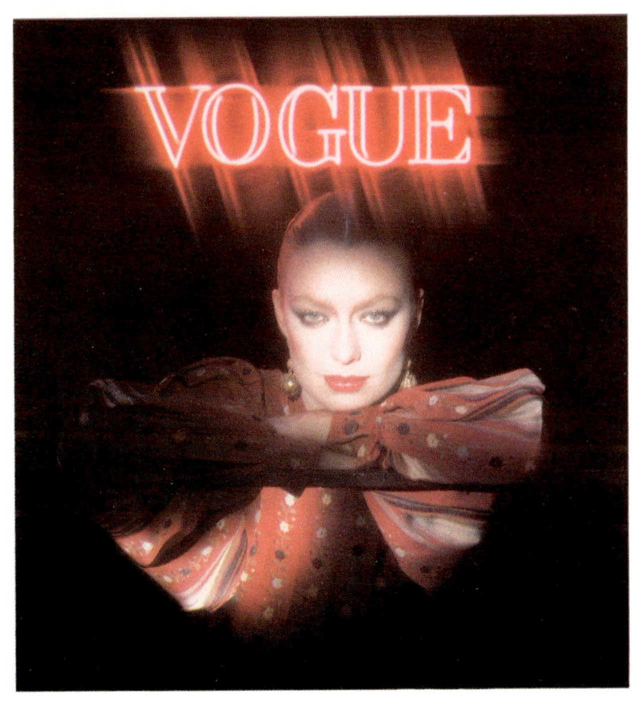
VOGUE
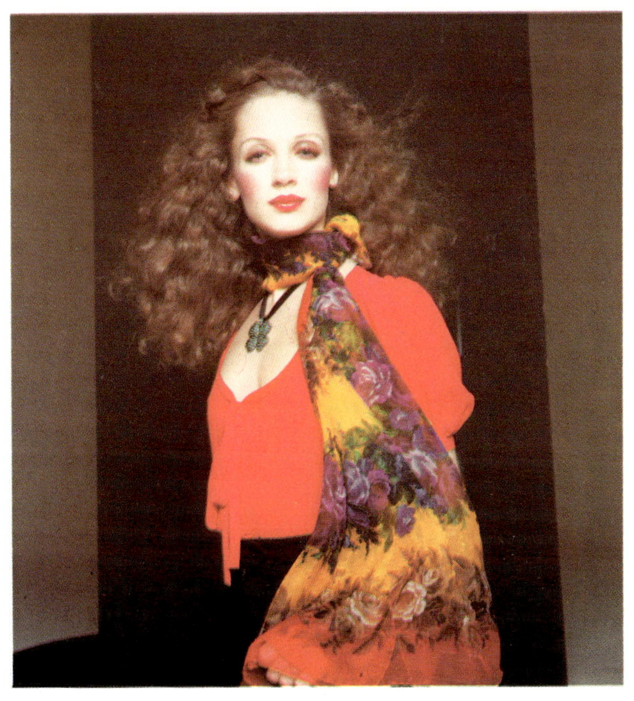

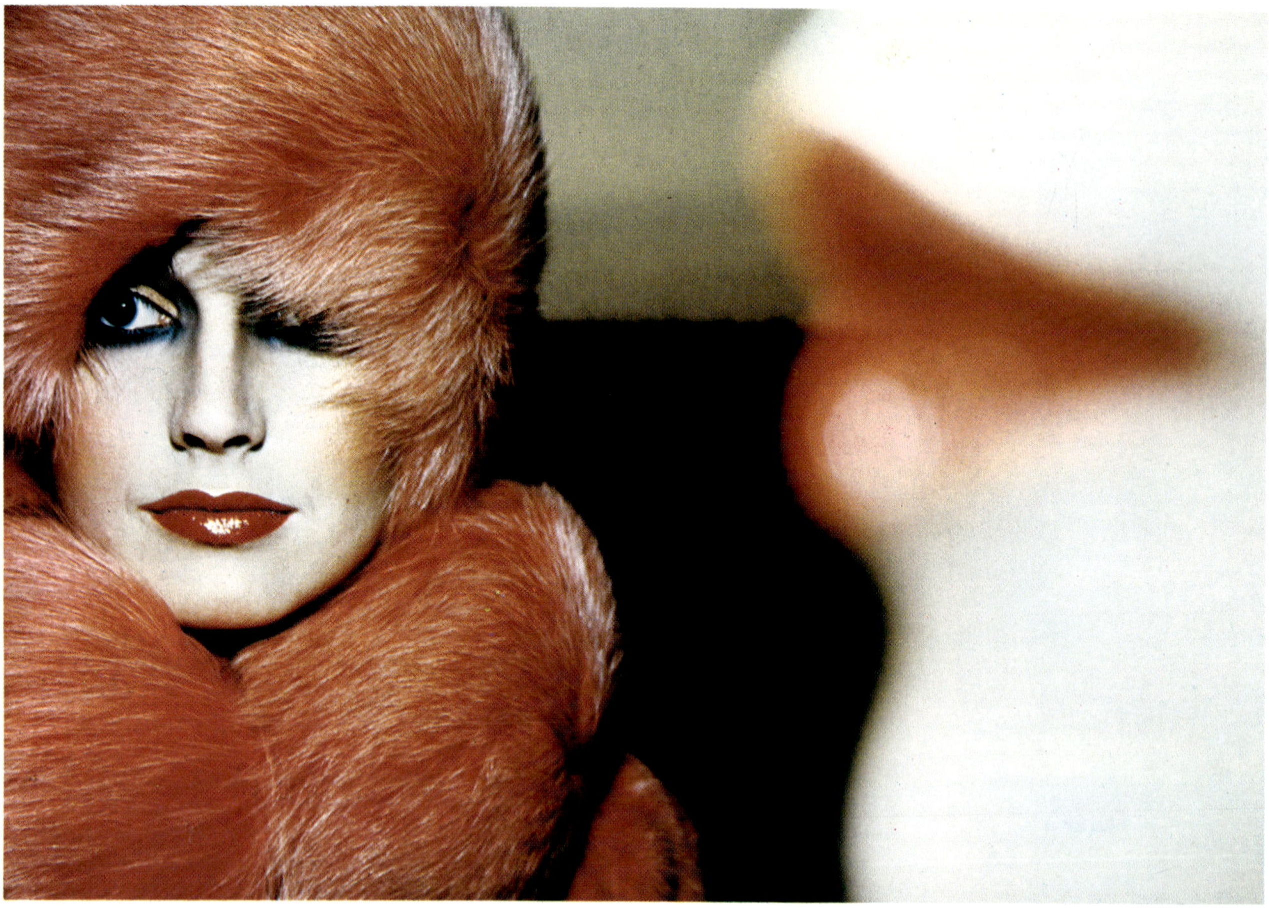

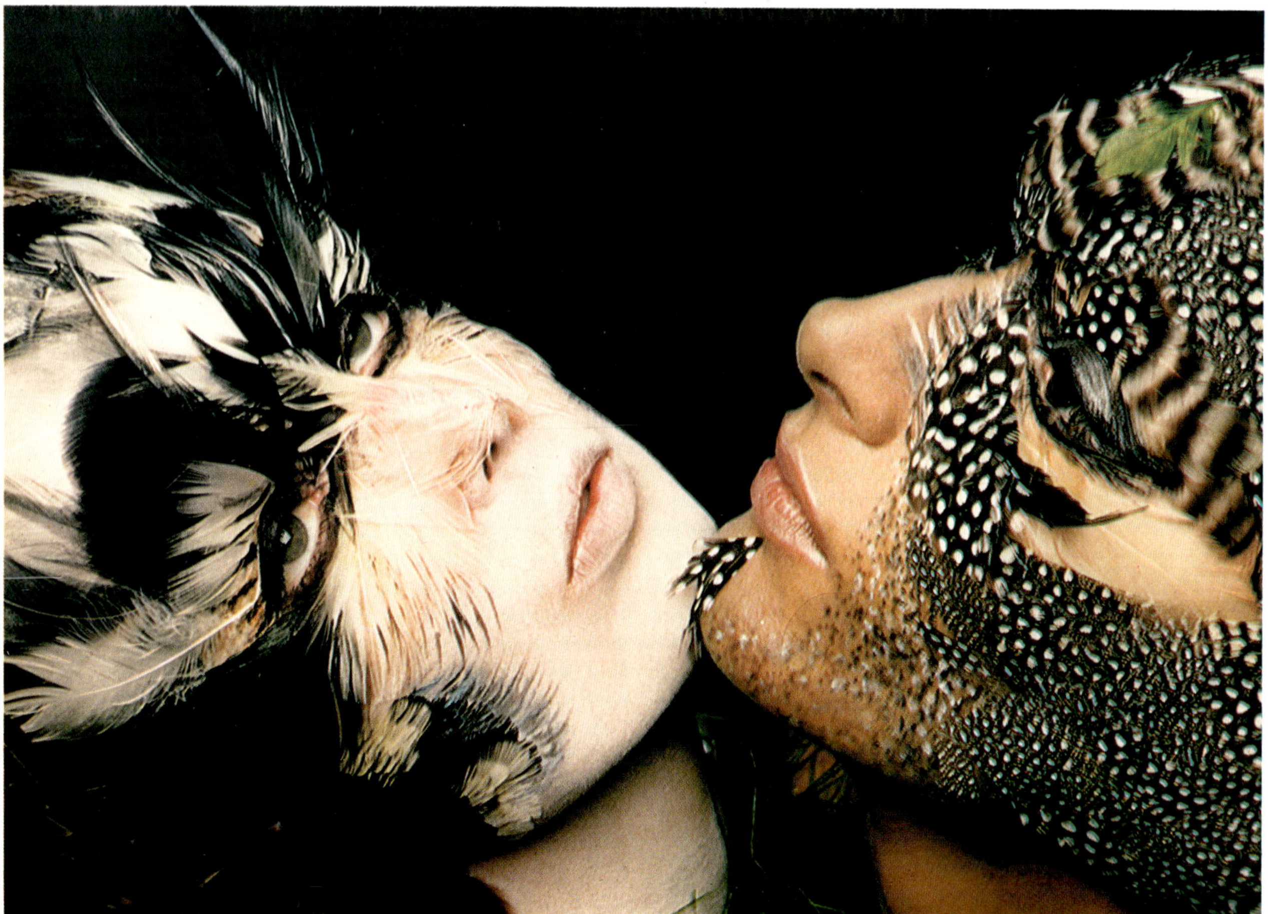

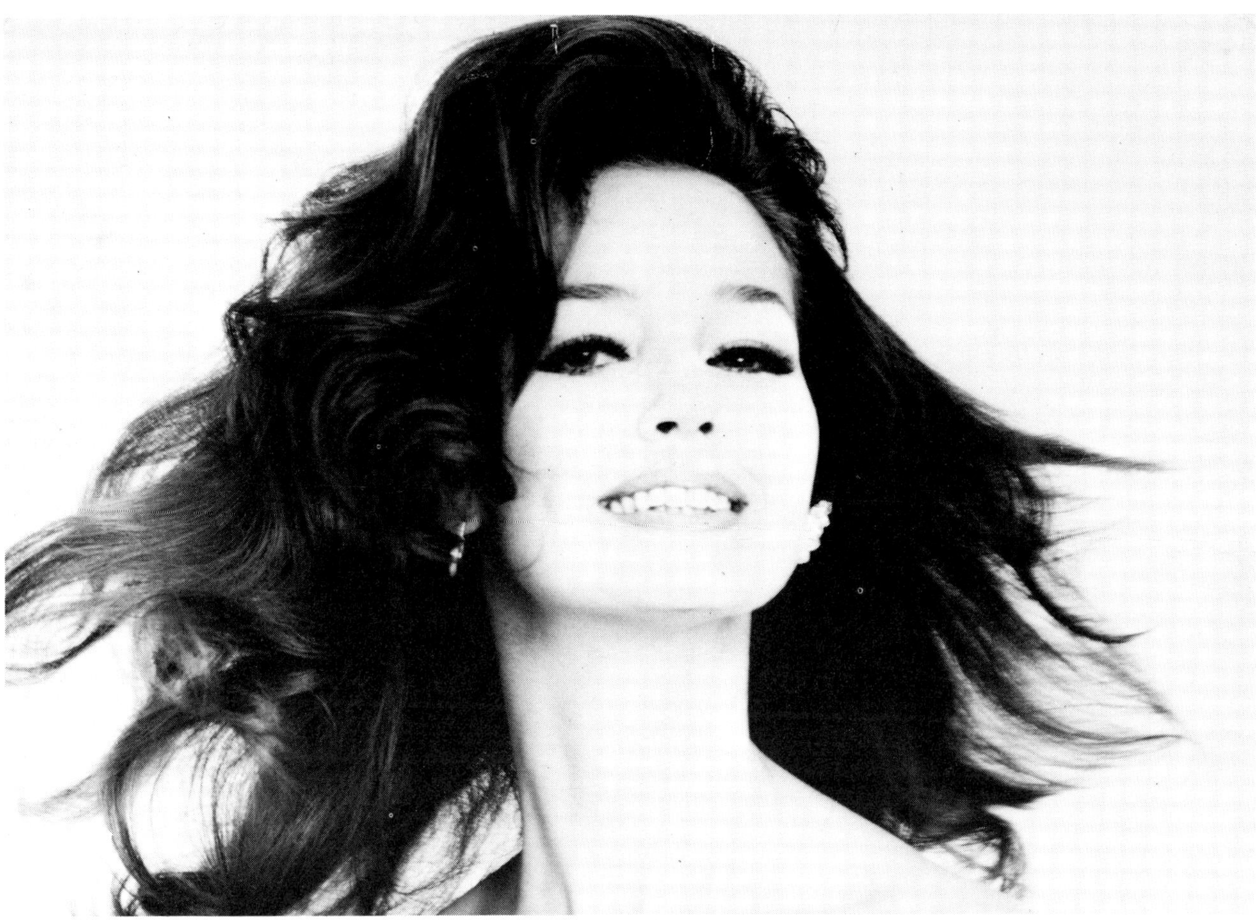

Above: Dolores Hawkins, photographed by Dick Hockman

Opposite. Above: Sue Purdy by Barry Lategan (By kind permission of Condé Nast Publications)

Below: Dorothea McGowan and Natty Abascal by Melvin Sokolsky

Dolores has long, dark hair and big eyes, a good full mouth, and a beautiful swan-like long neck. She moved and photographed well in all kinds of light. She has high cheek bones, with two exquisite little parallel bones on her right cheek.

Dolores Hawkins probably looks better today than she did when she gave up modelling thirteen years ago. 'That's because I think you look best when you're happier. I'm happier today than I was then', she said from her fashionable East-Side New York apartment, where she lives with her husband and two children. She has a couple of thoroughbreds on their farm in Middletown, New York, some seventy-five miles from the city. She still keeps her hand in by doing the occasional job. 'It's been a fabulous business for me', she adds. 'It changed my life. If a girl is lucky enough to know how to handle it all, it can be marvellous. Not to let it go to her head, and save her money. Enjoy it, and get something out of it. You put a lot into it; your time, professionalism and talent, and you're rewarded for it.'

In the sixties, young exponents of music, the arts, and fashion seemed to let themselves go. The ripple-effect of the pop explosion in Britain with Beatlemania, Carnaby Street, and Mary Quant spread across the Atlantic to America's big cities and, although the mid-West was saved from the holocaust, its citizens were all too conscious of it through the media. It was as though the young were shedding all the formality and good taste of the fifties, substituting for them long hair and gypsy-type clothes. They were drifting—looking for an identity of their own, but didn't find it until the seventies.

America's top model in the sixties, however, remained the personification of good taste, high class, and dignity. She was Dutch-born Wilhelmina, who was *Vogue's* top cover girl of all time with over two hundred and fifty major magazine covers to her credit—almost twice as many as Twiggy and Jean Shrimpton's covers put together. Although her modelling career lasted for as little as seven years, from 1960 to 1967 when she retired from modelling to open a model agency in New York, at her peak she earned over a hundred thousand dollars a year.

Born Wilhelmina Behmenburg, she

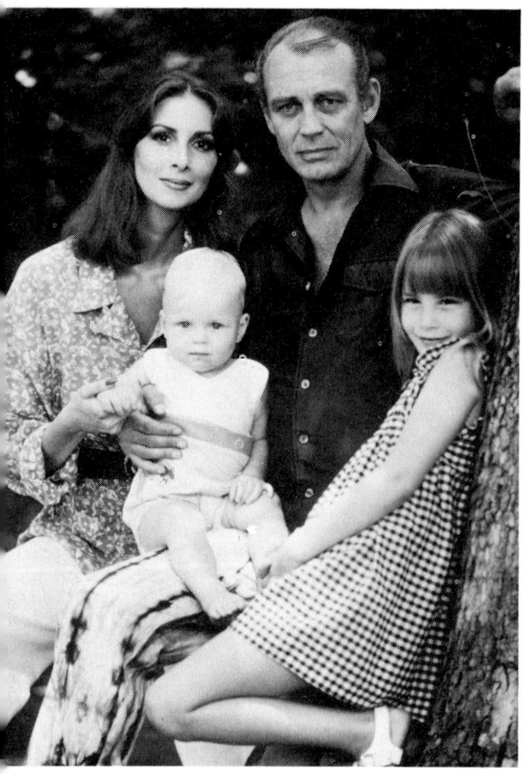

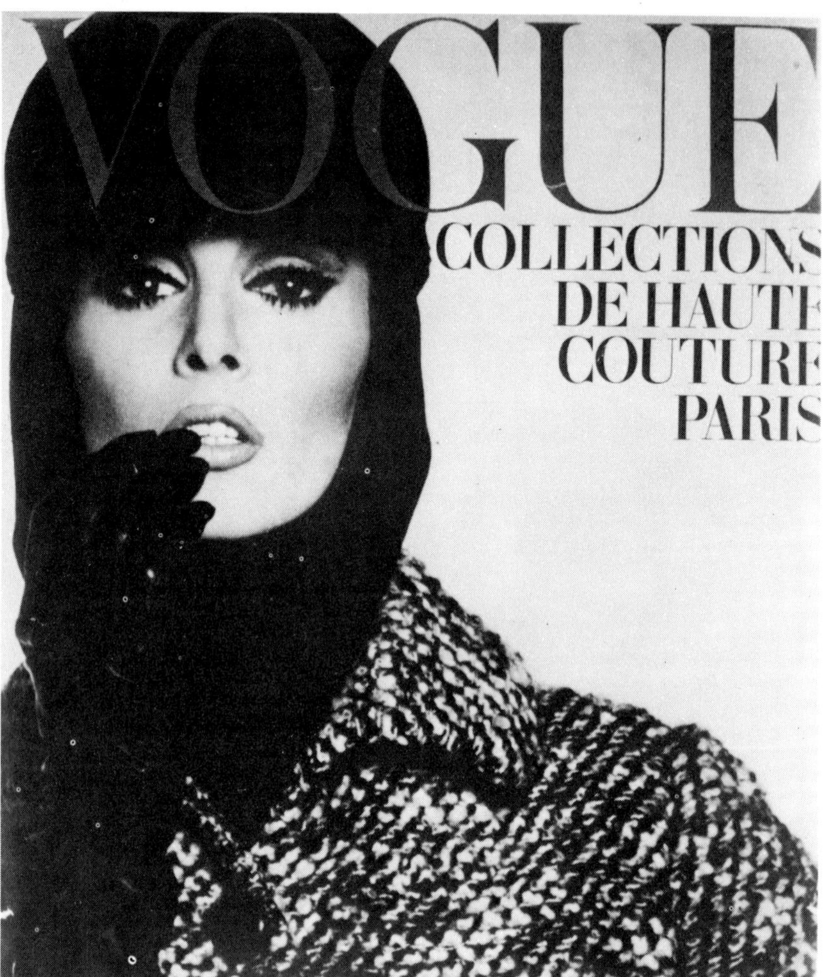

was raised in Holland and Germany. When she was fifteen she and her family moved to Chicago. At this time she couldn't speak English, and so was backward in her schooling. By the time she was nineteen, she had decided on a modelling career, and joined a model school. She began modelling, securing work through a Chicago model agency who decided to change her name to Winnie Hart, as her own name was difficult to pronounce; but when she discovered that the name of the agent's previous biggest moneymaker was Winnie Hart—and that she had died on him—she reverted to her own name, and became known simply as Wilhelmina! She moved to New York, joined the Ford model agency, and began work immediately—becoming one of the leading cover girls almost at once, working for *Vogue*. She travelled to Paris to be photographed wearing the French collections, and joined Dorian Leigh's

agency there. She handed her portfolio to Dorian Leigh who exclaimed that she had a most adaptable face, and could make herself look like anyone she wanted. Since Suzy Parker was Wilhelmina's idol, she tried to mould herself on her looks, but despite this she looked like a composite of Sophia Loren, Gina Lollobrigida, Suzy Parker—and Dorian Leigh herself.

'I used to use Wilhelmina for French *Vogue*', Henry Clarke says. 'But at that time, although she had this marvellous small head, her body was rather large. She liked her food. And so I used to photograph her in things like lingerie which floated, so you didn't see the body.' Clarke did trips with her to London, and took her and Veruschka—who is 6ft 1in—to India to photograph the French collection. Although Wilhelmina is 5ft 11in—she and Veruschka were decidedly tall by model standards (the preferred height is 5ft 9in in

America)—her height was a decided advantage to her, enabling her to show clothes with great style.

'Willy was incredible', echoed English photographer Richard Dormer. 'She had very large hips, but I've never, never known her not be able to wriggle into a dress. The entire zip would be undone at the back, but she always got in! And that was somebody who put a completely different face on. There was nothing there at all, to begin with, only good bone structure, but by the time she'd finished the paint-job, which she'd applied in the Cadillac going along the streets, you wouldn't recognise her.'

Wilhelmina lost a considerable amount of weight by the time she returned to New York, and there continued her phenomenal career.

Photographer Peter Fink recalls that when Wilhelmina worked with him, he watched her image change with every outfit she put on. A whole new person-

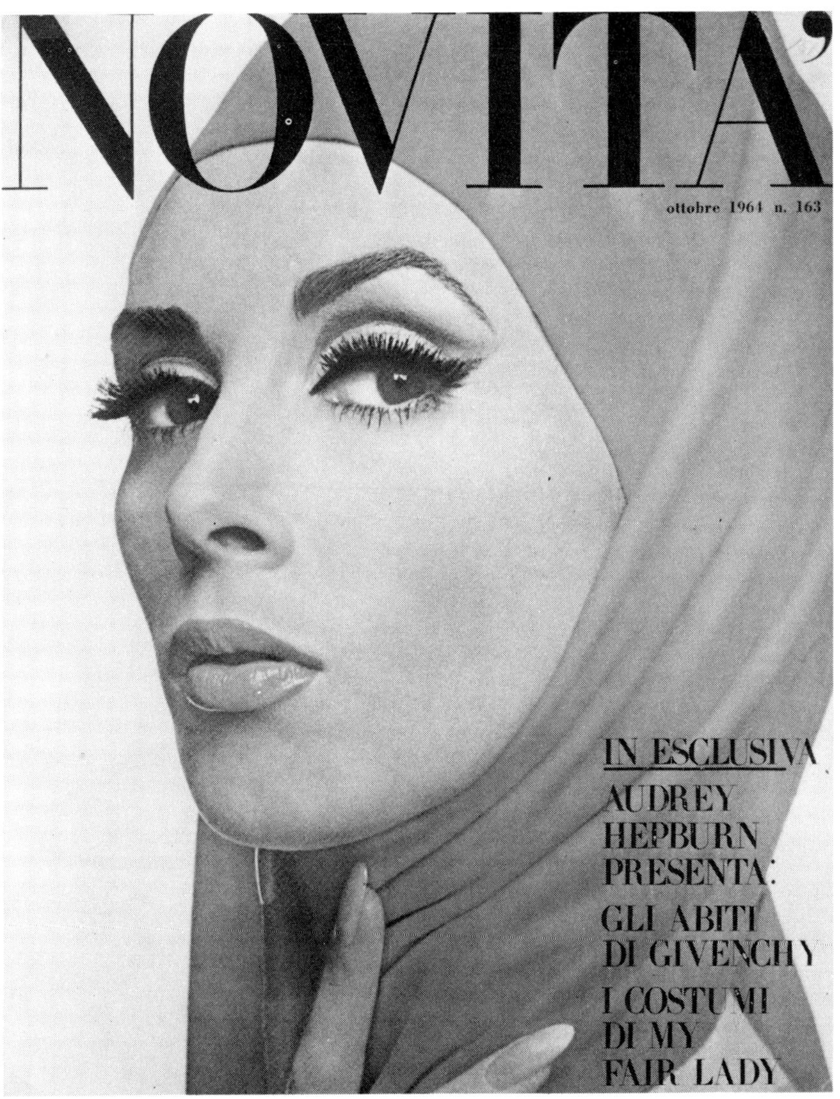

Above: Donna Mitchell the well known American model who was discovered—and photographed here—by Melvin Sokolsky

ality showed through the look in her eyes, or change of hairstyle. She could put on a fur and it would come to life. No animal ever looked as marvellous in its skin as Wilhelmina did in every fur she wore. All she had to do was model something and everyone in the country wanted one just like it.

Veruschka, Jean Shrimpton, and Twiggy were regarded as the superstars of the sixties, and although Wilhelmina earned more than they did and appeared on more covers than the three of them put together, her name was never really known to the public. She neither mixed with the jet-set nor engaged a public relations man and, as she stresses, 'I never used to jump around in the Place de la Concorde at four in the morning for the benefit of the sensational press. I was the conservative, strait-laced model. Although my name was never really known, my *face* certainly was!'

When she appeared on NBC's *Tonight* show, to be interviewed by Johnny Carson, she met production executive Bruce Cooper. They fell in love, married, and have two children, Melissa, aged nine, and Jason, two.

'I knew that I had up to seven years to really pile in the money as a model', Wilhelmina says. 'I realised the importance of doing editorial work for magazines, being good at my work and being liked, because one can take advantage of the editorial successes. But then somehow something was wrong. I worked every day for six months, and it got tougher to get out of bed and get myself together. I used to be the inventor of a lot of new poses; but suddenly I felt myself merely going through the same routine with my eyes closed and realised it was time to retire from modelling.' Her husband suggested opening an agency, and within three weeks the Wilhelmina Model Agency opened.

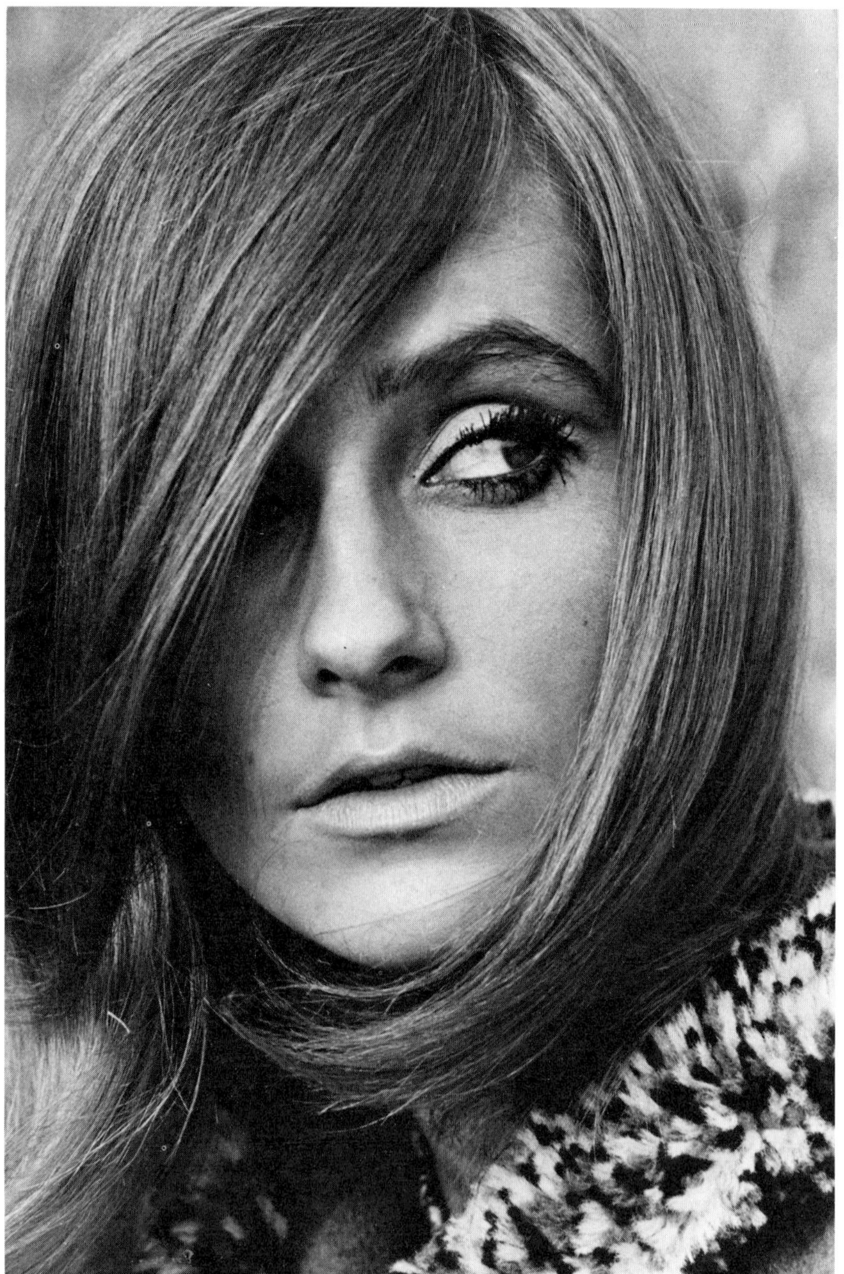

Left: Beate Shultz who is married to a top American photographer, James Moore. Photograph by Francesco Scavullo

Opposite: Beate Shultz and Agnetta Darren, photographed by Francesco Scavullo

After only ten years in business, it has become one of the largest model agencies in New York—second only to the great Ford agency.

In second league to Wilhelmina were Dorothea MacGowan and Tilly Tizani, but there were other top girls from the fifties who continued on the steady path of success during the sixties. Among the big earners were Dolores Hawkins, Marola Witt, Beate Shultz, Agnetta Darren, Evelyn Kuhn, Brigitta Bauer, Elsa Peretti, Ivy Nicholson, Iris Bianchi, Anne Saint Claire, Donna Mitchell, and Ushi. The newcomers who became sought after included Lyn Kohlman, Pat McGuire, Lyn Sutherland, Cathee Dahmen, and Maud Adams—all of them continued to work steadily into the seventies.

'Agnetta Darren didn't look like a model, but a countess', recalls Scavullo. 'With no make-up on, she was like a madonna. Strobe lights show the planes in her face. I liked her best in a satin shirt and jeans.'

Donna Mitchell was discovered by Sokolsky: 'She was a kid I took off the streets. She was only sixteen, and she had a long racoon coat held together with a big safety pin. I took her off to *Harpers Bazaar*, and they thought I was mad.' In those days Richard Avedon was Sokolsky's intermediary at *Harpers*, and before he could use anyone new, he had to seek Avedon's permission.

'He thought she was just a ruffian off the streets and didn't think anything of her until I did the Paris collections with her, and then he used her all the time.'

Although Donna Mitchell was rather ordinary looking, she was one of the finest models, appearing in more commercials on American television than any other model. She has brown hair and is rather plain looking, but, once in a studio, she transforms herself into a great beauty. She is a genius with make-up. 'I remember working with her', says model Jerry Hall, 'and when she came into the studio, everyone said, "What are we going to do with this ordinary looking girl?" and then suddenly she turned into this incredible beauty.'

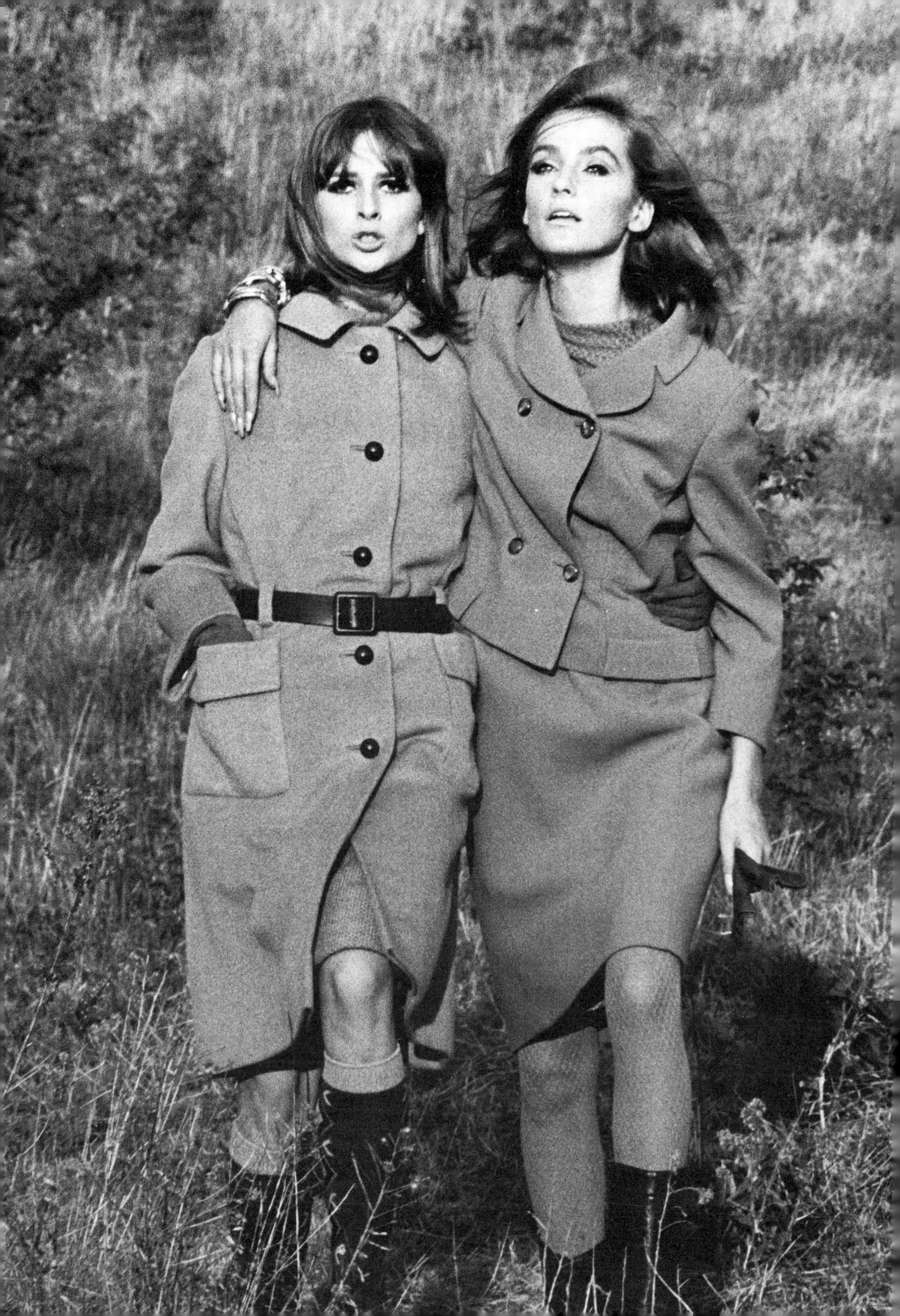

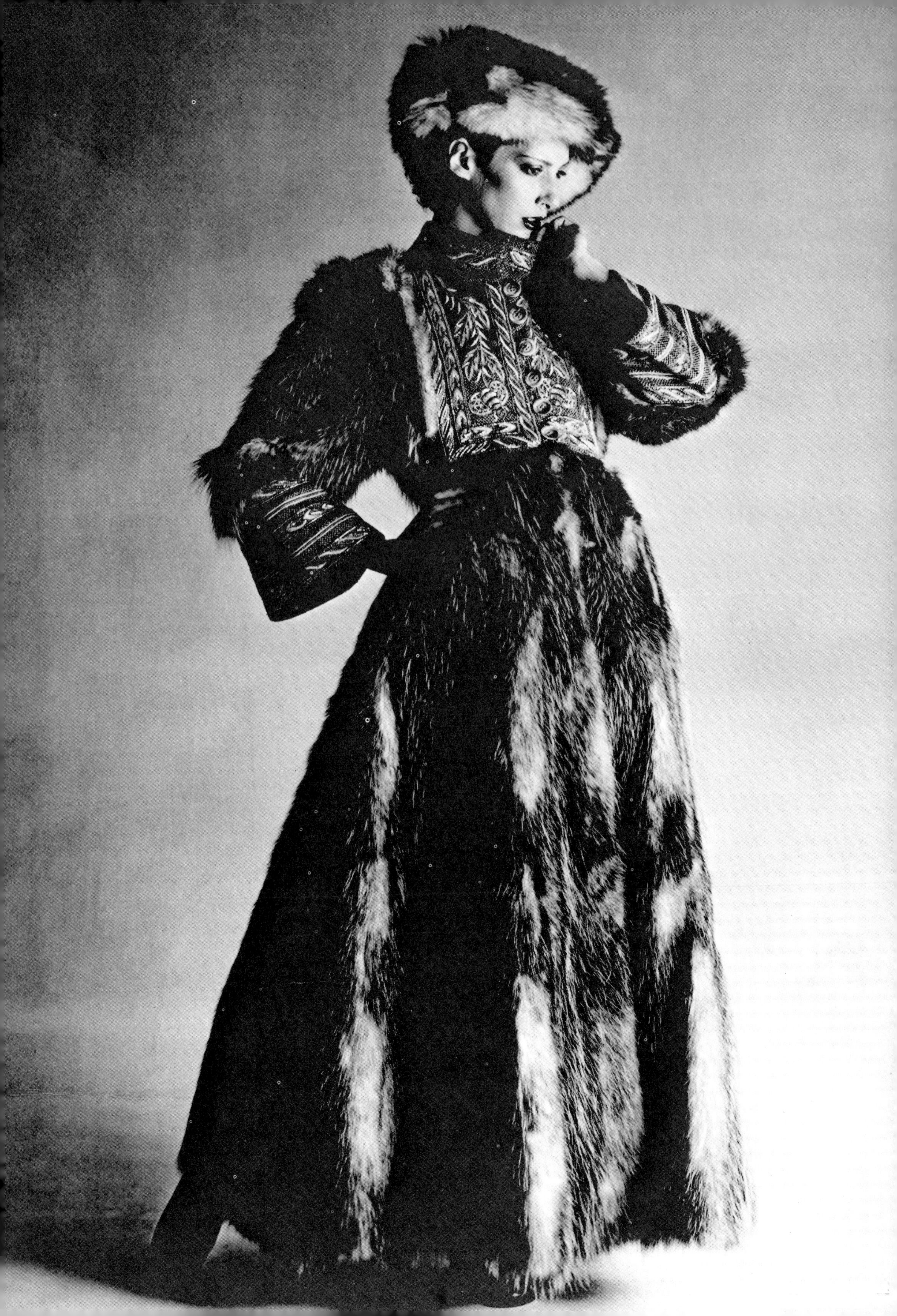

Top American Models in the Seventies

In America models now fall into three categories. There are the eccentric ones who are famous for creating beautiful shapes—the exotic fantasy girls of the Donyale Luna type who are discussed in a separate chapter. Then there are the all-American beauty girls, discussed later, who do the glossy covers and fashion editorials—they are beautiful, smiling, and look exceptional modelling mink coats and evening gowns. The third category are the 'personality' models who fall between the two types, one of whom is Dutch-born Apollonia von Ravenstein, who has done considerable work in Europe with photographer Norman Parkinson, with whom she started. She has worked a good deal for *Vogue* with Richard Avedon, but her appearance in a pornographic movie put paid to some of her connections in the higher echelons of the fashion field. The images clashed. Slim, with an elegant perfection, and 6ft tall in her bare feet, she is the fantasy girl who can sell anything. She has a China-doll-like face, high but flat breasts, and boyish hips. When she walks onto the studio set and the session begins, she is alive at once.

She does not merely move, she glides and dances as the background music inspires her mood. She turns and undulates, vamps and laughs. She actually seems to delight in the perfume and dress she is advertising. Suddenly she is the happiest, the most beautiful, the most successful girl in the world; she is inventive and exuberant. All this keeps her steadily in the hundred-thousand-dollars-a-year bracket.

Opposite: American-born Lyn Kohlman, former wife of photographer Barry Lategan, in a pose by Richard Dormer

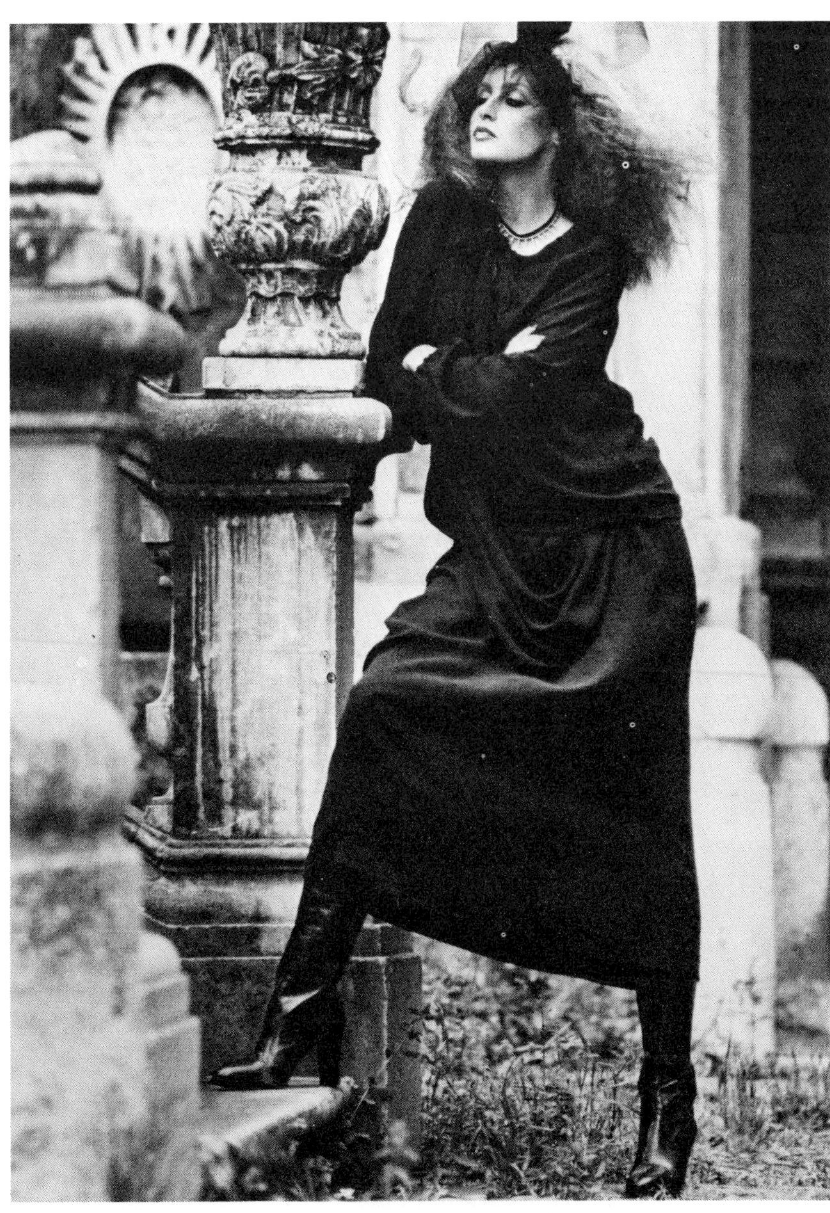

Right: The 6ft tall, Dutch-born Apollonia von Ravenstein who specialises in fantasy roles

Shelley Smith is completely different from Apollonia. Shelley has the fresh, clean look that *Vogue* and *Harpers* like for their covers, and she has appeared on covers of both simultaneously without the other knowing, because her looks are so versatile. She seems completely different in almost every photograph she takes; she can never be typecast.

She began modelling by accident on holiday in Paris and, after learning her craft in Europe, returned to New York. She and Jerry Hall went to India together, for French *Vogue*. 'We went for three weeks', says Jerry, 'and they paid us $500 a day each, every day. We travelled first class, stayed in a luxury hotel, and when I met Shelley for the first time, I thought, "This girl looks so strange. Why did they pick her for this job? Paying her all this money?" And then I knew. As a person she is very quiet and unassuming, but once she's in front of the camera, she's sensational. She's a great model.'

Patti Hansen is the top American photographic model of 1977, followed closely by Lisa Taylor, Christie Brinkley, Roseanne Vella, and Rene Russo; all leading *Vogue* and *Harpers Bazaar* cover girls.

'The reason I consider Patti Hansen the best', says Scavullo, 'is that everybody can photograph her. She's not so special, like Margaux, that only one person can photograph her. Anyone with a camera and a light meter can

Below: Shelley Smith

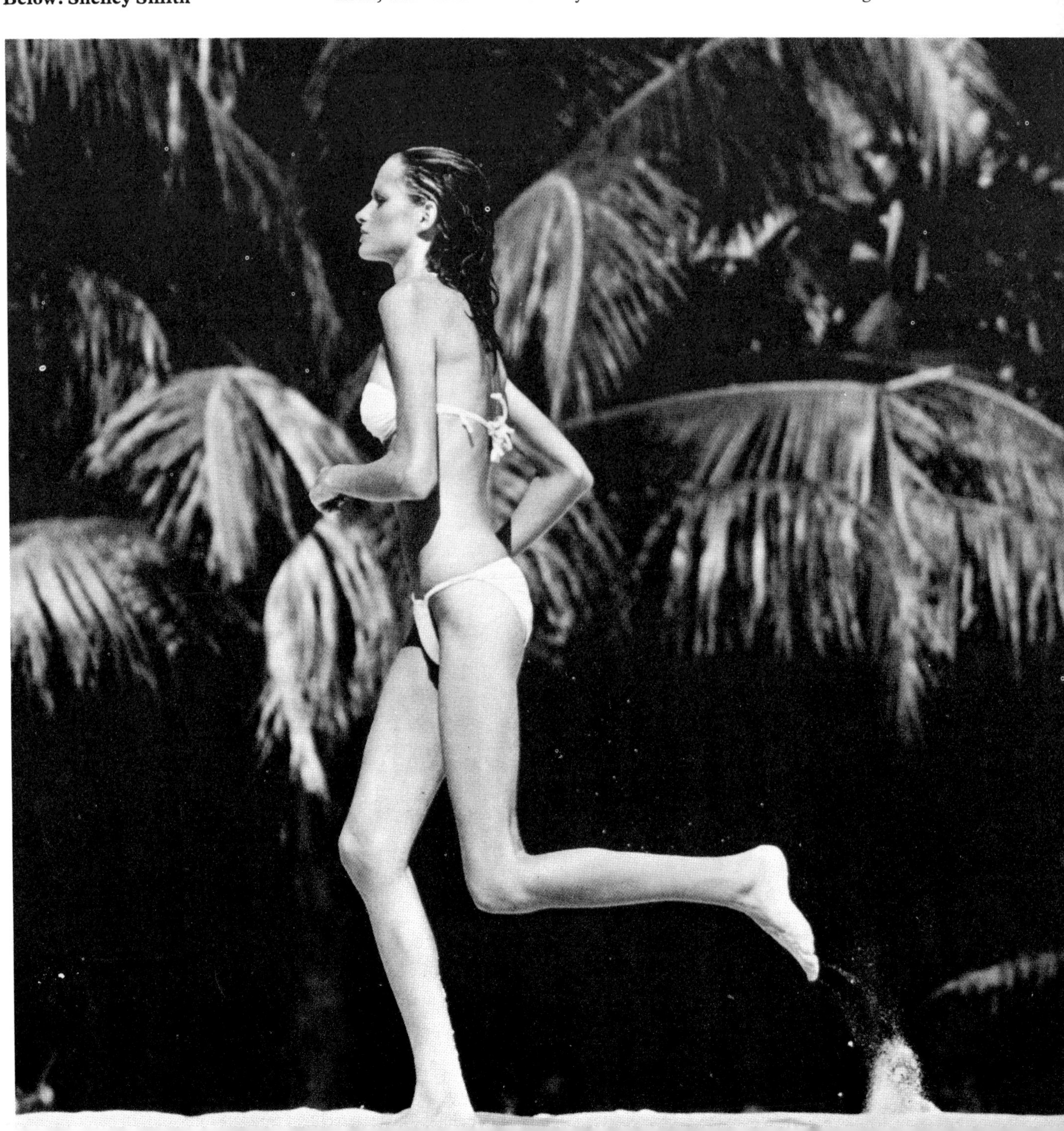

photograph Patti, and make her look good. I was the first to photograph her for *Vogue*. I took her along to them and did three covers for them. They love her.'

Californian Rene Russo has that clean, healthy, not-overdone look. She looks as if she did it all by herself; her hair, her clothes, her make-up, even when she's being her most sophisticated.

Scavullo admits that he cannot photograph Lisa Taylor because her eyes are too deep set and disappear in his light. She is best photographed by Helmut Newton because he uses a ring flash that makes her look fabulous.

'Christie Brinkley is sexy', says a top photographer. 'I love her. I'd like to spend a whole week with her!'

Jane Hitchcock is a beautiful girl. She is movie material more than anything else, excelling in her new movie, *Nickelodeon* directed by Peter Bogdanovich, and also starring Ryan and Tatum O'Neal and Burt Reynolds.

In New York the three types of photographic modelling are 'money-work' or advertising; catalogue work, and editorial work. The other, more specialised type of modelling is television commercials. 'I prefer doing photographic modelling for magazines', Shelley Smith says. 'It's the most fun thing to do. It's imaginative, you're always selling a product and you always have certain restrictions about how you can look and how much you can move.'

Lyn Kohlman is one of the more

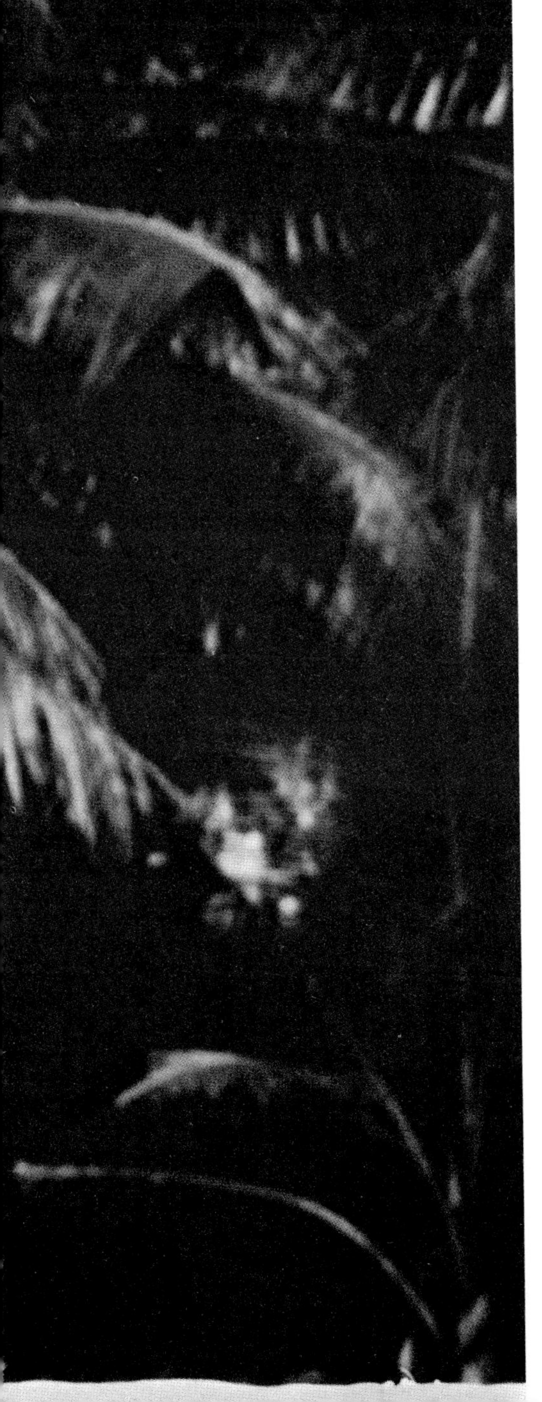

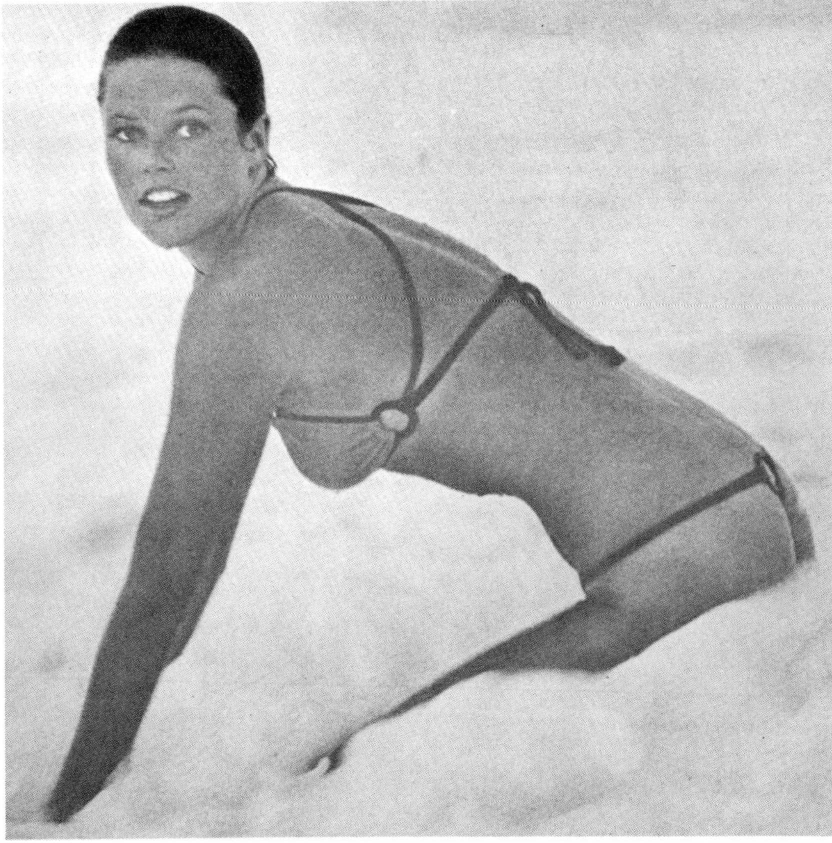

Below: Christie Brinkley, by Walter Loos Jr

established New York models. She specialises in fashion photography and beauty advertising, and there isn't a photographer of note throughout the world with whom she has not worked. Once married to top British photographer Barry Lategan, she has lived and worked in London, and although she is based in New York, spends a great deal of time working in Europe as well as America.

Lyn does not consider modelling the humdrum business it is cut out to be. 'I was an art major at college for five years', Lyn says, 'and I do consider myself to have a creative eye. I can sense lines and shapes and composition from my end of the camera. That's how I think of modelling; as a creation of moods and lines. I like to think with the photographer and I like to get on their wavelength. But you're not given time to do that in America, nor is the photographer. There is very little creativity in New York. There is when I'm working with certain people, but it doesn't happen as often in New York as it does in Europe, where the model can take part in the creativity. In New York the photographer just has to produce pictures, and is only very rarely allowed creative flair.'

Opposite: The top American model, Roseanne Vella, photographed by Francesco Scavullo. Courtesy *Vogue* **USA**

Above right: Barbara Carreras, one of the leading young black models of the seventies, photographed by Francesco Scavullo. Courtesy American *Cosmopolitan*

Right: Patti Hansen who appears regularly on *Vogue* **and** *Harpers Bazaar* **covers. Photograph by Francesco Scavullo**

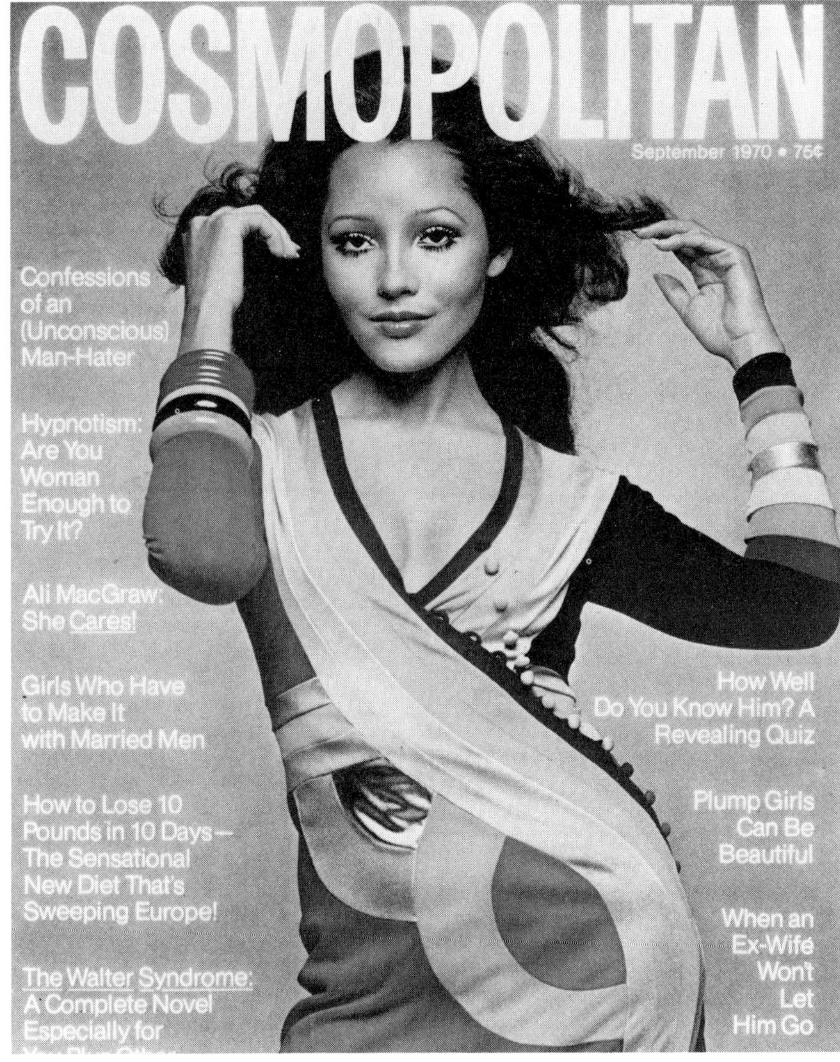

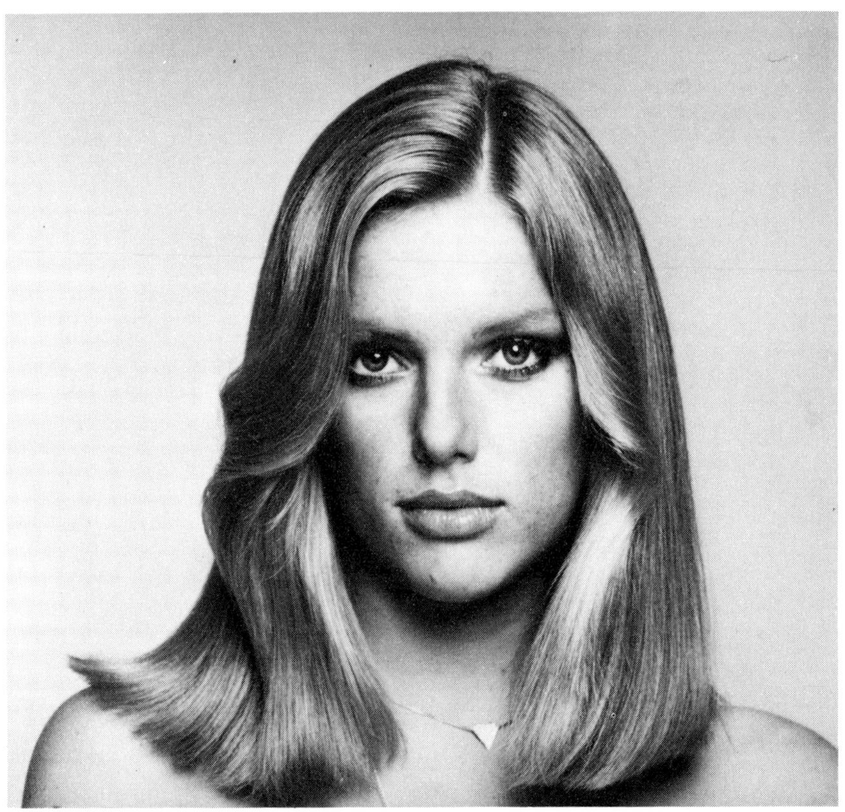

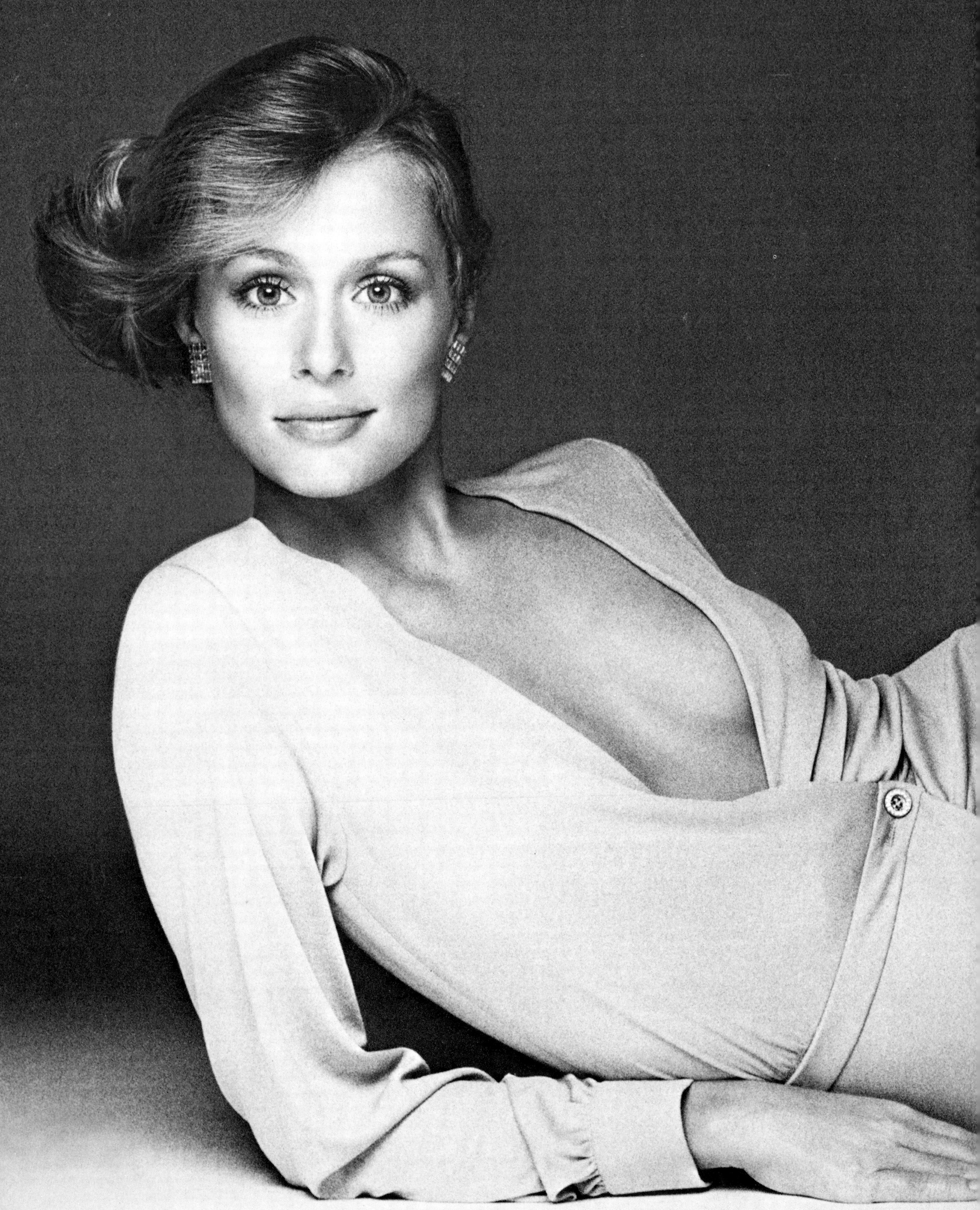

Cosmetic Queens

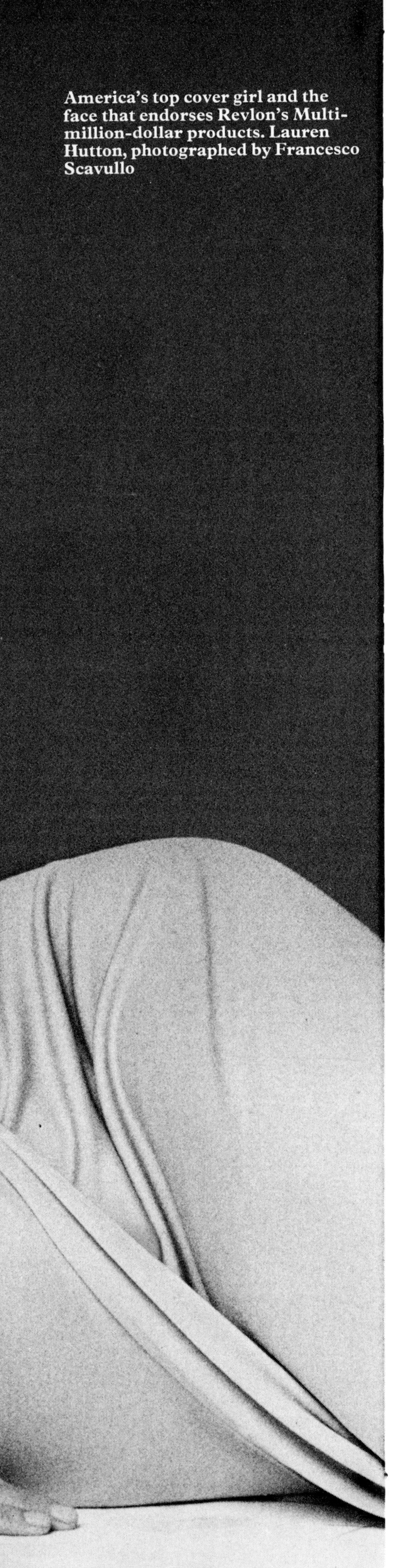

America's top cover girl and the face that endorses Revlon's Multi-million-dollar products. Lauren Hutton, photographed by Francesco Scavullo

There are only a handful of top models in America who command gigantic fees under contract to the top cosmetic manufacturers. The highest paid is Margaux Hemingway, but her rise is recent compared with Lauren Hutton, who has been under contract to Revlon since the beginning of the seventies, and has now given up modelling for movie-acting. In her thirties, tawny-blonde Lauren Hutton has been America's top cover girl for more than ten years. Born in Charleston, South Carolina, her career as a model in the seventies is unequalled. Her movie career to date, however, has gone practically unnoticed with relatively inconsequential roles in *Paper Lion*, *Little Fauss and Big Halsy*, *The Gambler*, and *Gator*. Her most recent movie is *Welcome to L.A.*

There is hardly a glossy magazine anywhere in the world advertising Revlon that doesn't carry her image alongside its products. Charlie is one of the latest campaigns, with Lauren striding along in the open with her fresh, sexy face glowing from the pages.

Horst was the first to photograph Lauren Hutton when she posed for an underwear feature for *Vogue*. Yet although she is incredibly attractive, she has facial disadvantages that do not detract from her beauty; a crooked nose, a gap between her front teeth, and a largish jawline. 'Richard Avedon and I are the only ones to have done good photographs of Lauren', says Scavullo, who secured his *Vogue* contract through Lauren's recommendation. 'Not everyone can photograph her. She is scrubbed, sexy, intelligent, real—the way women should look now. She is the best model in the world, and she is my favourite.'

But now that Lauren's contract with Revlon has expired, a strong contender as her successor has appeared—tall, slender, and childlike, with cascades of yellow hair and a little pink face, Deborah Raffin personifies the model craze. Revlon and the huge Japanese cosmetic empire, Kanebo, both vie for her services, with $500,000 contracts as bait. Michael Viner, Deborah's husband, is an able negotiator and will no doubt secure the best contract.

Although Suzy Parker was Revlon's first number-one model, earning $500 for each day she worked for them,

Evelyn Kuhn, married to television commercials producer and photographers' representative, Stanley Sokolsky, was the first model to be put under contract to them—or to any company. Evelyn had worked for every cosmetic company in America and Europe, scoring a tremendous sales success for the new Love-Lemon eau de cologne. Revlon had been struck by the sky-rocketing sales of a competitor's product and, realising that it was because of Evelyn Kuhn's participation in the advertising campaign, wanted her to work for them exclusively. Her manager, Nat Markowitz, and the Ford agency negotiated a contract with Revlon guaranteeing her a certain figure for working a certain number of days. In the first year alone, with Evelyn Kuhn as their new brand image, Revlon's sales rose by 37 per cent. They were onto a winner, and their competitors, Estée Lauder and Max Factor, followed suit by formulating similar contracts with Karen Graham and Christina Ferrare.

Consumers began relating models to the product, identifying Evelyn Kuhn as the Revlon Girl. However, fearing over-exposure of the model's face, time limits were imposed on the use of Evelyn Kuhn's picture in advertising campaigns. Contracts were signed for three- or six-monthly exposures of the photographs in various territories— different American states, Europe, or Britain. This system is now being applied to most cosmetic and cigarette advertising campaigns, strengthening the model's position in America.

Texan-born Jerry Hall, 5ft 11in, a top international model, was proposed as Lauren Hutton's successor for the Revlon campaign, but she was finally turned down. 'They tried me for months with every different photographer in New York', Jerry explains. 'They paid me a fortune in trying, but they kept saying that I looked too un-American in my pictures. They'd say, "Smile. Look casual." They tried me with make-up, and then without make-up.' She was chosen for a Revlon advertising feature in Europe but her looks weren't American enough for the American campaign. 'They wanted me to look more American! Me, a girl from Dallas, Texas. I couldn't be more American if I tried, and here they were

Right: Margaux Hemingway, a niece of the great American novelist, has become the highest paid girl in model history advertising Fabergé's beauty products. Photograph by Francesco Scavullo. Courtesy *Vogue* USA

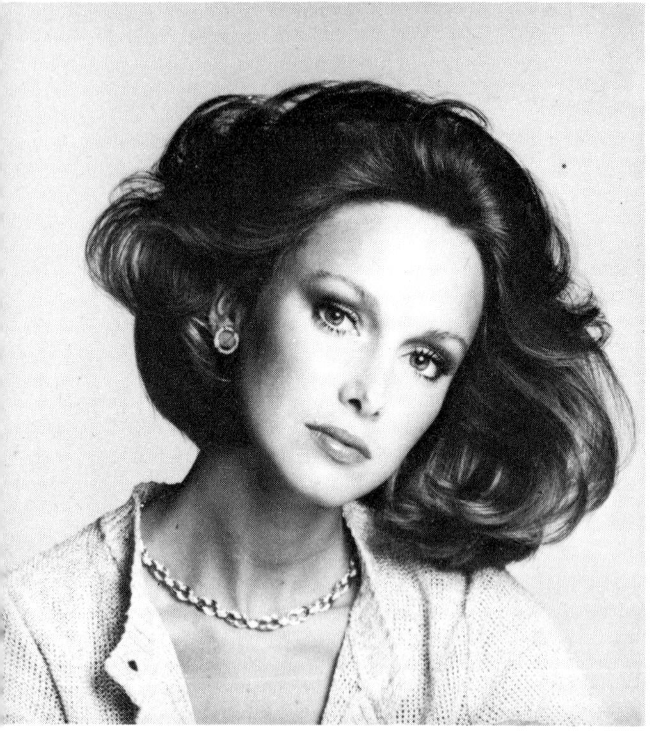

Above: Karen Graham, the model who endorsed Estée Lauder's internationally known beauty products until her retirement in 1977 from her exclusive contract. Taken by Francesco Scavullo. Courtesy *Vogue* USA

Right: Christina Ferrare who endorsed Max Factor's products until she moved into films. Photographed by Francesco Scavullo for American *Cosmopolitan*

Opposite: Revlon and the Japanese cosmetic giant Kanebo both vie for the services of Deborah Raffin. Photographed here by Francesco Scavullo

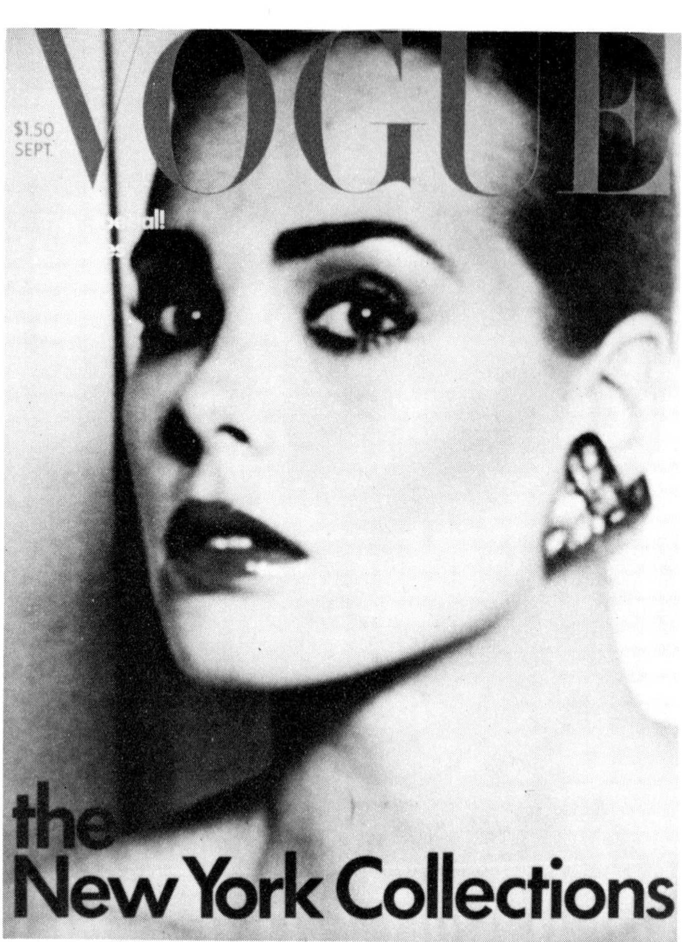

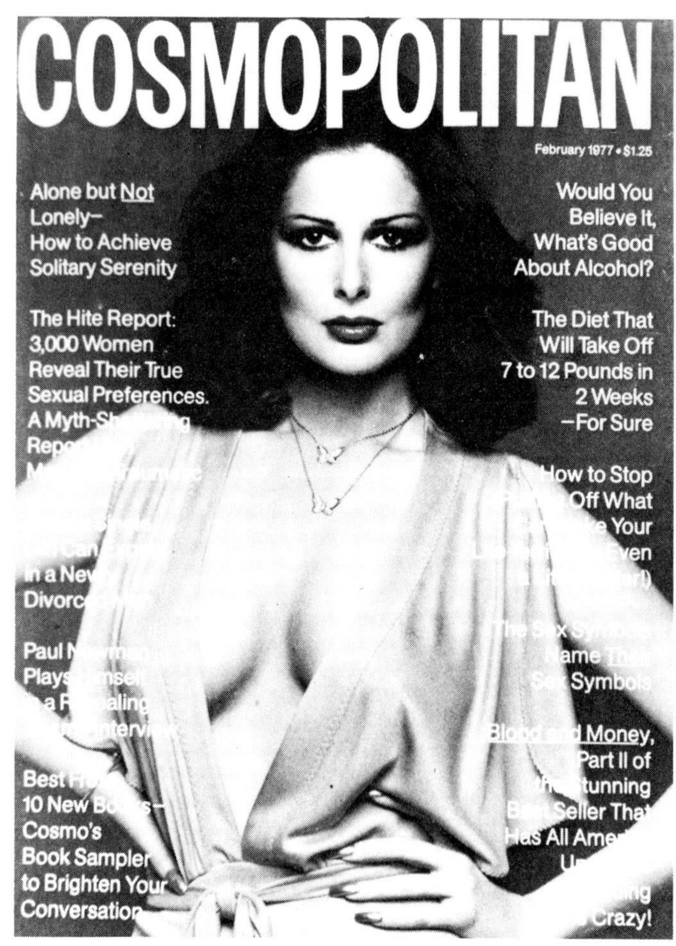

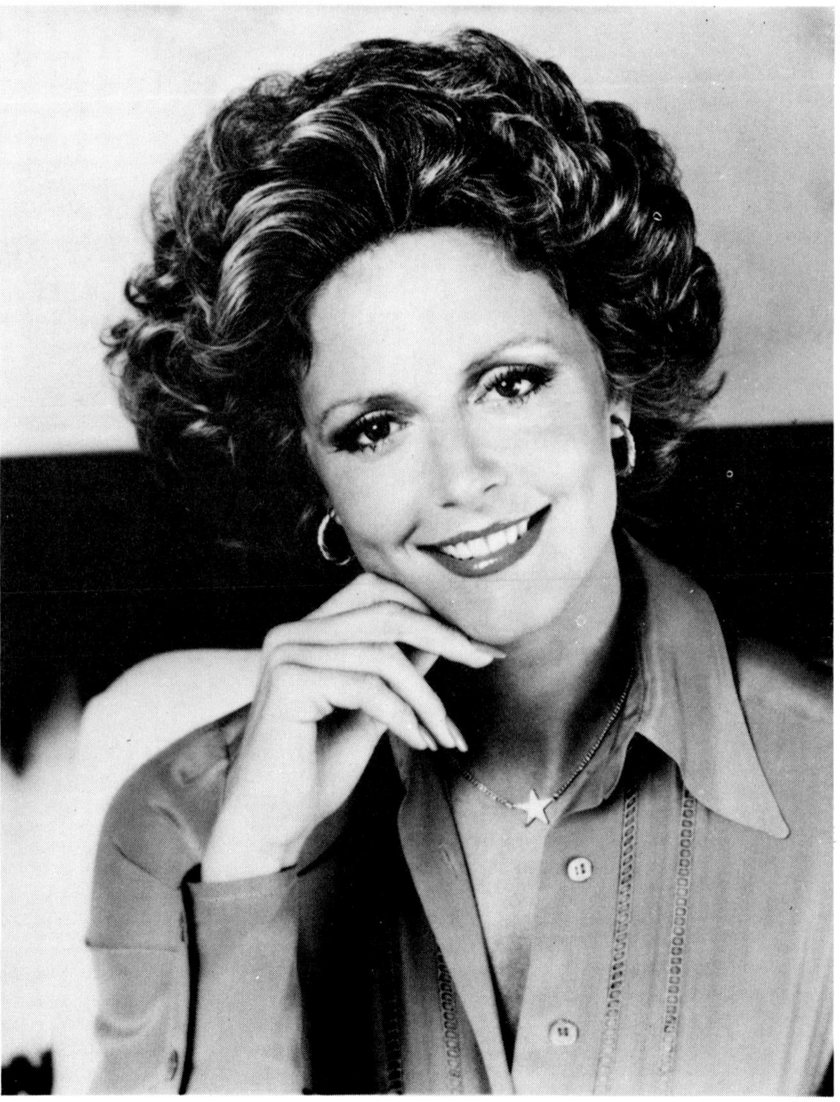

Below: Sunny Griffin, Avon's beauty and fashion director, who travels across America as spokeswoman for their world-famous products. Photographed by Gary Gross. Courtesy Avon Products Inc

saying I didn't look American enough!'

Margaux Hemingway's vibrant quality is her strength. When she smiles and her hair is left wild, she has an animal quality; like a Californian version of Anna Mangani. Margaux caused a sensation when Fabergé announced that they were paying her a million dollars to endorse their 'Babe' range, making her the highest paid model in the world. Fabergé, however, reaped more than four times that amount in free advertising when the deal was announced in five-minute items on national television and radio news coverage throughout the world.

Margaux's father, Jack, was born in Paris, the eldest son of novelist Ernest Hemingway, and the family lived in Cuba with him for a short time. In 1967 Jack and his wife, Puck, decided to settle in Sun Valley, where they could lead an outdoor, sporting life. The three Hemingway daughters, Muffet (a former tennis champion and co-author of suspense-novel-turned-movie *Rosebud*), Margaux, and young Mariel were brought up to hunt, fish, shoot, and ski. Margaux became an expert skier, specialising in free style, and it was the promotion of women's skiing that first took her to New York in September 1975.

On the day of her arrival in New York, she met Errol Wetson, a sophisticated entrepreneur who founded the Wetson Hamburger chain when he was just eighteen. Margaux was whisked into fashion's jet-set. She began modelling, and Fabergé, who were searching for a particular girl to represent an exciting new fragrance, a girl who was fresh and natural, warm and sexy, found Margaux their ideal choice for 'Babe'. She was signed on an unprecedented contract, and began making headlines across the world, even receiving the ultimate tribute, a *Time* magazine cover story. To celebrate it all, Margaux and Errol married in Paris, and returned to Ketchum to begin planning their first home.

Margaux took up dancing, singing, and acting lessons in preparation for her Fabergé 'Babe' commercials and her up-and-coming career as a film star. The film *Lipstick*, in which she plays a model who is raped, with Anne Bancroft as her co-star, was reasonably successful.

'I did the screen test for Margaux right here in my studio in New York', Scavullo recalls, 'and out in California they had to send for the tests to put in the beginning of *Lipstick*.' He feels that his are the finest photographs of her— that the photographs taken for her 'Babe' campaign don't do her justice. 'I think Margaux's a most exciting model at the moment, but unfortunately for her, I am the only one that can photograph her. A supermodel must photograph great in bright daylight and Margaux does. She's not the evening glamour fantasy. She's a far cry from European vampires. Other photographers don't use the right technique for her.'

Cheryl Tieges, the tall model with the fresh, healthy outdoor look, is under contract to the Noxell Corporation, for whom she advertises their popular make-up called Cover Girl. Her face appears as well on posters throughout

Outdoor girl Cheryl Tieges, Noxell's brand image for their Cover Girl make-up range. She is also the face which appears on Virginia Slims posters throughout the world

America, advertising Virginia Slims cigarettes.

The Avon girl is the beautiful Sunny Griffin, however, the role of these exceptionally striking women is not merely to appear in glossy magazines endorsing multi-million dollar products, but, as in the case of Sunny, to travel as spokeswomen for the companies, as beauty and fashion directors. Although based in New York, at Avon's executive headquarters, Sunny's home is in California, where she lives with her husband, Richard Wagner, one of the top CBS reporters on the West Coast.

'Sunny is an absolutely marvellous model', says one of the photographers with whom she works frequently. 'She's a good commercial model, but I can only laugh when I think of her, because she talks and talks and talks throughout the photographic session, and never shuts up. She gives me a headache with

the talking! But she's worth it. S'hes great!'

Christina Ferrare, of lush sensuality and raven hair, is the inviting face that gleams from Max Factor's advertisements. Scavullo, who photographed her for the cover of *Cosmopolitan*, says: 'She's such a perfect lady, she'd make the perfect wife for a millionaire. She deserves diamonds, furs, the lot. She's fabulous.' Her role in *J. W. Coop*, as Cliff Robertson's leading lady, created considerable interest and, now that she has given up her Max Factor contract, an interesting movie career lies ahead of her.

The third cosmetic-contract girl to go into retirement is Karen Graham, another great beauty, with all-American sophisticated looks, contracted by Estée Lauder to endorse their products. The strongest contender for Karen's contract is the beautiful newcomer, Lyn Brookes.

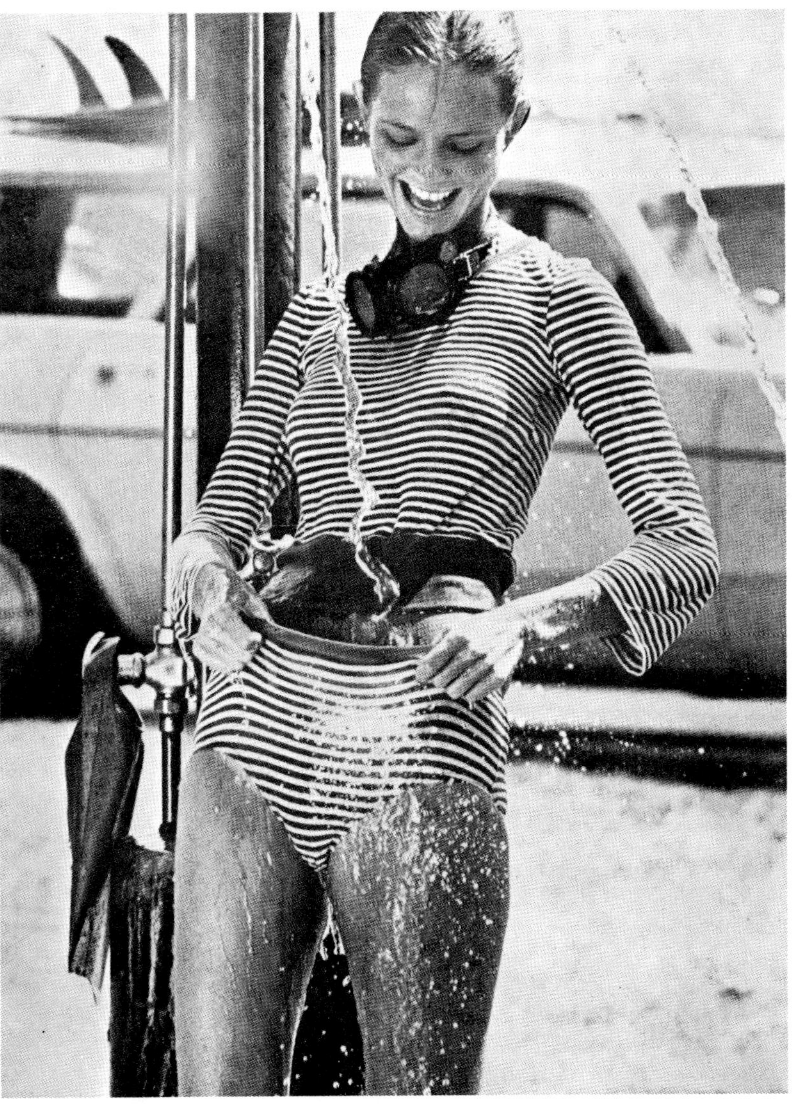

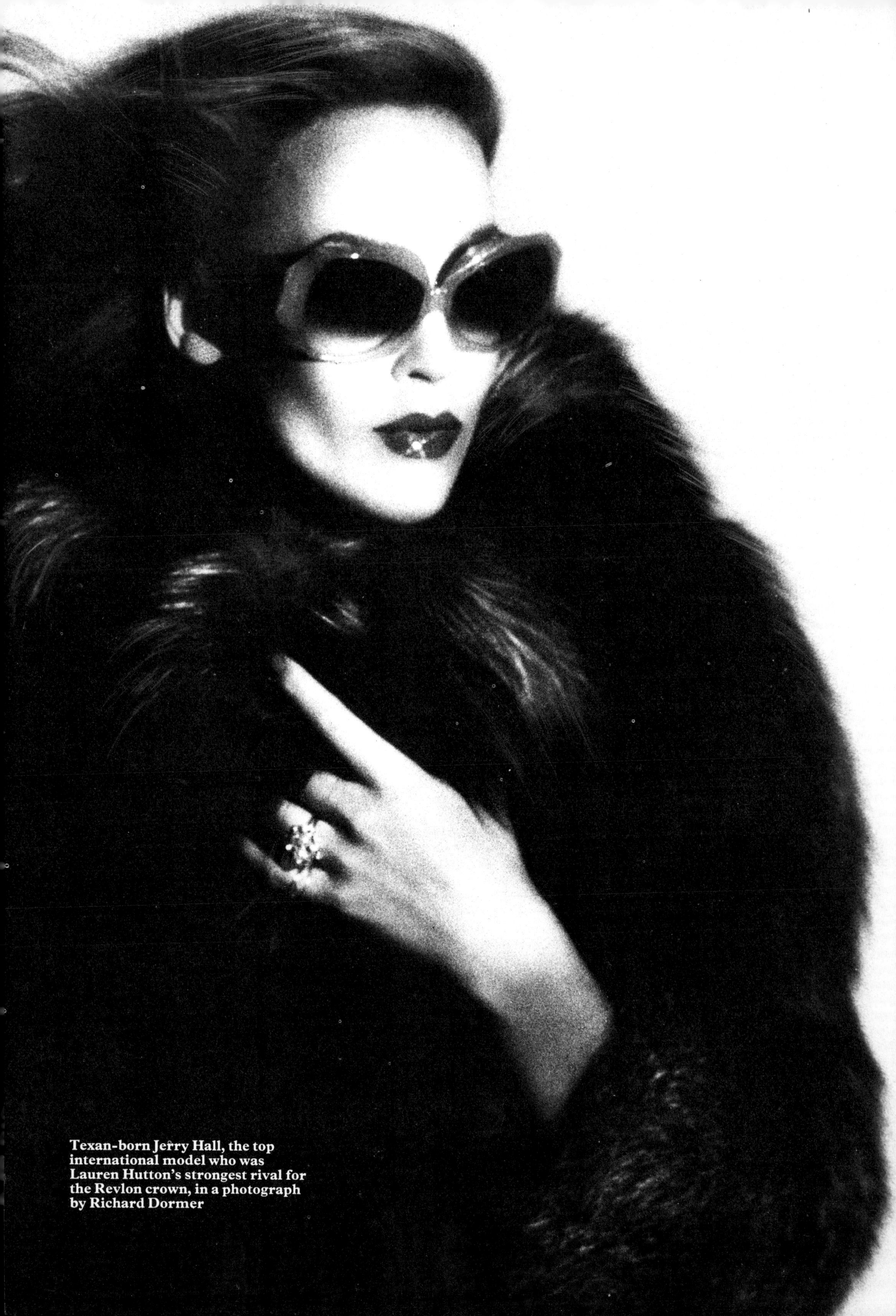

Texan-born Jerry Hall, the top
international model who was
Lauren Hutton's strongest rival for
the Revlon crown, in a photograph
by Richard Dormer

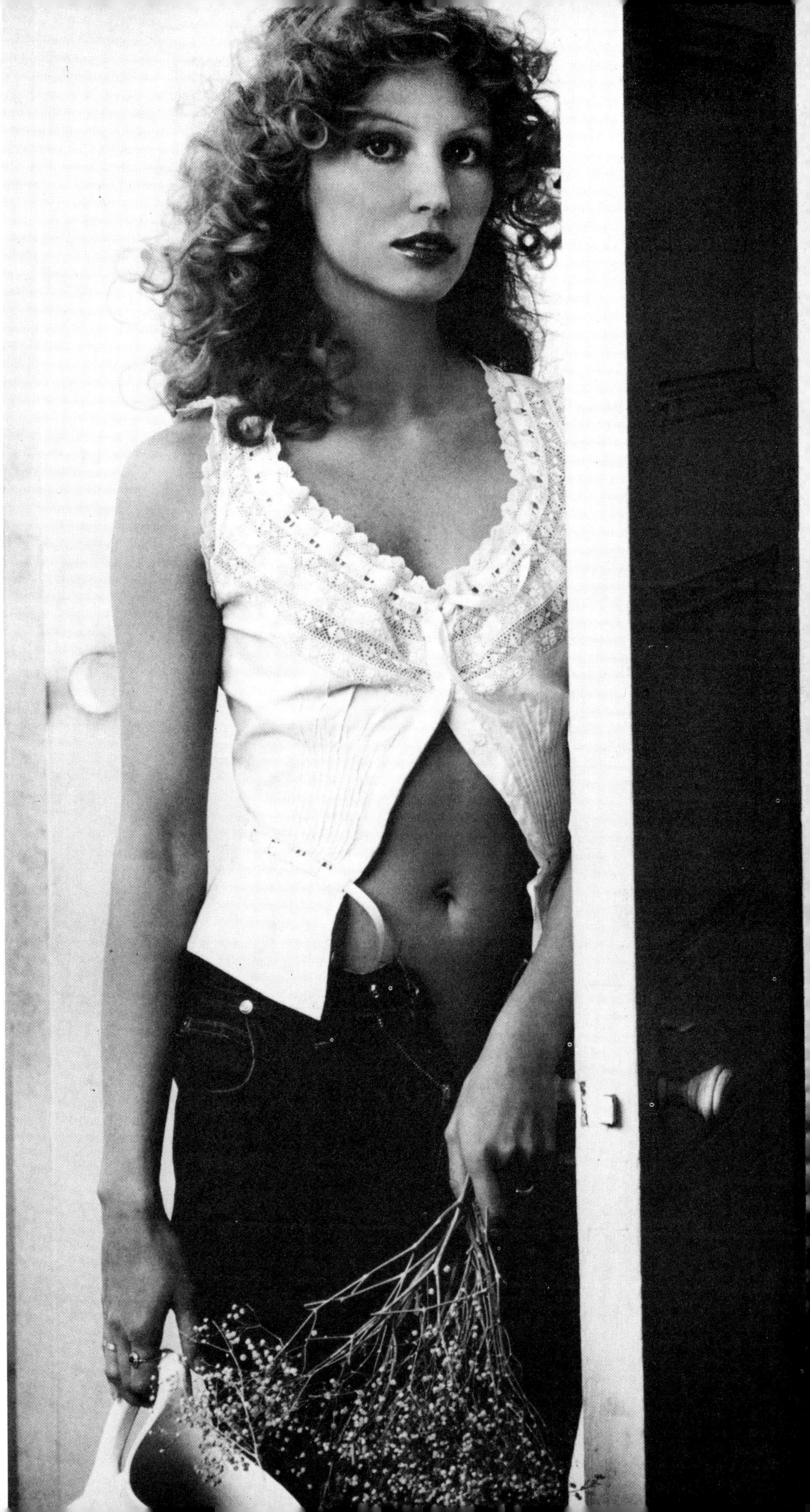

Evelyn Kuhn who was
the first model to be
put under contract to
any company. In her
first year as Revlon's
brand image their sales
rose by 37 per cent

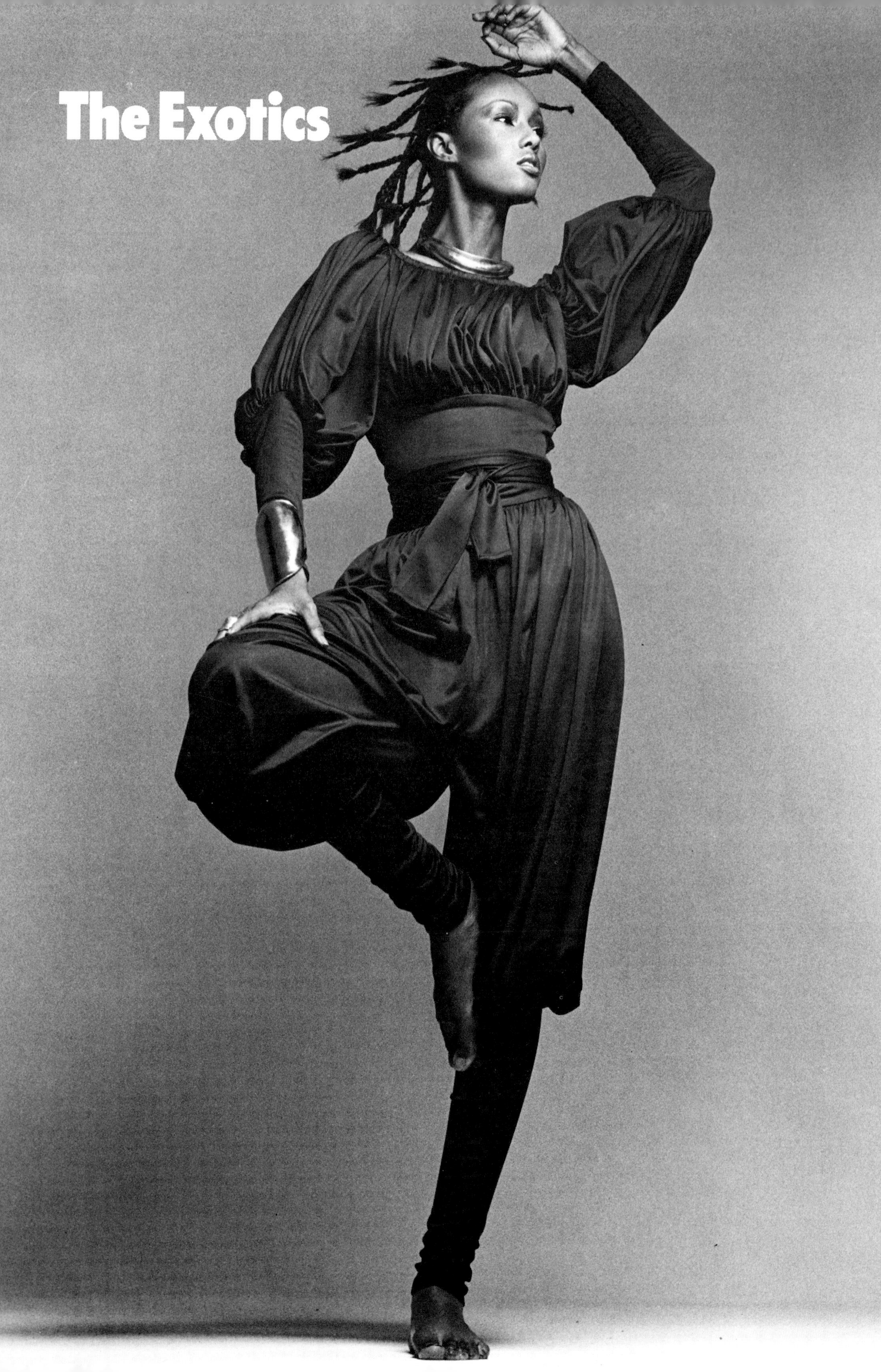
The Exotics

Exotic models specialising in fantasy and eccentric work are uncommercial, and rarely make the sort of money that the top girls in New York can earn. In this category there are a handful of girls, mainly black. Black models have style and energy and an incredible ability to move. They also seem to have an exceptional feeling for the clothes, and flair for creating moods and line. One of the few Caucasian models with the same ability is the slim 6ft 1in model Veruschka.

Born Baroness Vera von Lehndorff, Veruschka's parents were rich German aristocrats from East Prussia, who were driven out and their castle and possessions confiscated.

There had always been a taboo about top models posing for underwear, and when American *Vogue's* editor, Diana Vreeland, asked photographer Horst to arrange a photographic session for underwear, she told him, 'We don't want any underwear-girls. We want *real* girls.' And so he asked Veruschka, who agreed to do it on condition that they used her name in the advertisement. Girls who were photographed in underwear usually preferred to remain anonymous, but Veruschka's insistence on the use of her name formulated her career. 'I made her pose like the Africans with her foot on her knee and her bottom sticking out; very muscular', says Horst. 'And that was a big hit.'

American photographer Henry Clarke was impressed with what he saw and wanted to photograph her too. Thereafter Veruschka's reputation as a model was made, but although she continued to work throughout the world, few other photographers had access to her once she met and fell in love with an Italian, Franco Rubartelli. Veruschka became part of the international jet-set, favoured by the press, photographed careering about on the back of Rubartelli's motor-bike in the early hours. They worked together earning top money in every country, but she became over-exposed, and when their relationship dwindled after five years, other photographers refused to work with her. Her career as a top model came to a regrettable end. These days she works occasionally in Paris.

The fantastic, strong, professional Baroness could wear the most ghastly

Opposite: The exotic African Imen, top black model of the seventies, as she appears in one of Revlon's advertising campaigns. Photograph by Francesco Scavullo. Courtesy Revlon Inc, USA

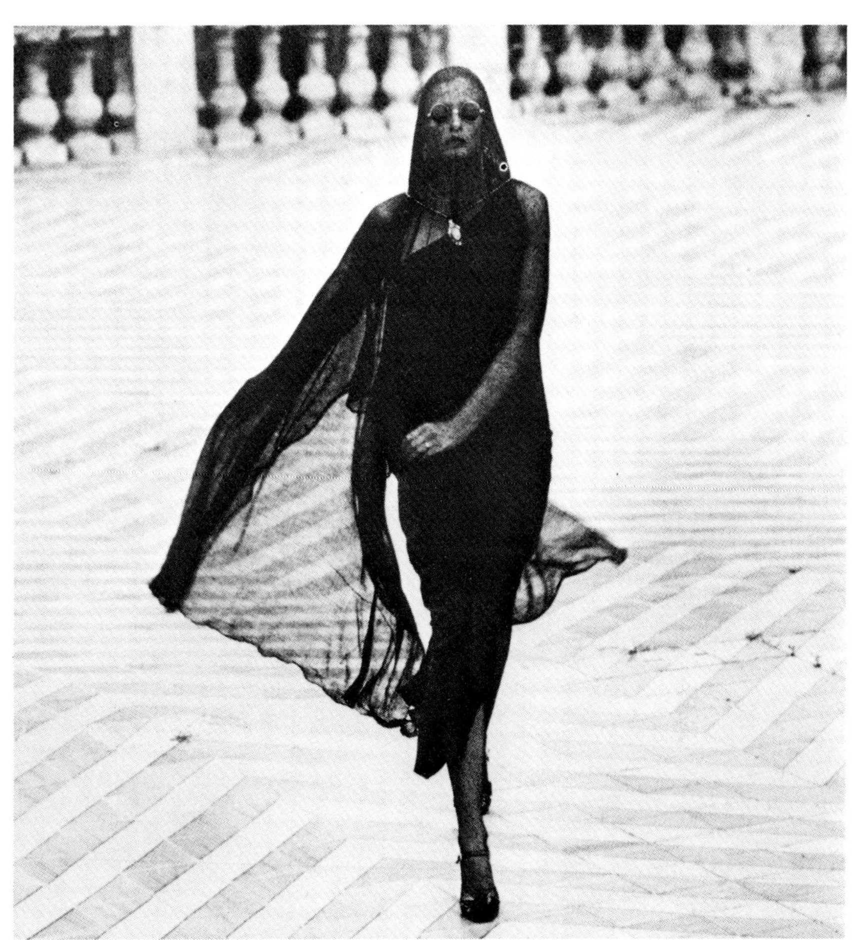

Apollonia von Ravenstein, photographed by Hans Feurer

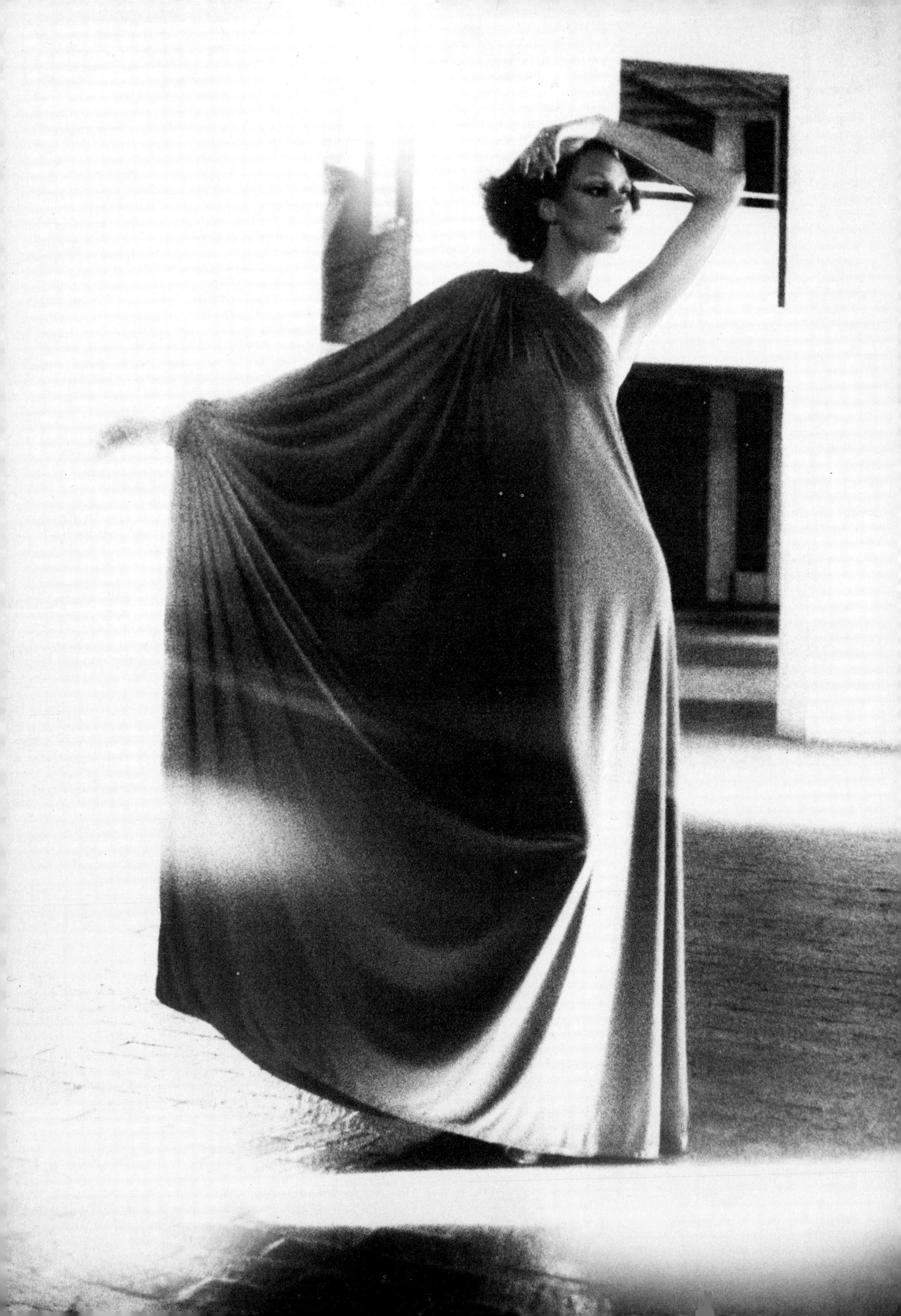

Opposite: Jan Stevenson who was
the first black model to appear in
English *Harpers Bazaar* editorial
pages. She was photographed here
by Richard Dormer for one of
London's leading fashion stores,
Harvey Nichols

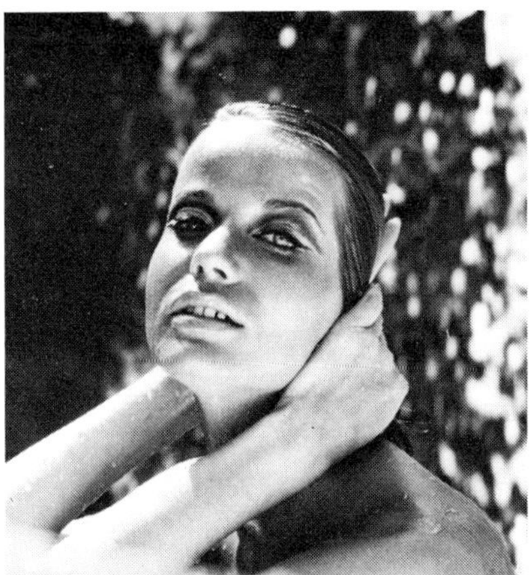

**Above: The fabulous Veruschka,
photographed by Henry Clarke**

'A clothes horse joins the stardom
race', trumpeted the Press
Association in 1970 when it released
this picture. 'Fashion model
Donyale Luna, 22, 6ft tall, and a
mixture of Negress, Irish, French
and Mexican ancestry, has turned
her talents to film making. Donyale
has made a dramatic impact as
Oenothea, the sorceress, in
Satyricon. She is not likely to be
overlooked, even in a film as
crowded with exotic images as
Federico Fellini's controversial
story of pagan Rome.'

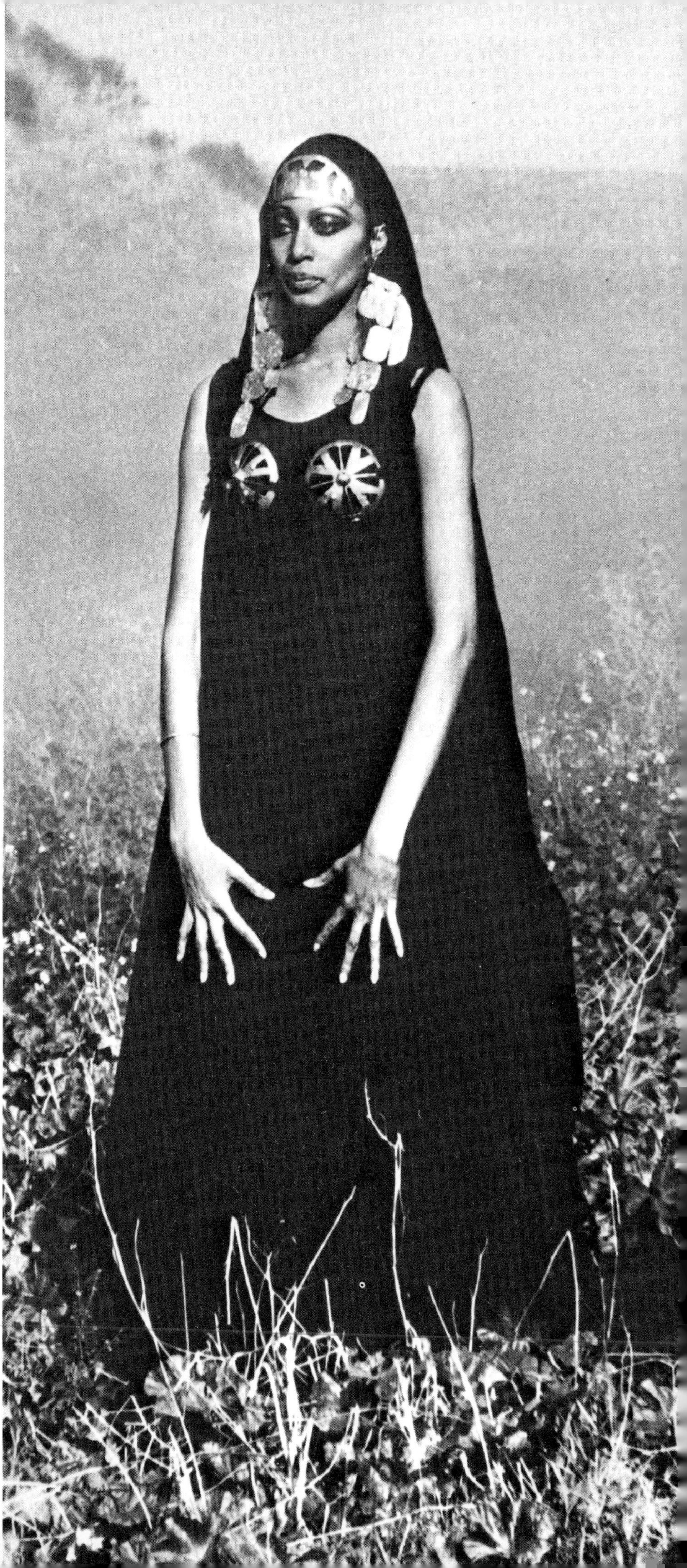

clothes and make them come alive with her innate sense of chic and ability to move. (It is said that her feet were so large that she had the middle bones of her toes removed to make her feet smaller!)

Donyale Luna, Pat Cleveland, Jan Stevenson, and Imen are black models with exceptional flair. Theirs is a specialised, fantasy brand of modelling, completely different from Beverly Johnson, who was the first black girl to appear on the cover of American *Vogue*. Beverly Johnson is not as ethnic looking as the others, and because of her refined features and lightish complexion she stands apart.

'Donyale Luna is mad as a hatter', laughs a close friend. Nobody ever knows where she lives, or where she goes to. She appears at parties looking exotic with a red dot in the centre of her forehead. She is extremely tall, well over 6ft, very beautiful, with black eyes. 'I'm from the moon, darling', is her stock reply, but it is thought that she stems from the Bronx. 'She's on another planet', comments a confidante. 'The last time I saw her she was crawling on the floor trying to get through an opening!' A mixture of negress, Irish, French, and Mexican ancestry, she made a dramatic impact in her first movie, as Oenothea, the sorceress in Federico Fellini's *Satyricon*, the controversial story of pagan Rome, which was crowded with exotic images. She was used as the model for many of the exotic looking shop-window mannequins in London's Oxford Street.

Pat Cleveland is another exotic black model with an incredibly long, slim body. A born extrovert, she has been seen taking off her clothes in Italian restaurants, displaying her pubic hair shaved in a heart-shape. Her outrageous, fun loving nature has made her comparatively popular in the model world, where she is admired for her incredible beauty and modelling skill, but she is not commercial enough to become known to the public, or to make a great deal of money.

In Britain, black models were taboo for a long time. They were used in fashion shows, but the glossies refused to have them until Richard Dormer photographed Jan Stevenson for Harvey Nichols, who were courageous enough to break new ground, and won a seventeen-page spread in *Harpers Bazaar* editorial pages. American Jan Stevenson has a tremendous feeling for clothes, and, to prove her essential worth as a model, one tends to look at the clothes she wears rather than at *her*.

Left: Beverly Johnson who broke new ground by being the first black model to appear on a *Vogue* cover. Photograph by Francesco Scavullo. Courtesy *Vogue* USA

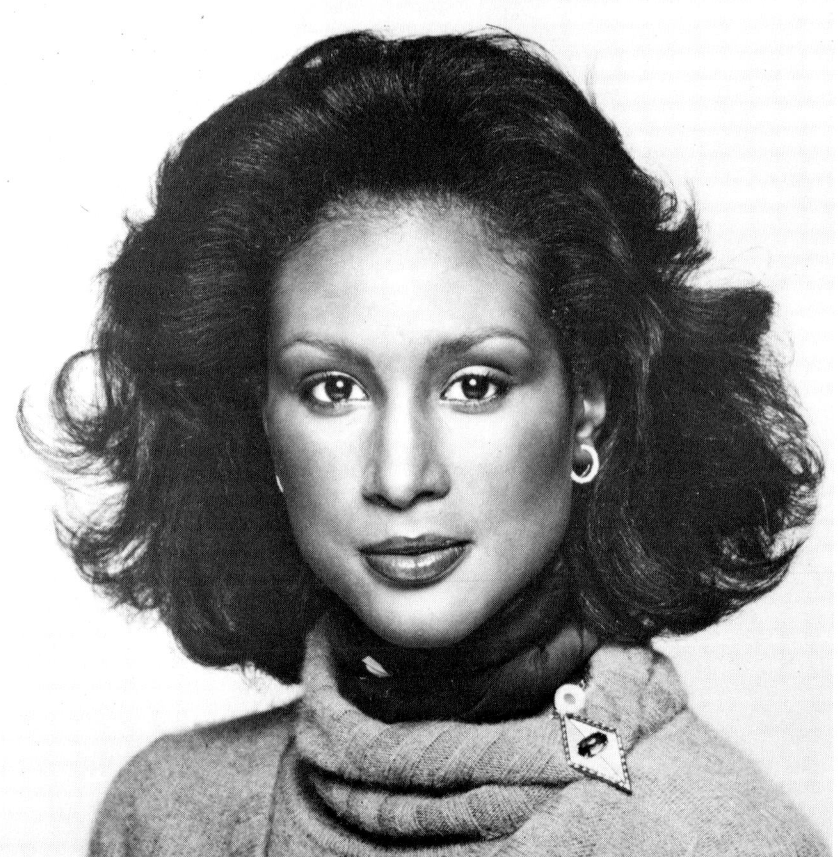

Opposite: Veruschka, photographed in an oriental setting by Henry Clarke

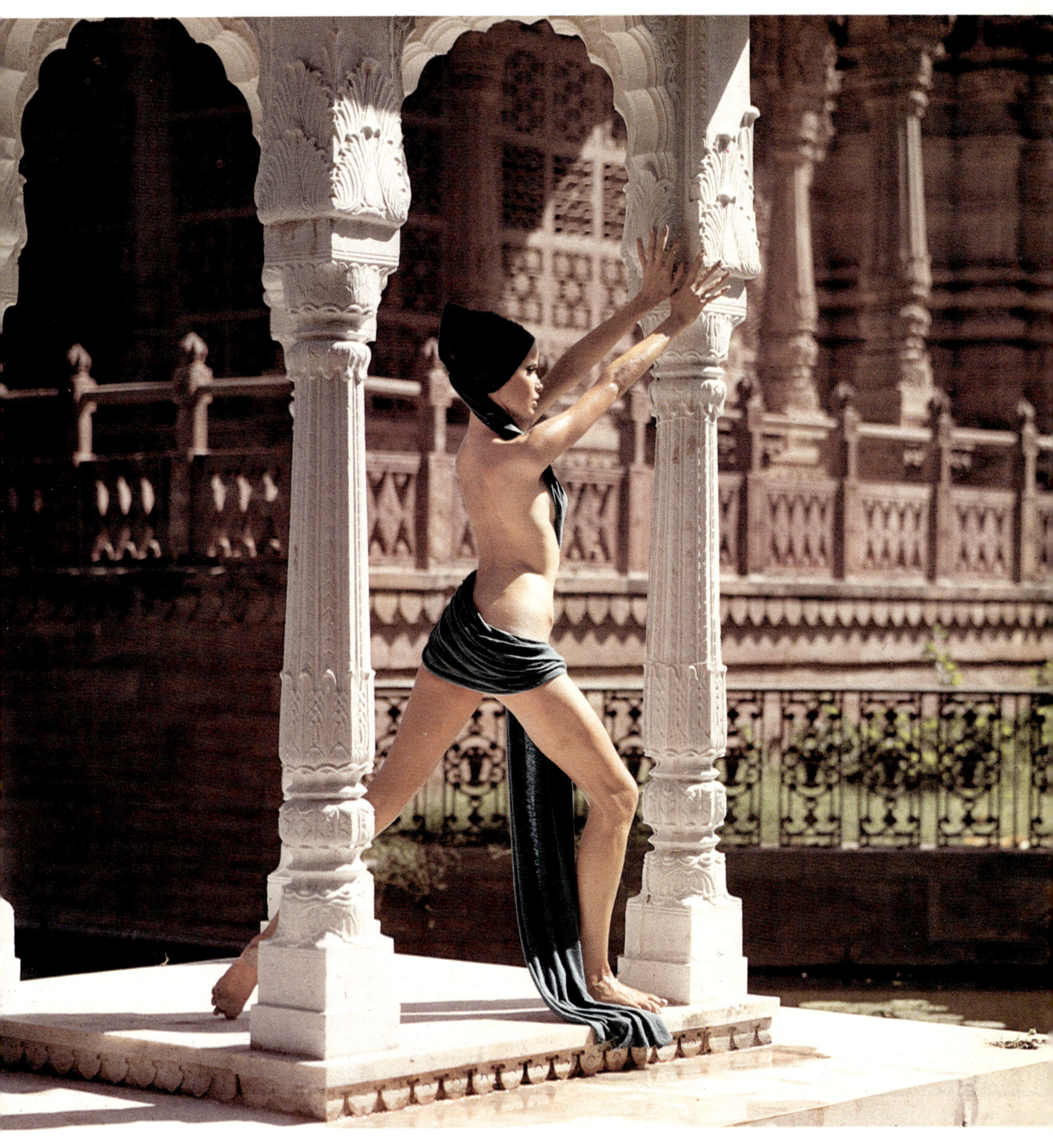

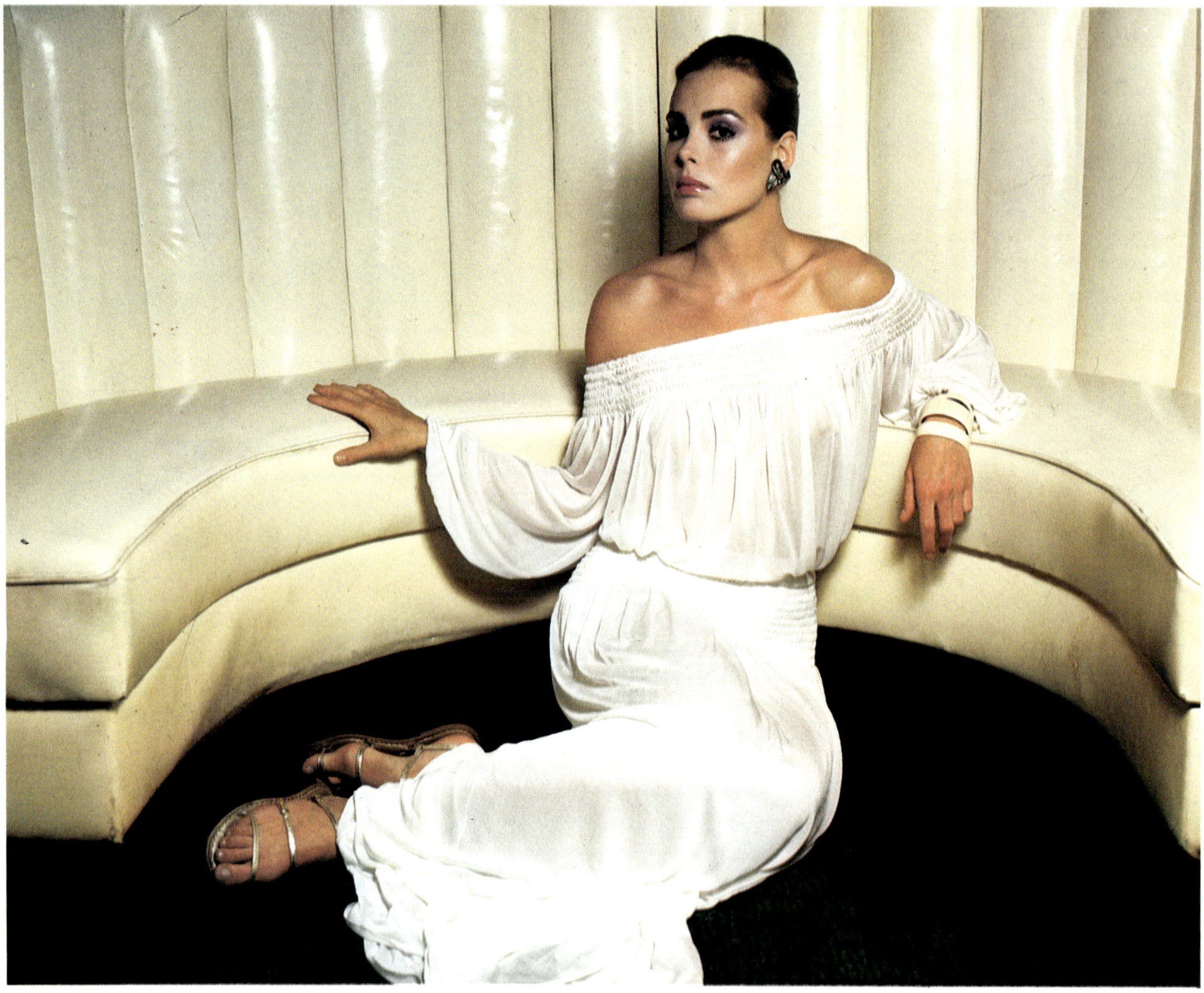

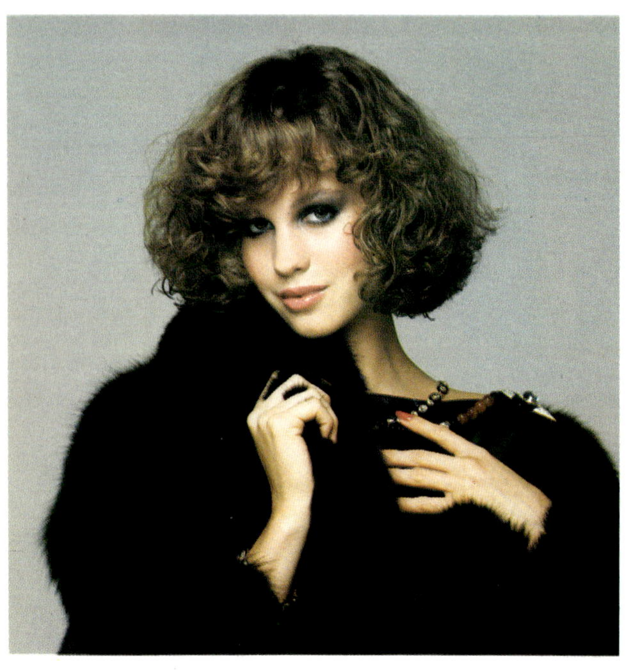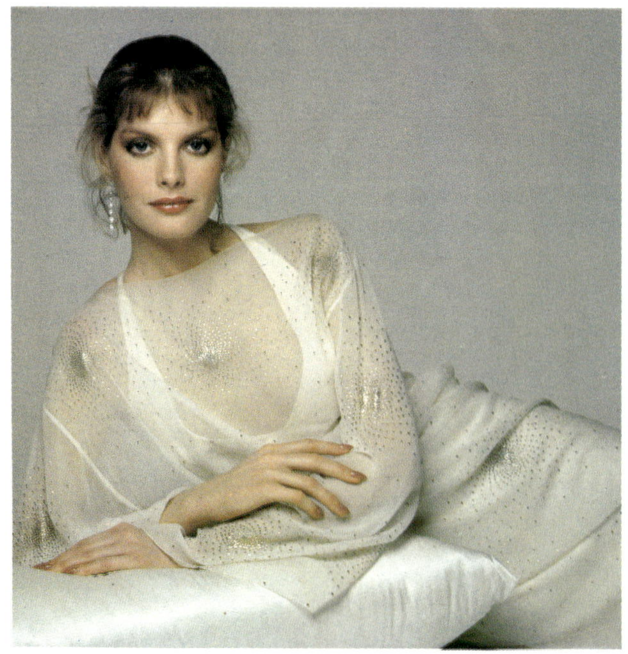

Model to Movie Star

Just as cover girls are the star models of today, many movie stars were once top-line models who graced the covers of glossy magazines. Their beauty is instantly recognisable from their commercial exposure, yet some are never quite identifiable. 'I know the face', we say, but seldom know—or remember—the name. Movie audiences are now able to put labels on faces that stare out at them from news-stands on street-corners, railway stations, airports, and bookshops throughout the world. Modelling has long been a stepping stone to the screen for aspiring young beauties—not least of them Lauren Bacall, who was one of the first models to make the big time. With Lisbeth Scott, whilst appearing in an off-Broadway show, she used modelling as a vehicle for the journey to Hollywood.

Francesco Scavullo was assistant on a job when Lauren Bacall came into the studio to be photographed in the fifties: 'Her voice was so low, that next to her, I sounded like a girl!' She didn't have a good body for modelling in those days, but she was extremely beautiful, and still is. She was doing an editorial for *Harpers Bazaar* and then veteran photographer Louise Dahl Wolf did a cover of her. Soon after becoming a top New York model, she went to Hollywood to make *To Have and Have Not* with Humphrey Bogart—whom she married, and the rest is Hollywood history.

Lucille Ball was a Seventh Avenue showroom girl before she left for Hollywood to join the Samuel Goldwyn chorus line as one of the famous Goldwyn Girls. While Suzy Parker, who began her own dazzling modelling career as a New York model under the tutelage of her top model sister, Dorian Leigh, became Revlon's pet image-maker before embarking on her own road to film stardom.

It is well known that Grace Kelly appeared in commercials, not so much as a model but as a demonstrator of refrigerators, motor cars and the like, before the lure of Hollywood rocketed her into international stardom, culminating in her marriage to Prince Rainier of Monaco.

Long before she became famous and married Rex Harrison, Kay Kendall modelled for *Harpers Bazaar* in London. She had a beautiful, amusing face, but at that time her body was rather large, and so when she was photographed, the dresses were open at the back tied together with bits of string. She was tremendous fun and used to make the most original remarks, such as: 'You know, in life it's never difficult to be laid; the difficult thing is not to be laid.' She had such small nostrils that she slept with tiny balls of cotton-wool stuffed into them, in the belief that the cotton-wool would stretch them.

She toured the halls with her parents, who were on the stage, and struggled to make it in films. 'I wasn't exactly born in a trunk', she confessed, 'but I damn well nearly was.' She didn't succeed with a theatrical career to begin with, and, in order to save herself from both boredom and starvation, took up modelling when she was in her early twenties. It was a tremendous game to her, and it came extremely easily to her, because she was so natural and sweet.

Photographer Richard Dormer recalls taking her to be photographed in Madeira for *Harpers Bazaar*. She was the girlfriend of a rich gentleman whom she referred to as 'Mr Sausage'; never by name. She was terrified of flying and on the way to the airport she plied herself with huge quantities of Mr Sausage's brandy to pluck up courage for the flight. Once on the aircraft, she could not remember the word 'steward', and whenever she wanted another drink, she would call out, 'Waiter, dear! Waiter, dear!' And he would dutifully pour more brandy down her throat.

On their arrival at the majestic Reid's Hotel in Madeira, Kay settled in for hard work, but after four days found the formal atmosphere of the hotel oppressive and suggested to Dormer that they go down to the local town. When they got down to Funchal, she

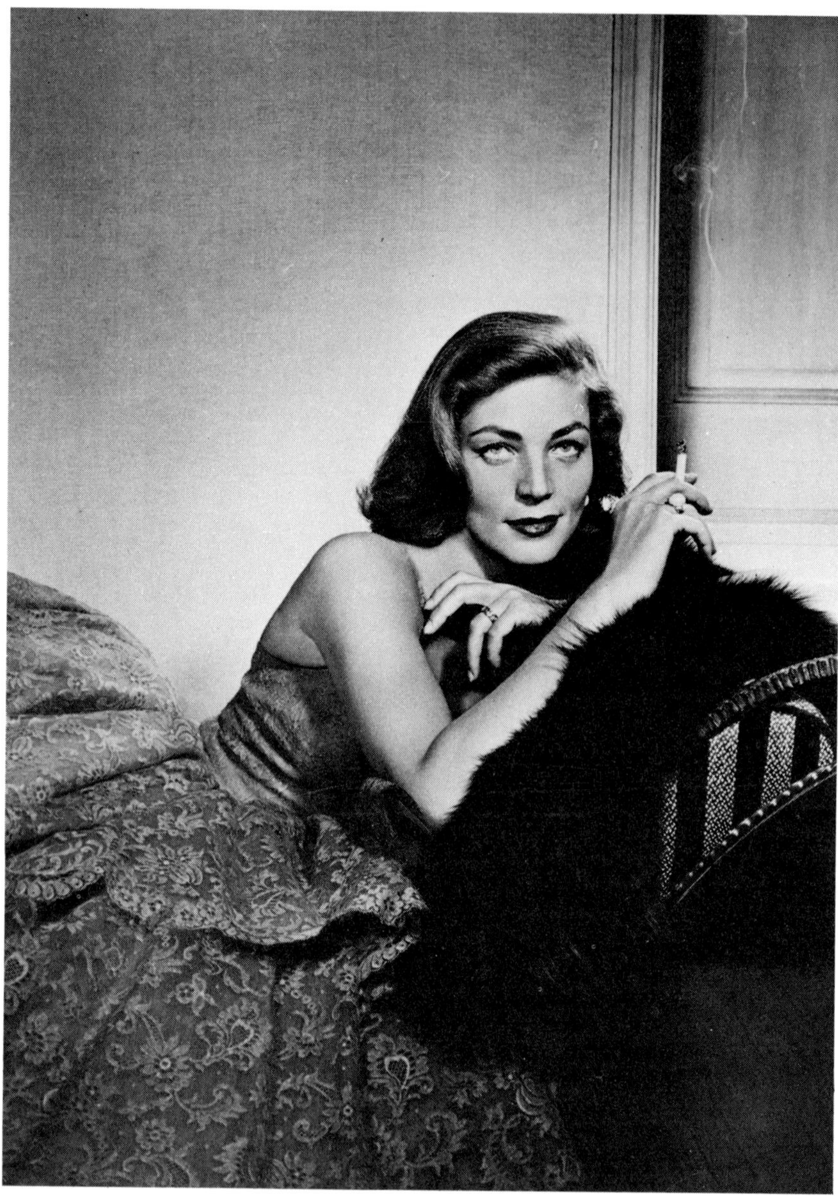

Right: Lauren Bacall, who was a New York model for *Harpers Bazaar* before her first movie role with Humphrey Bogart. This study of Miss Bacall is by Karsh of Ottawa

immediately asked, 'I wonder where the local brothel is ?' They found out, and she marched in, keen to meet the Madame and the 'girls of the house'. She showed the 'girls' some of the clothes and shoes she had come along to model in Madeira, and said to them: 'Now, you've all to come to Reid's Hotel for tea with us, tomorrow.'

Nobody in the hotel knew who they were, except the waiters who were their most ardent visitors, and when they saw the trollops marching in, their eyes almost popped out of their heads. And then Kay shocked everyone by asking for Worcester sauce. 'You've never tasted avocado pear until you've had Worcester sauce in it', she said, and then called out, 'Waiter, darling! Worcester sauce, please!'

Audrey Hepburn, who had suffered from malnutrition during the German occupation of her home town, Amsterdam, in World War II, was slim and waif-like as a consequence. She and her mother, the Baroness van Heemstra, moved to London where Audrey worked in a nightclub. Dressed in a tutu, she displayed the cards announcing the various nightclub acts. She managed to secure parts as a movie extra and became a chorus dancer at the London Palladium. She modelled clothes in her spare time to boost her income. When on holiday with her mother in Monte Carlo one year, Colette, the famous French novelist, discovered her sitting in the lobby of the Palace Hotel. Colette knew at once that she had found the perfect *Gigi* for the movie version of her famous novel, and Audrey Hepburn's remarkable film career had begun.

Jean Simmons was another aspiring young actress who modelled in order to eke out a living. Although she was a young Rank starlet, she had no money at all when she was seventeen, and modelled sweaters for 'young' magazines and for knitting patterns.

Two of Britain's great models of the sixties failed in their quest for stardom. Jean Shrimpton, with her long brown hair, big eyes, and luscious mouth changed the model-girl look of the sixties with her sexy, youthful image. Her only movie, *Privilege*, with pop star Paul Jones, was only a mild success, and her movie-star potential petered out.

Twiggy, too, although adept as singer and dancer in Ken Russell's *The Boy Friend*, failed to make the grade, and except for a couple of 'B' pictures, her movie career was short-lived. Her

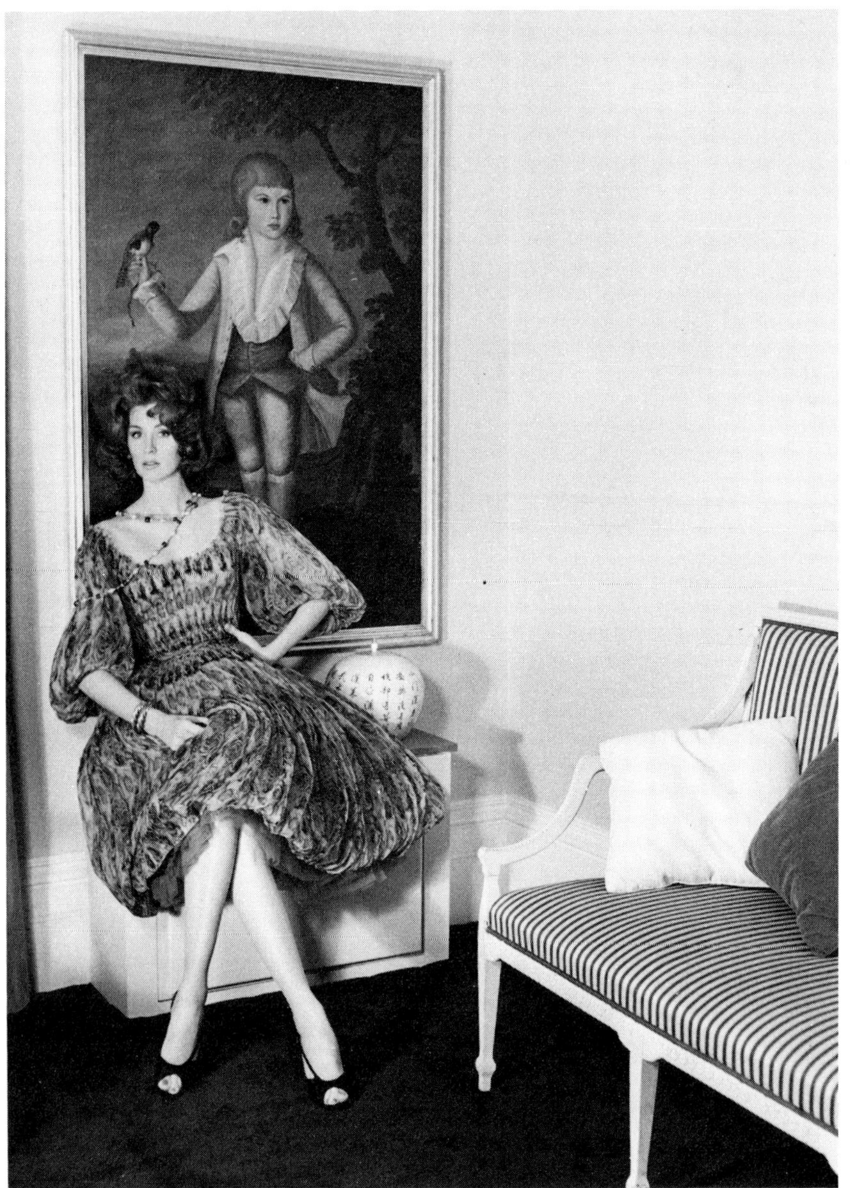

Left: Suzy Parker, probably the most famous model to have become a film star. Photographed by Henry Clarke

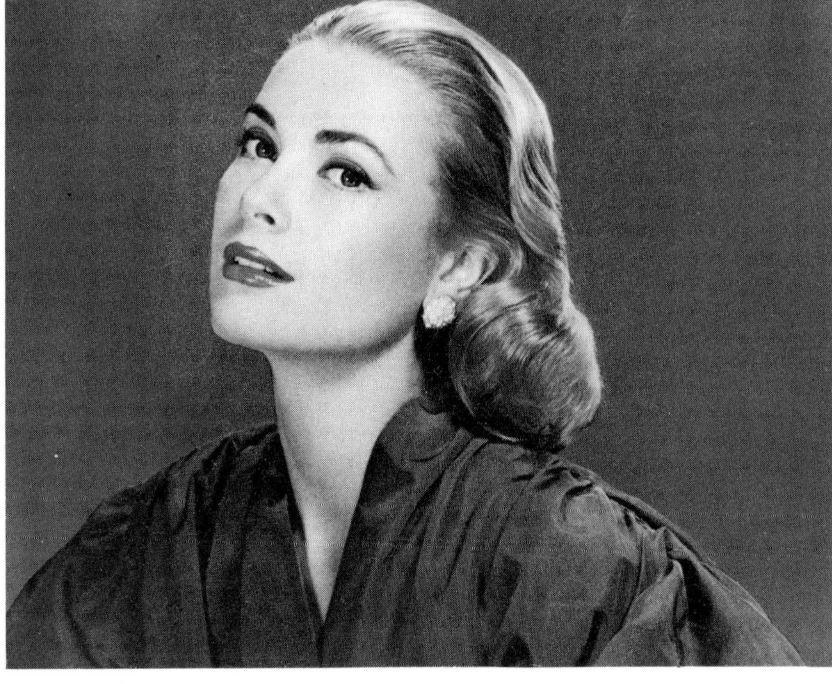

Left: Grace Kelly who appeared in commercials before moving to Hollywood

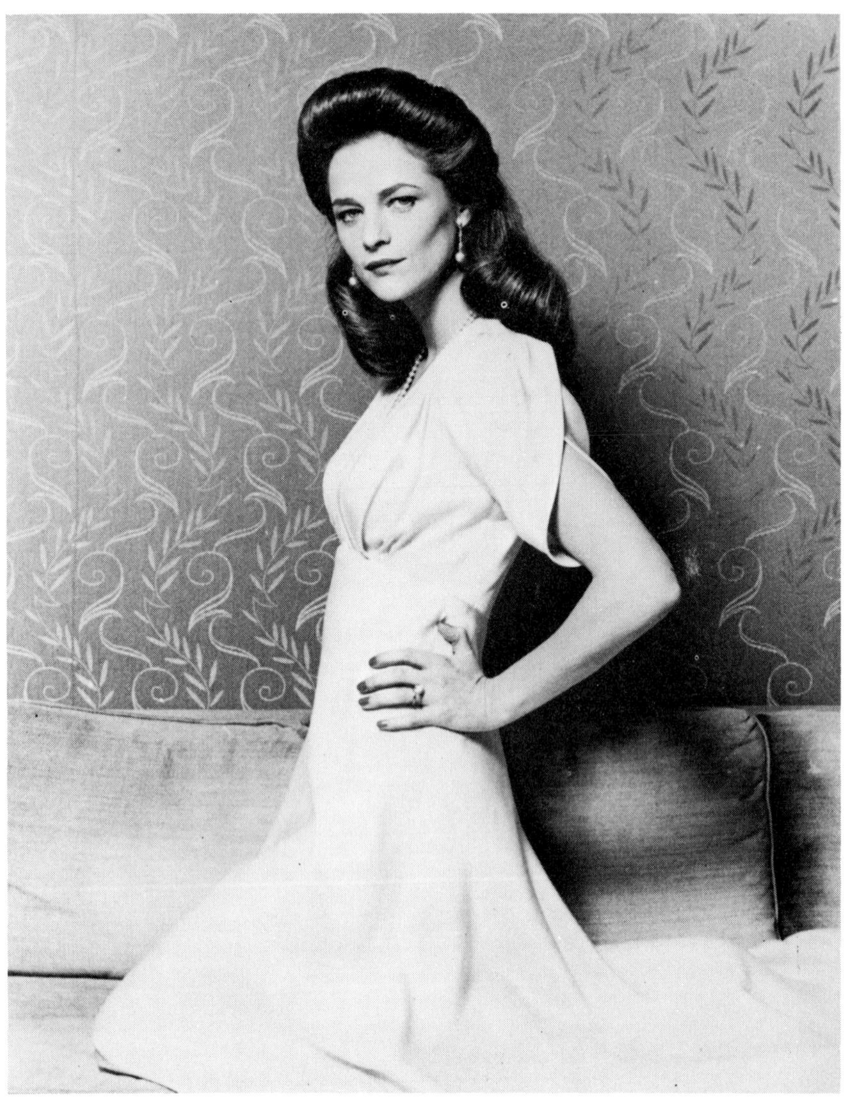

Left: Charlotte Rampling, who gave up modelling for a movie career, seen here as she appeared as Robert Mitchum's leading lady in the classic remake of Raymond Chandler's *Farewell My Lovely*. Courtesy Fox/Rank Distributors

appearances in her own musical shows for BBC television have, however, scored, and her new career as pop singer is well on the way, with two albums to her credit.

Tania Mallet, another British top model of the sixties, made her film debut with Sean Connery in *Goldfinger*; but when she was killed off by the baddies in the second reel, it seemed to kill off her chances for more movies, too.

One English model who did make the big time was Jacqueline Bisset. 'We used to use her for corsetry adverts because she had wonderful bosoms', comments a top photographer, 'but she had a terrifically sexy face; marvellous big lips—much more suitable for films than for fashion.' For fashion, models require an asexual quality and they need to be slender; but for films they're often too thin and tall for leading men of the small stature of today's Paul Newman's, Robert Redfords, and Dustin Hoffmans.

Ann Turkel, a top model in London, retired from modelling for a movie career—and marriage to rumbustious film star Richard Harris, whose former wife, Elizabeth, later married—and divorced—Rex Harrison. While another English movie actress who began her career as a model is Suzy Kendall, one-time wife of Dudley Moore who is now married to Tuesday Weld and living in Beverly Hills.

Italian-born Marla Scarafia, who worked in London as a model in the fifties and sixties, appeared in many movies and frequently on television as Marla Landi.

One fashion model with film-star potential was introduced in Scott Fitzgerald's *The Last Tycoon*, with Tony Curtis and Robert Mitchum. Ingrid Boulting, the possessor of a haunting, mystical beauty, plays Kathleen, the enigmatic girl with whom studio mogul Monroe Stahr (Robert

De Niro) becomes obsessed. Her performance has an almost misty quality about it.

Ingrid Boulting was born in South Africa, the daughter of a Dutch solicitor called Munik, her parents separated when she was a child. Her mother, former fashion model Enid Munik, married film producer Roy Boulting who adopted Ingrid. Boulting left her mother for actress Hayley Mills, who in turn left Mr Boulting for actor Leigh Lawson. Ingrid's mother left London for Paris where she became a fashion editor on *Elle* magazine, and later married—and left—Lord Hardwicke.

After training to be a ballet dancer at the Royal Ballet for nine years, Ingrid was discovered by fashion photographer Richard Avedon in New York. He photographed her. *Vogue*, and many covers followed. After ten years of modelling, she attended the Lee Strasberg Drama School, and later read that the film, *The Last Tycoon* was being planned. She promptly informed the film's producer, Sam Spiegel, that he could make a star of her, pretending to have met him socially. She was given a screen test, got the part—and now awaits stardom.

Of the French movie stars, Capucine began as a model. She was a very pretty French girl with a strong face, rather like Joan Crawford. She had an exquisite nose and profile and wonderful liquid eyes. 'She had one of the most beautiful heads I've ever seen in my life', says one of the photographers with whom she worked, 'but the body was not so hot. Her breasts were too large for modelling and so we used her for hats and beauty shots.' She thinned down considerably when she got to Hollywood—and fell in love with William Holden.

Anouk Aimée was another French movie star who began her career as a model. She was once married to English actor Albert Finney.

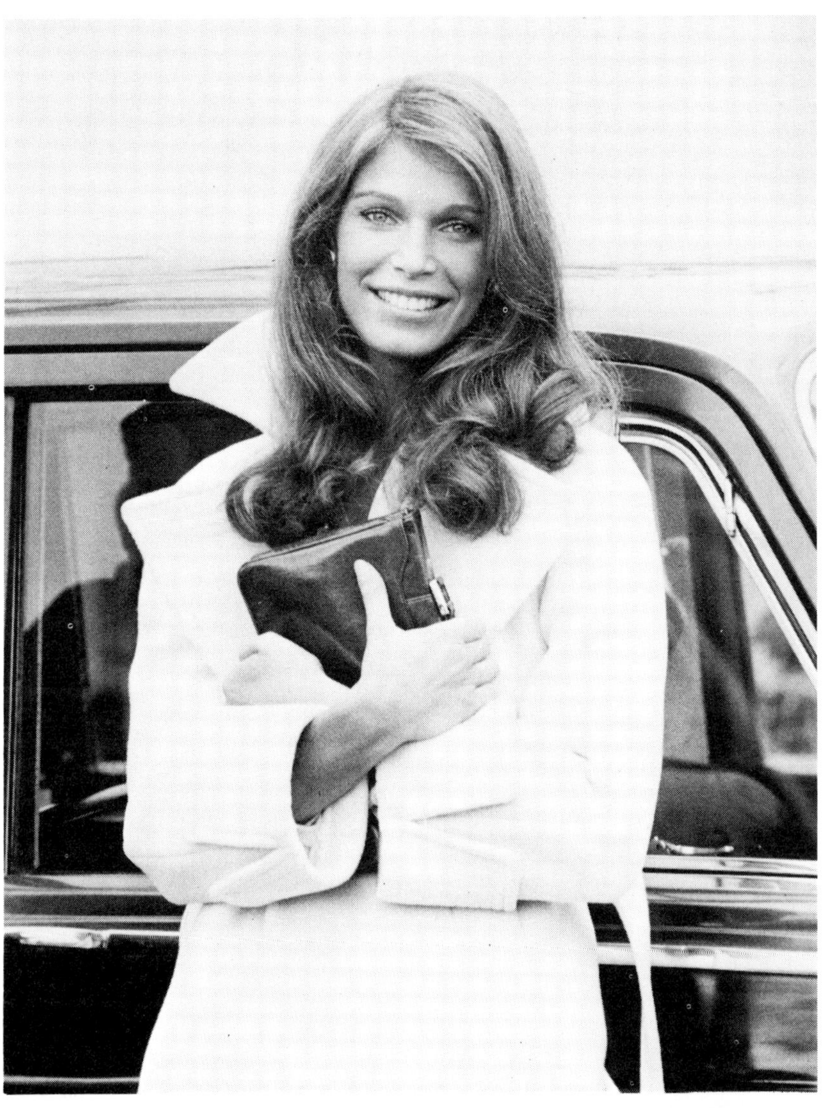

Left: Former model Ann Turkel as she appeared with her husband, Richard Harris, in John Frankenheimer's *Call Harry Crown*. Courtesy Fox/Rank Distributors

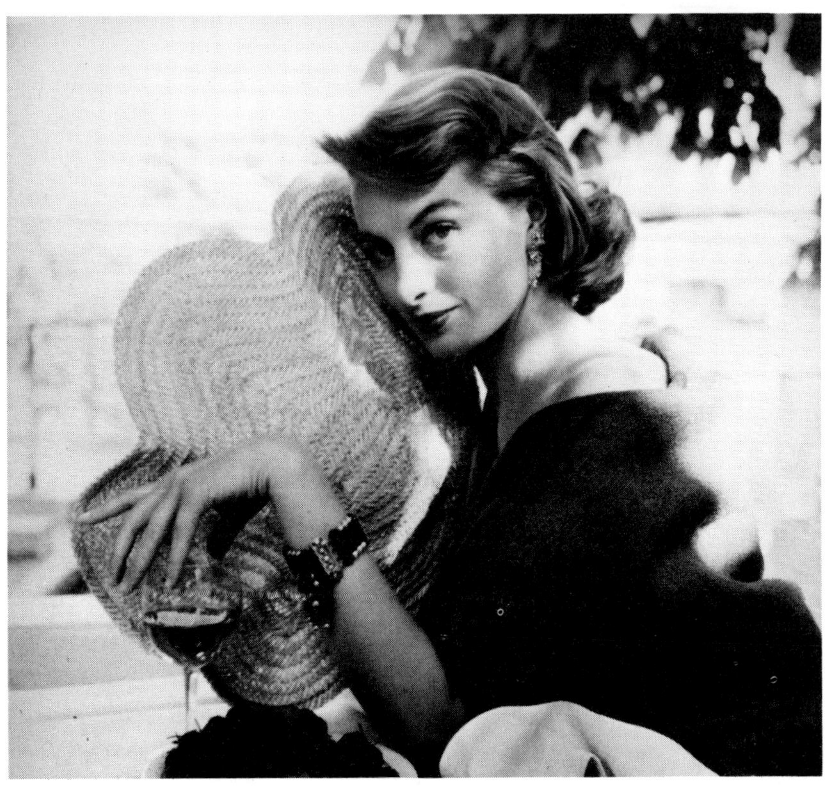

Below left: The former French model Capucine, photographed by Henry Clarke

French movie star Aurore Clement, star of *Lacombe Lucien*, modelled in the early days too, as did Sylvia Kristel, who bared more than her breasts in the French-made *Emmanuelle* and *Emmanuelle II;* she had been a Dutch cover girl before giving in to the lure of the flesh.

Of the Italians who modelled, Gina Lollobrigida, Silvana Mangano, Elsa Martinelli, and Sophia Loren are perhaps the most famous.

Sophia Loren is regarded as one of the most professional of stars, and this was true of her modelling career as well. She modelled furs for French *Vogue* on one occasion, and Henry Clarke, who conducted the photographic session, recalls her arrival at the studio at eight in the morning, fully made-up and ready for work. She wouldn't stop for lunch because she wanted to complete the day's work without interruption, and in the boiling August weather, when

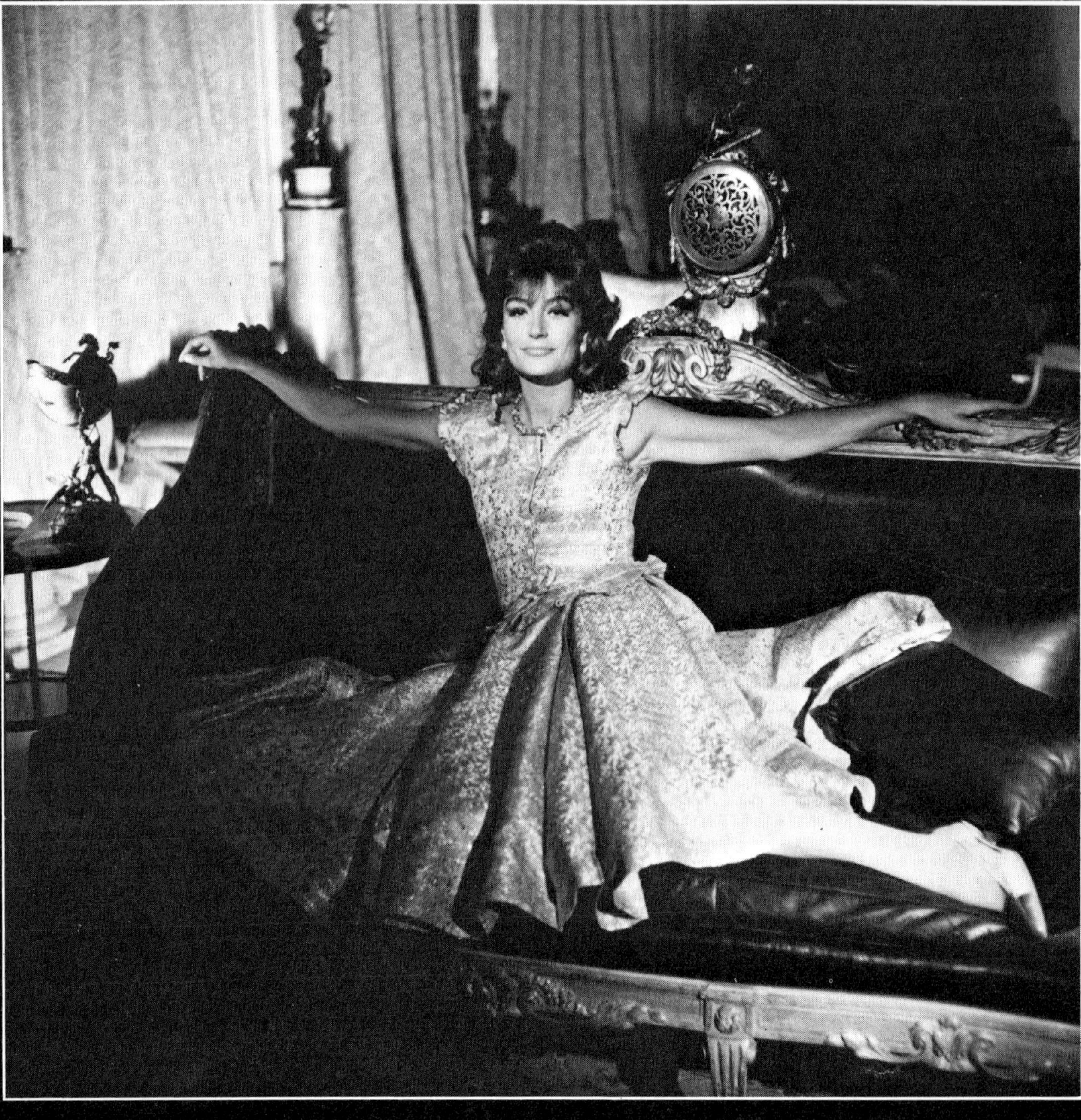

The beautiful French movie star
Anouk Aimée who was formerly
married to English actor Albert
Finney. Photographed in a Chanel
dress by Henry Clarke—*Vogue*
France

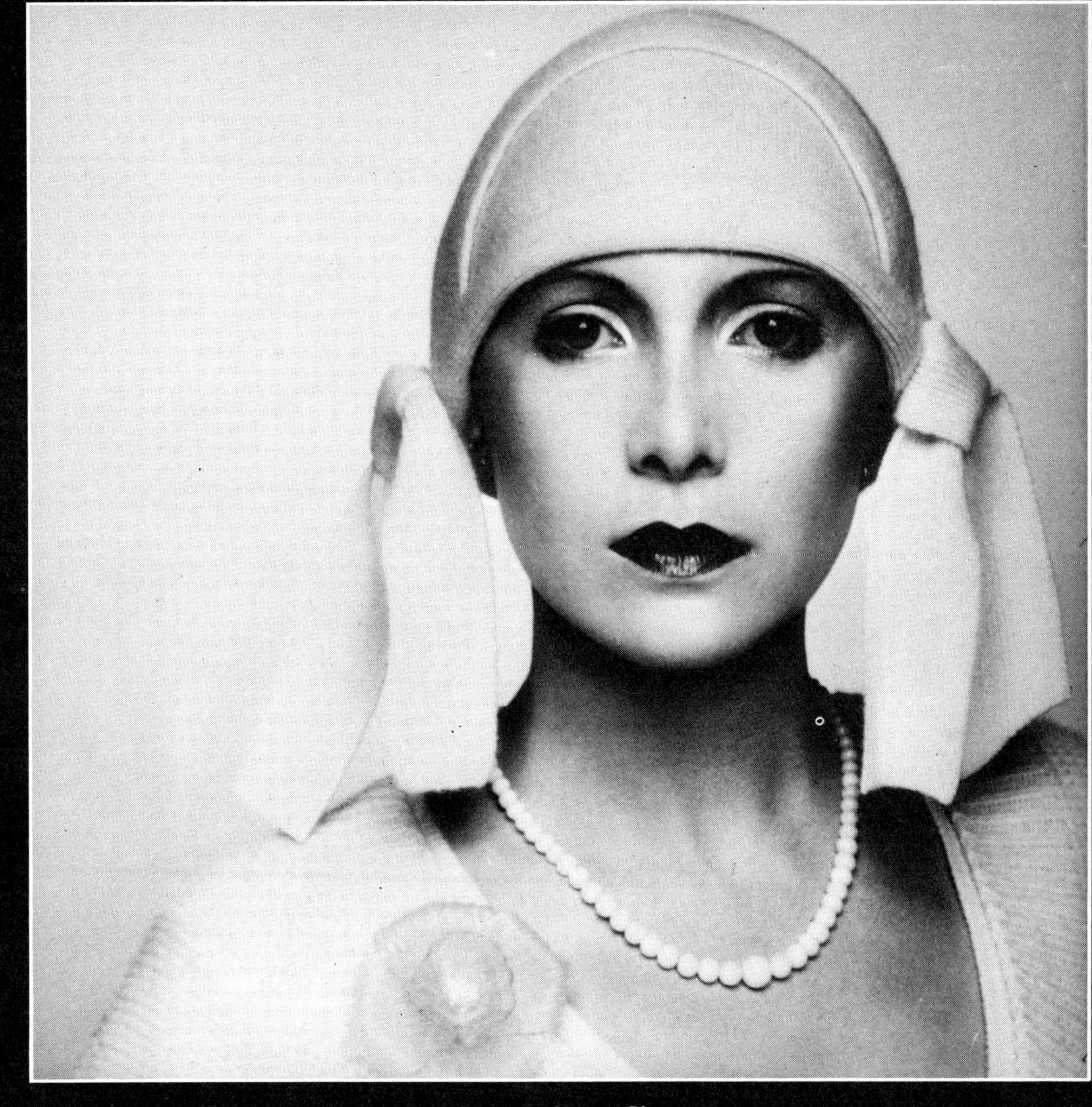

French actress Aurore Clement,
star of *Lacombe Lucien* in which
she looked entirely different
from this glamorous study by
Barry Lategan. By kind permission
of Condé Nast Publications

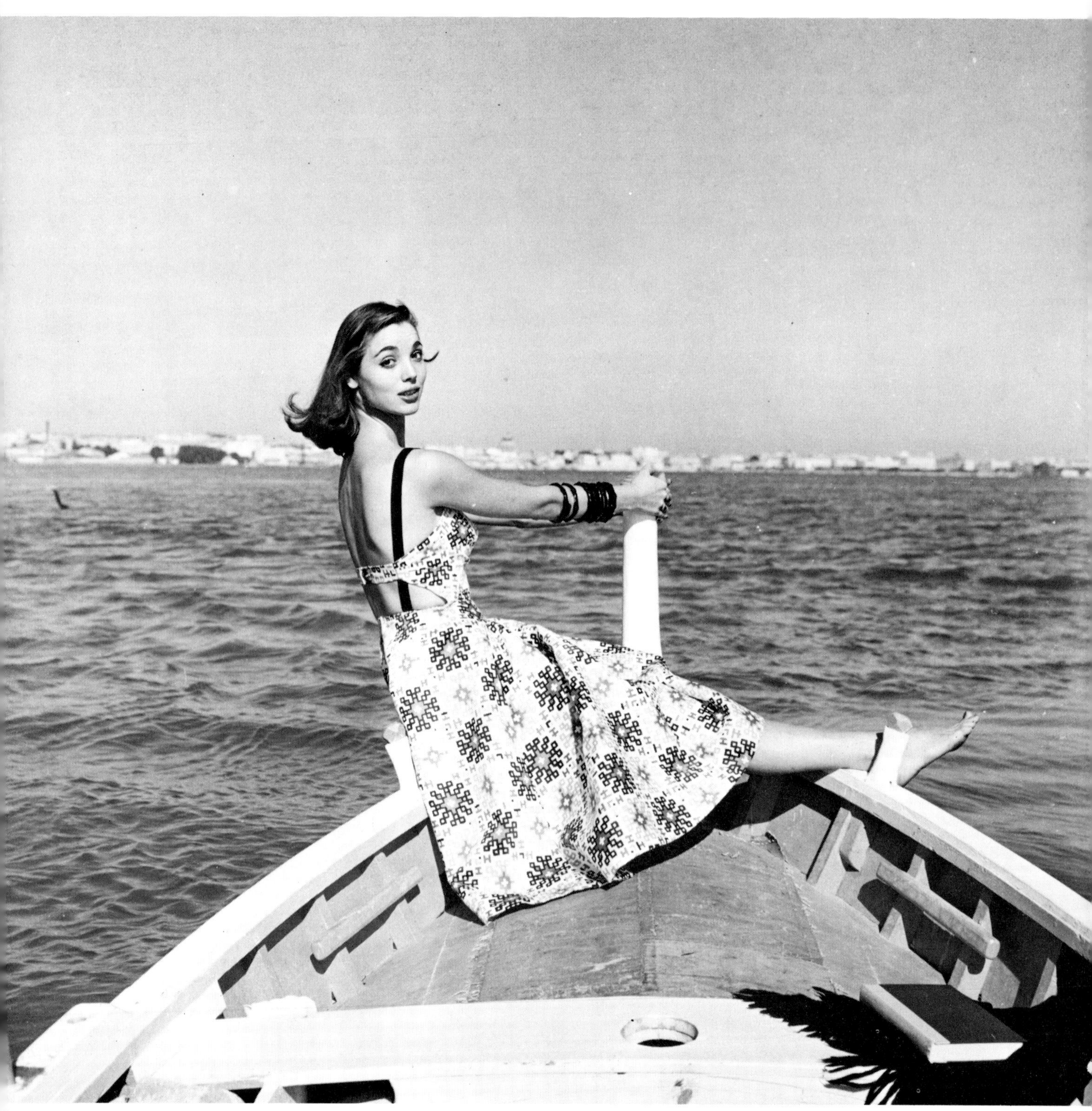

Clarke was using blazing spotlights instead of strobe lighting, she posed in the sweltering furs with sweat pouring from her brow, with never a complaint or comment about the heat. She remained perfectly calm and composed as the make-up assistant periodically mopped the sweat from her brow.

Another model turned film star who stemmed from Europe was Marisa Berenson. The grand-daughter of the great haute couturier Schiaparelli, she worked in London when she was very young, where David Bailey was the first to photograph her for fashion magazines. She travelled to Iran, Italy, and Sardinia for *Vogue*, but although sweet and considerate when young, she became spoiled with too much praise, and success turned her head. She lost her softness to an extent when she became more concerned about herself than for the people with whom she worked who helped mould her career, and a certain hardness in her looks replaced her gentle femininity. Her beauty, however, is undeniable, and although she played a rather 'plain Jane' in the successful movie *Cabaret*, the photography in the tediously long *Barry Lyndon* captured and took advantage of her beauty superbly.

English-born Jane Birkin started her

Opposite: Elsa Martinelli in her first pose as a model in Syracuse, Sicily, photographed by Henry Clarke for American *Vogue*

Below: Greta Garbo who, as sales-girl Greta Louisa Gustaffson, modelled hats in 1922 for a store in Stockholm, before being discovered by director Mauritz Stiller

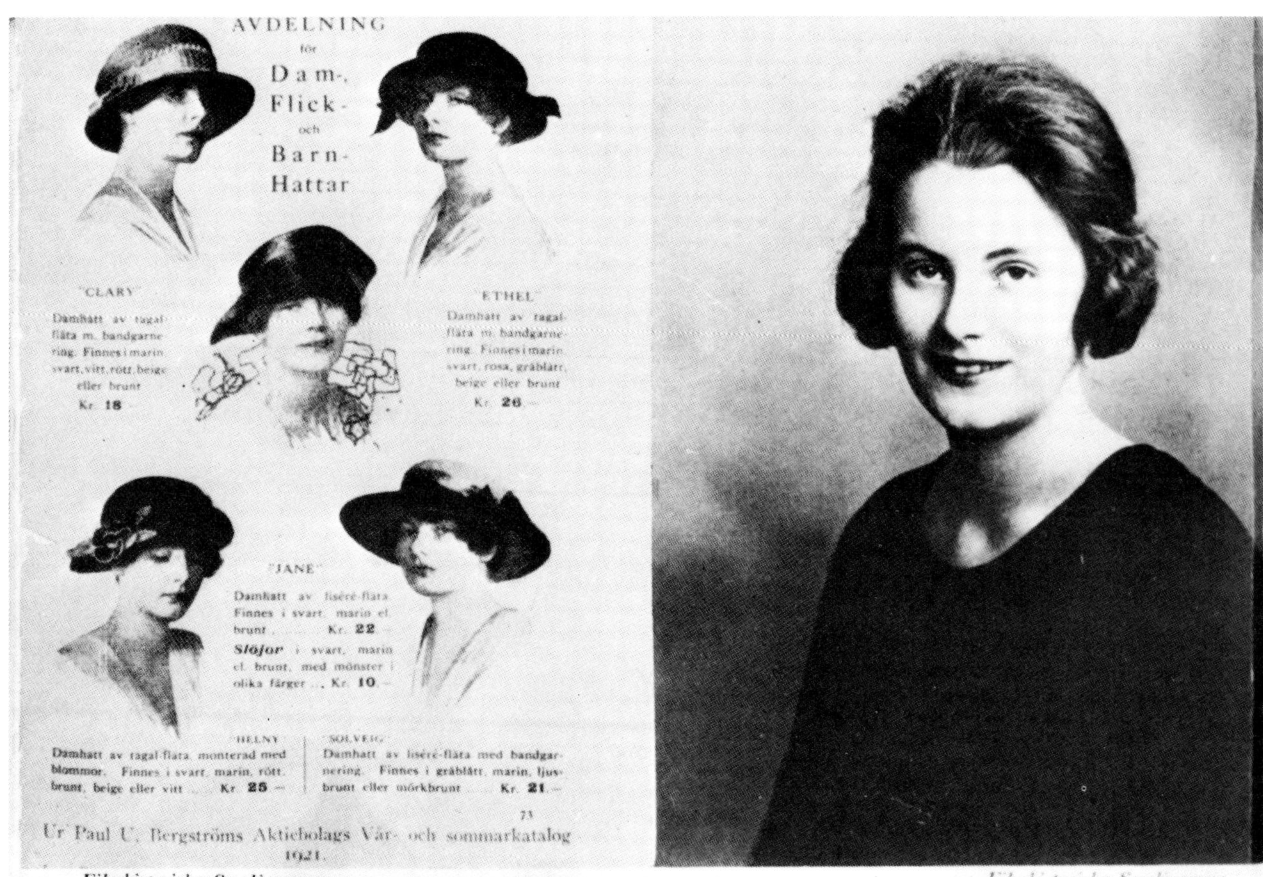

career as a model, with David Bailey once again being the first photographer to help her to success. She has become France's top sex symbol, rivalling Brigitte Bardot, who has become a little worn after wearing the crown for quite so long.

Henry Clarke photographed Bardot in Paris when she was very young. Her family knew the director of French *Vogue* and wanted her to be photographed modelling a bride's dress. They went to Notre Dame, where Clarke photographed the young and inexperienced girl, long before she developed the long, golden hair and film-star sex appeal. 'Even then she had a pussy-cat face', Clarke recalls. The photograph appeared in French *Vogue*.

It was inevitable that advertisers should decide that if models could become movie stars, then movie stars could become models—if only for a day, and Bardot resumed her modelling career recently when she was paid an astronomic sum for lending her image in press and television commercials to promote a new men's after-shave lotion.

French movie star Catherine Deneuve, once regarded as one of the most beautiful women in the world, one-time wife of English photographer David Bailey, and also French film producer

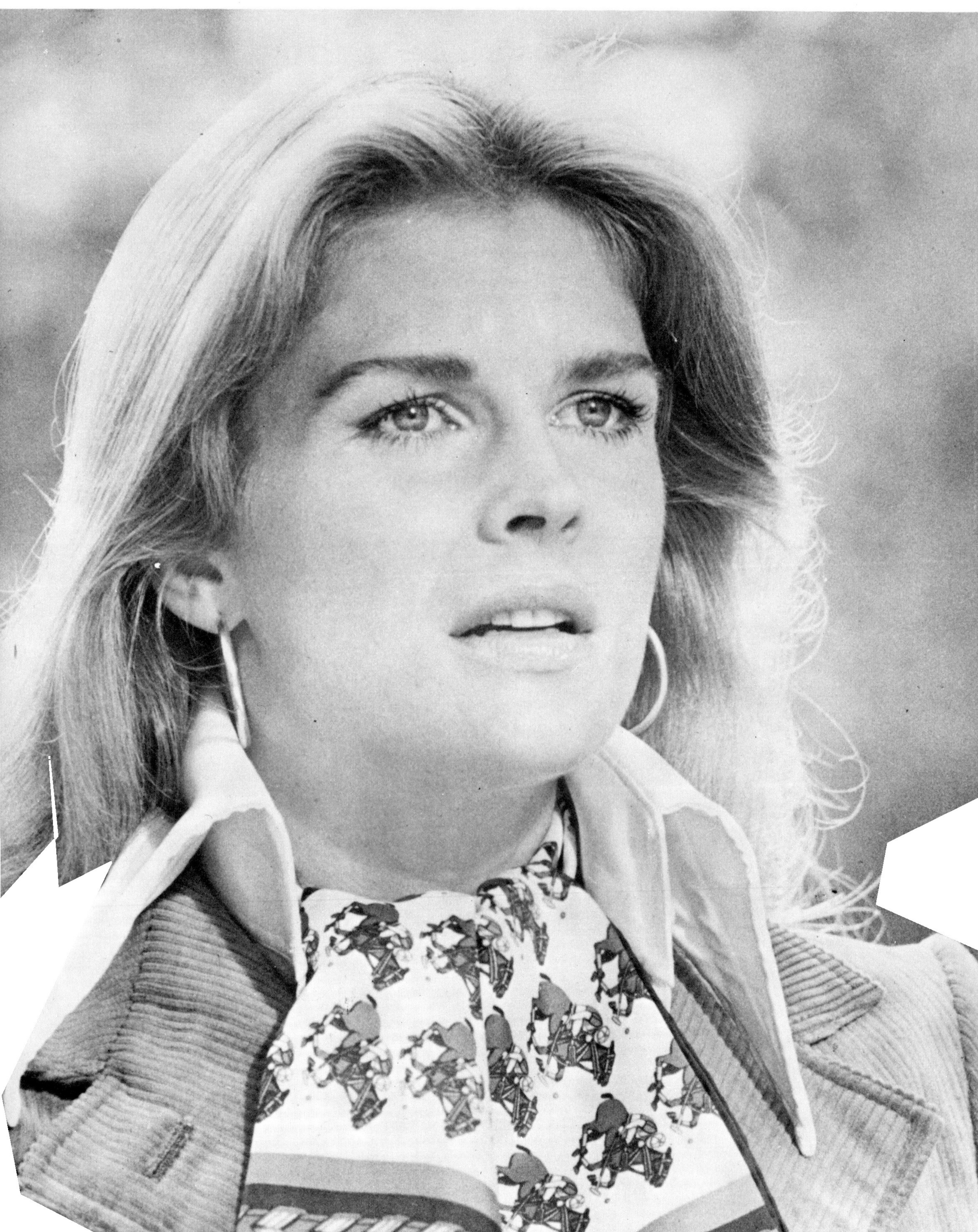

Candice Bergen as she appeared in
11 Harrowhouse

Roger Vadim, whose wives have included Brigitte Bardot and Jane Fonda, was another internationally known star to endorse a well known product. Her continental sophistication never registered with American audiences, who seldom take to a foreign actress at the box office. (Even Garbo was a bigger draw in Europe than in America.) More Americans know Catherine Deneuve as the symbol of Chanel through advertising and commercials than through her great European pictures—Luis Bunuel's *Belle de Jour* and Roman Polanski's *Repulsion*.

Even Garbo, at one time, turned her hand to modelling. In 1922, as a young salesgirl, Greta Louisa Gustaffson modelled hats for the store where she worked, and was photographed in Stockholm; a year later she was discovered by the great Swedish director Mauritz Stiller, and the rest of Greta Garbo's story is cinema history.

Another international star to lend her name to advertising was one of Garbo's co-stars in *Grand Hotel*, the late Joan Crawford. When her acclaim dwindled in the fifties, she married Pepsi-Cola chief Alfred Stecle, and carried her movie-star image and professionalism into the boardroom, travelling worldwide with her husband, endorsing Coke's multi-million dollar rival.

Not least of the world's top stars who returned briefly to modelling was Marlene Dietrich, who posed for a poster in the 1960s advertising the comforts and leg-room on British Airways.

Margaux Hemingway is perhaps the highest-paid model in the world with her million-dollar 'Babe' contract spread over five years; but her first movie, *Lipstick*, though heralded by much publicity, failed to draw expected audiences.

Other American stars who started out as models were Ann-Margaret and Ali MacGraw. Ali was a fashion stylist for years, assisting American photographer Mel Sokolsky in New York, with props and accessories. She lost weight, began modelling for teenage magazines *Glamour* and *Mademoiselle*, and, after taking acting lessons, soared to instant movie fame with *Goodbye Columbus*, *Love Story*, and *The Getaway*. Then she left her husband, Paramount chief Bob Evans, to marry Steve McQueen, and disappeared from the movie screen. Bob Evans had previously been married to another model, Camilla Sparv, a top model in the sixties, who had also a considerable movie career. Her most notable role was playing opposite Robert Redford in *Downhill Racer*, before settling down to become Mrs Herbert W. Hoover III.

Cybill Shepherd was a hard working model, appearing on numerous covers before being spotted by Peter Bogdanovich for *The Last Picture Show*. They fell in love, and he went on to cast her in the disastrous *The Heartbreak Kid*, which the critics panned. He tried and tried again; she played the title roles in *Daisy Miller*, failing again in the thirties type musical, and in *At Long Last Love* —a dismal attempt at a Ginger Rogers role. That seemed, at long last, to be the parting of the ways, and whilst she went on to create mild interest in *Taxi Driver*, he pressed on with his new discovery, Jane Hitchcock, a top New York model, for his latest film, *Nickelodeon*.

Of the top New York models to achieve movie stardom through actual acting ability, praised by the press and acclaimed by audiences, Jane Fonda is perhaps the best example of the model made good. Even though her political beliefs have often won her more press headlines than her movies and marriage to Roger Vadim, she is, nevertheless, an actress with a remarkable range.

The list of American models to appear before movie cameras is endless; Revlon's top image builder, Lauren Hutton, although little known to the general public, has several movies to her credit: *Paper Lion*, *Little Fauss and Big Halsy*, *The Gambler*, and *Gator*. Her latest, *Welcome to L.A.*, might change her luck. Swedish-born Maud Adams, ex-wife of British graphic designer Roy Adams, is one of America's top models today. Star of hundreds of Revlon and Clairol commercials, with her dark blonde hair and magnificent cheek bones, she has appeared in a string of forgotten movies. *Rollerball*, with James Caan, and the James Bond movie *Man with the Golden Gun* are perhaps the two notable exceptions.

Christina Ferrare, Max Factor's cosmetic symbol until the lapse of her contract with them recently, has also had a go at movie acting, playing Cliff Robertson's leading lady in *J. W. Coop;* with

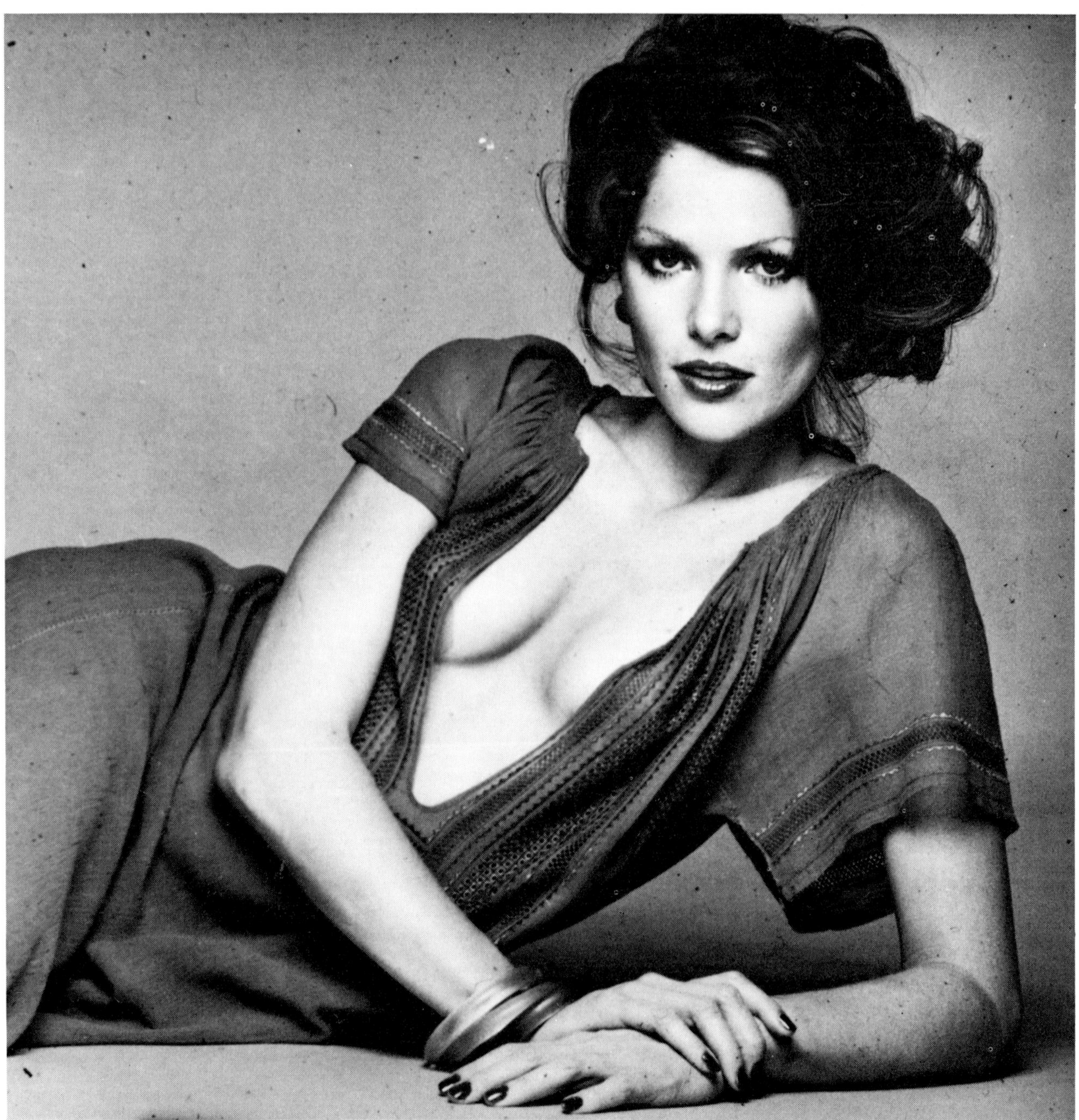

her million-dollar looks, she is almost certain to be back on the big screen.

The latest of the cosmetic contract girls to make the move from model to movies is Deborah Raffin, a strong contender for Lauren Hutton's Revlon contract. She first appeared in *Forty Carats* as Liv Ullmann's daughter, directed by Milton Katselas, and then the film produced by Gregory Peck, *The Dove*, co-starring Joseph Bottoms. The critics slaughtered her next movie, Jacqueline Susann's *Once is Not Enough*, with Alexis Smith, Melina Mercouri, Kirk Douglas, and David Janssen. Although she has two more movies, *God Told Me* with Sandy Dennis, and *The Sentinel*, in which she plays a super-star high-fashion model, she has far from given up her modelling career, and can frequently be seen looking out from the pages of *Vogue*, *Seventeen*, and *Mademoiselle*.

With the opening of the remake of *King Kong* came another actress taken from the ranks of modelling—Jessica Lange in the Fay Wray part—and another, Lois Chiles, who also appeared in *The Way We Were* and *The Great Gatsby*. Farah Fawcett-Majors, the golden-haired, pearly-toothed beauty, wife of television star Lee Majors, is the girl in the Wella Balsam advertisements; her performances in *Logan's Run* and

Above: Lois Chiles, photographed by Francesco Scavullo. Courtesy *Vogue*/USA

Opposite: Margaux Hemingway, also by Francesco Scavullo

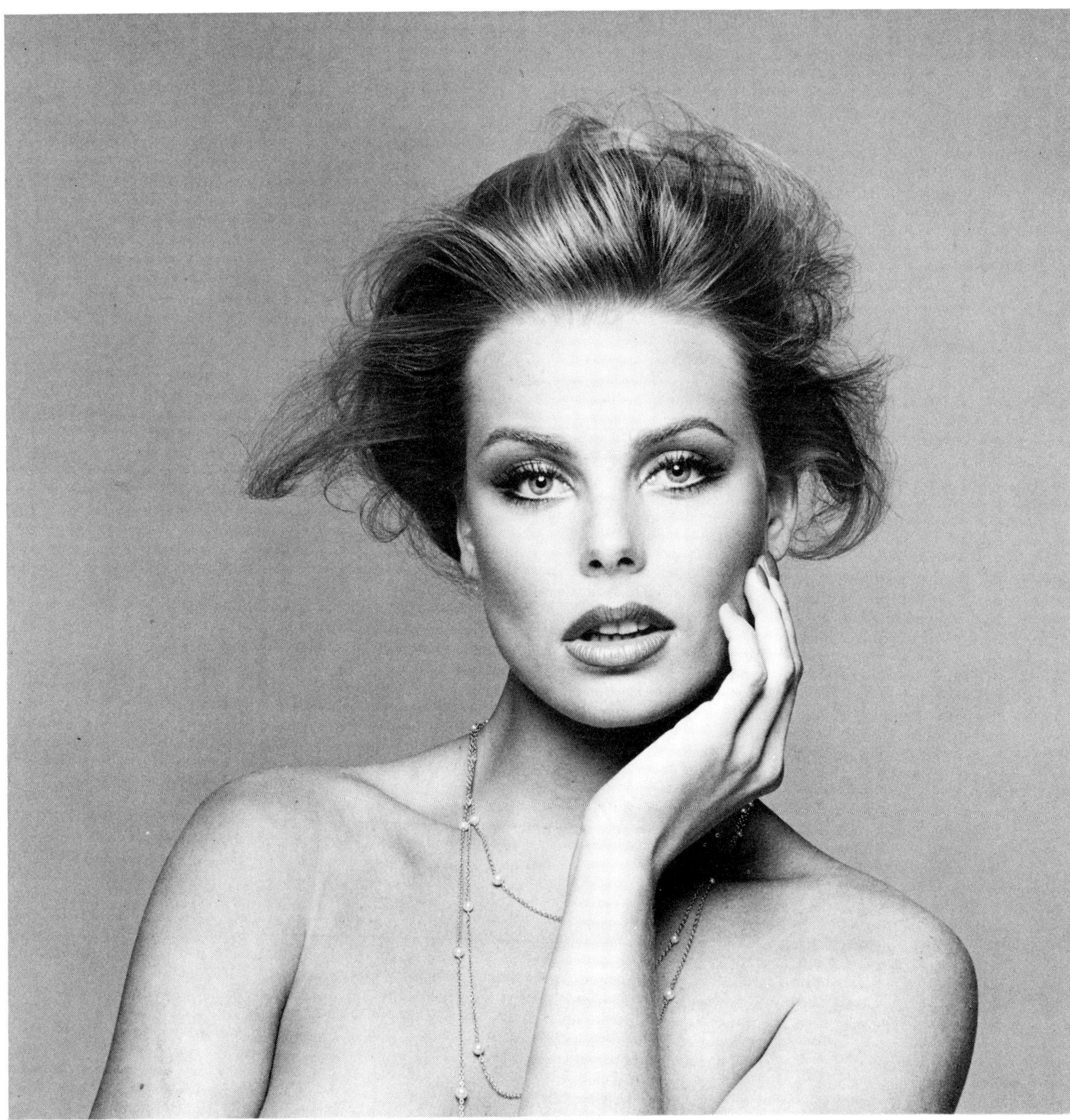

the television series, *Charlie's Angels*, a sort of girlie James Bond escapist spoof, prove that she *is* better to look at than a great many others who act better but don't look as good.

Of the models who seem likely to make the grade as movie stars, Dayle Haddon's prospects are brightest. Canadian-born, she began her career as a ballet dancer, and took to modelling to supplement her income. Modelling led to roles in Walt Disney's *The World's Greatest Athlete* in Los Angeles, and with Keir Dullea and Elizabeth Ashley in *Paper-back Hero*, back home in Canada. This beautiful dark-haired, blazingly blue-eyed Canadian then made an Italian movie, and turned down a role offered by Roger Vadim because she didn't like the story. Whilst in Paris, she was photographed for *Vogue* by Guy Bourdin and Helmut Newton, the top and most controversial fashion photographers in the world today. Her latest role in the French movie, *Madame Claude*, in which she, and Europe's top model, Vibéké, play whores in a political scandal set in Madame Claude's bordello for kings and politicians, seems bound to elevate her into international stardom.

But how many of the models who aspire to movie stardom will make the grade enough to be remembered as well as Lauren Bacall and to reach Grace Kelly's heights? The list of the models who have appeared in movies, whether good or bad ones, is impressive, and continually on the increase: Susie Blakely, Barbara Carreras, Tamara Dobson, the gorgeous black karate queen who appeared in *Cleopatra Jones*, and *Norman . . . is That You?*, and Angelica Huston, whose famous father and relationship with Jack Nicholson might help her. But, cast as playthings for the heroes, as girl-friends, wives, or protagonists, their roles are rarely more than secondary. They do, however, add a much needed touch of glamour to movies today.

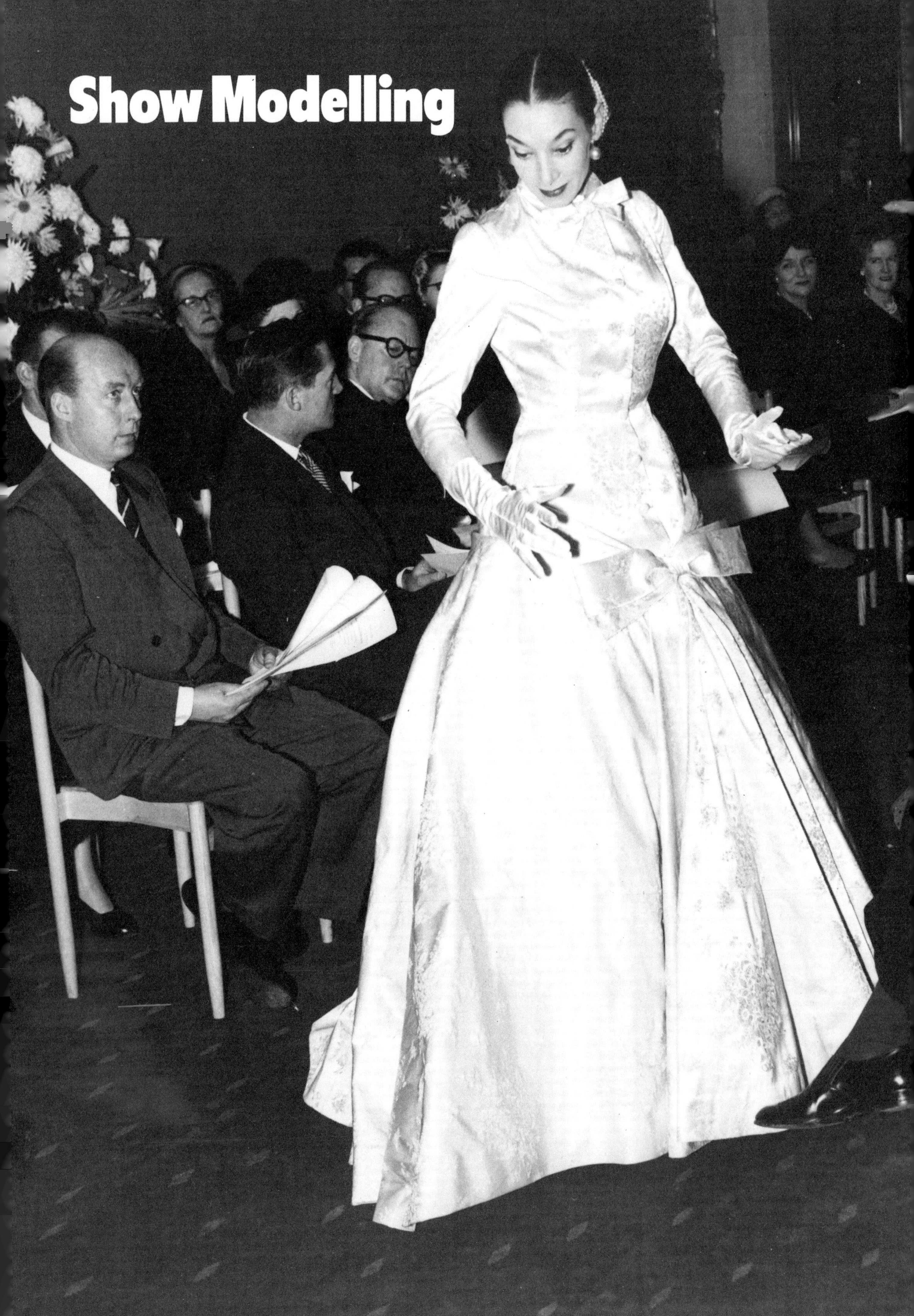
Show Modelling

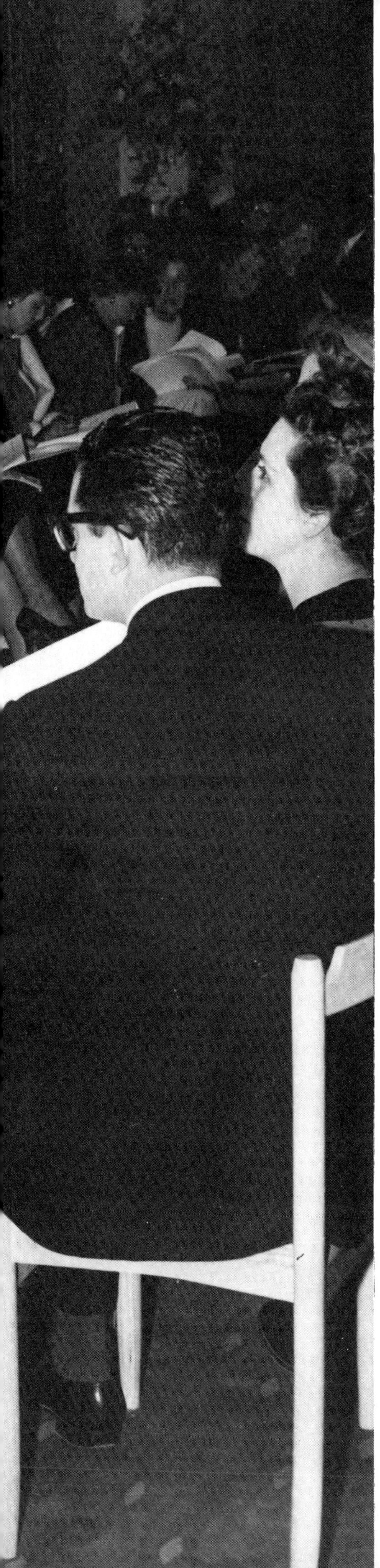

Show modelling is the least well paid, but the most rewarding form of modelling. No *Vogue* covers and editorial spreads here for the hard-working girl with striking looks and slender proportions, but satisfaction from wearing beautiful and expensive clothes and enjoying the admiration and applause more usually reserved for beautiful and talented actresses on stage. Yet, like acting, there are different levels of modelling, from the girl showing clothes to hardened buyers on Seventh Avenue, New York's dress manufacturers' centre, or London's equivalent, Great Titchfield Street, to the star models at Dior in Paris. Showing clothes in department stores can be a thankless chore, hard on the feet and unsatisfying to the ego, but for the girl with the right proportions and the right mental approach for the job, it can be an exciting and rewarding profession.

In years past, models got a certain satisfaction from wearing beautiful clothes they could never afford. Top designers lent them their latest creations to wear at Ascot and Henley. Couturiers believed that the model played a vital part by seeing seen at elegant public and social functions in his latest clothes. She was as important to the dress as the cutter, the fitter, and the vendeuse in clinching a sale. The model was an integral part of the creation. If fashion were an orchestra, the designer was the conductor and the model girl the first violinist.

Where productions at fashion shows are of the highest level, it is not only because of the spectacular and original clothes, consisting of some of the finest fabrics and textures, but because of the dramatic and theatrical flair lent by stunning and glamorous models who create an atmosphere, an aura of exaggerated movement and poise; luring, challenging, and defying onlookers to respond effectively. The model makes the clothes *live*, being ever-conscious, not only of the reputation of the fashion house, but of the expensive garment she is showing. She inspires designer, photographer, and fashion writer alike and plays a fundamental part in presenting to the public the beautiful and expensive creations.

Many designers create the dress on the model, rather than at the drawing

Norman Hartnell's leading model Dolores, perhaps one of the best known British show models

**Opposite: Marisa Berenson,
photographed in Sardinia by
Henry Clarke**

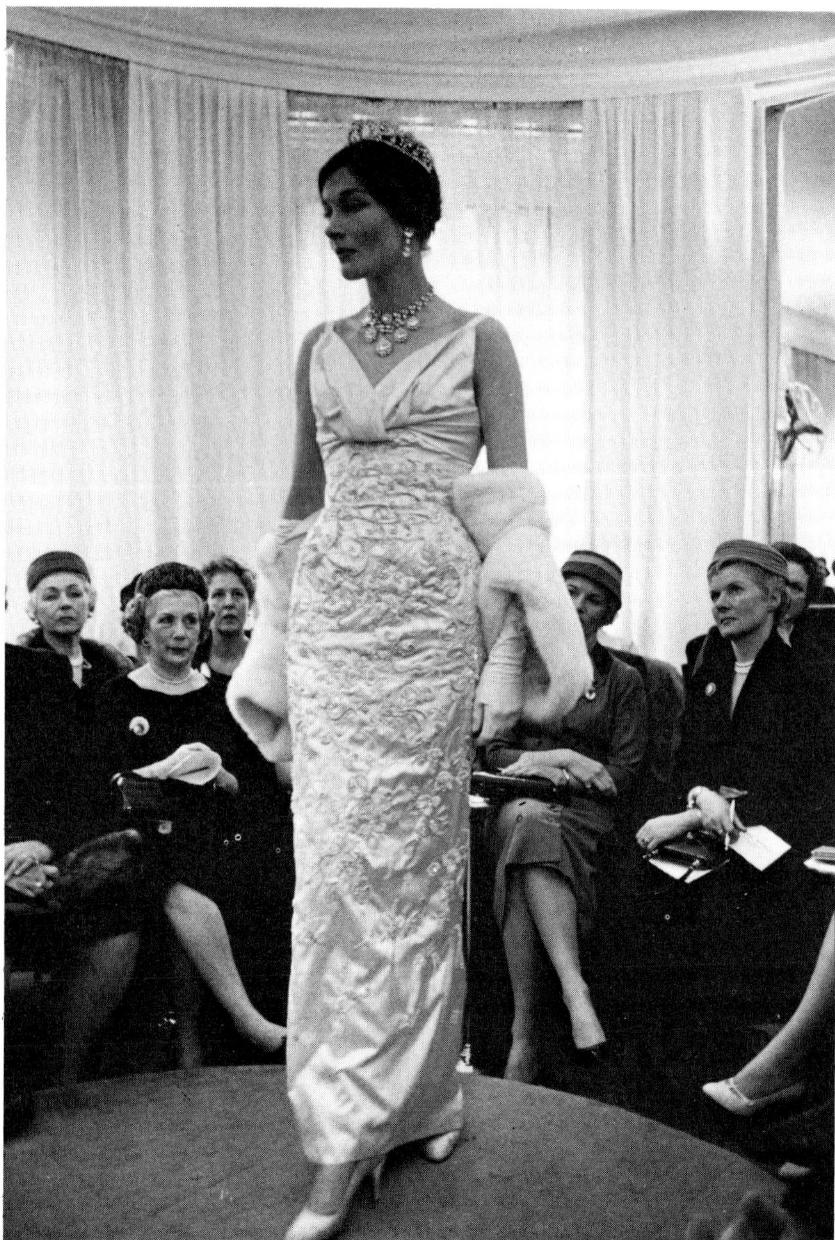

**Above: Bronwen Pugh modelling
for Balmain in Paris in 1957**

board, and in so doing find out at once how the fabric and design respond to shape, form, and movement.

Show models must be attractive, elegant, and intelligent. They need to be even-tempered in order to be helpful to the saleswomen and junior during the rush of the season. As fitting rooms are usually small, it is essential for models to get on well with one another.

Each fashion house has its own style of model and is careful to employ only those in keeping with it. In London, John Cavanagh's models were young and sweet-looking, in harmony with his pretty, feminine clothes, whereas the Courrèges models were like sun-tanned Amazons with broad shoulders in order to show his futuristic-looking clothes-with-holes effectively. Some models know instinctively how to wear a dress, others ruin it. The best models inevitably achieve recognition and stardom.

The spring and autumn collections are shown in January and July. Four girls are the barest minimum for a show because by appearing in rotation they have just enough time to change without causing delay. There are invariably eight to sixteen models showing at the big collections. On the first day of the season, there may be two or three shows, but, after that, only one show is held daily, at three o'clock in the afternoon. It takes an hour-and-a-quarter to show sixty-odd creations. The girls model privately for individual customers who return later on to examine the clothes more closely.

Models in the top couture houses in Paris enjoyed fleeting fame during collection times: amongst the greatest were Bronwen Pugh and the late Praline at Balmain; Sylvia, Sophie and Alla at Dior; and the most famous Parisian model of all, Bettina, at Jacques Fath.

The blonde, 5ft 8in American model, Sue Blair, who now works in the showroom of the new Nina Ricci boutique in the Avenue Georges V in Paris, used to be a model for the Nina Ricci fashion house in the fifties, in the days when there were fourteen to eighteen models employed by most designers. Today, there are four models permanently employed by the few remaining high fashion houses. The majority of the well known designers have turned to *prêt-à-porter* (ready to wear) for obvious econ-

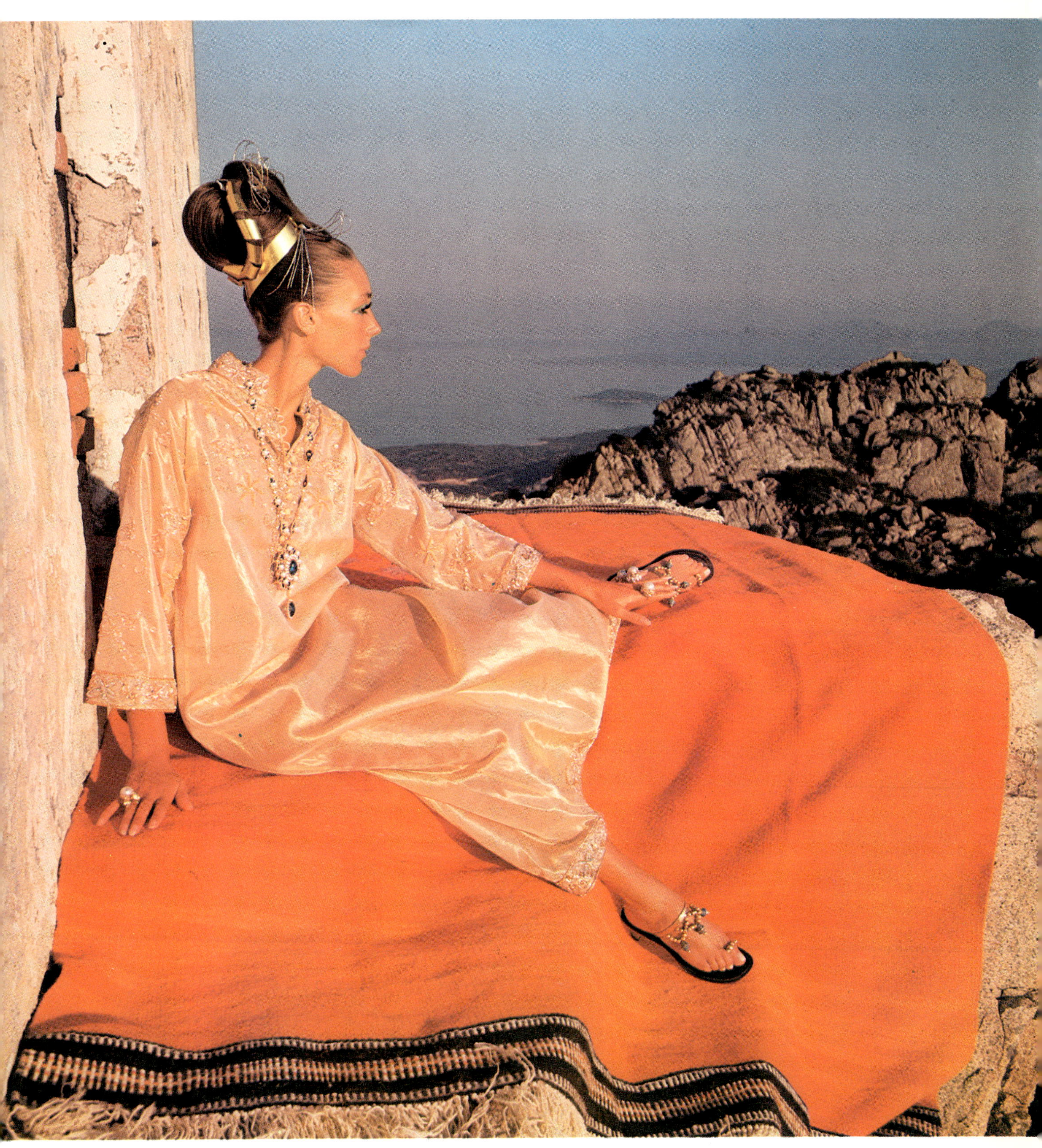

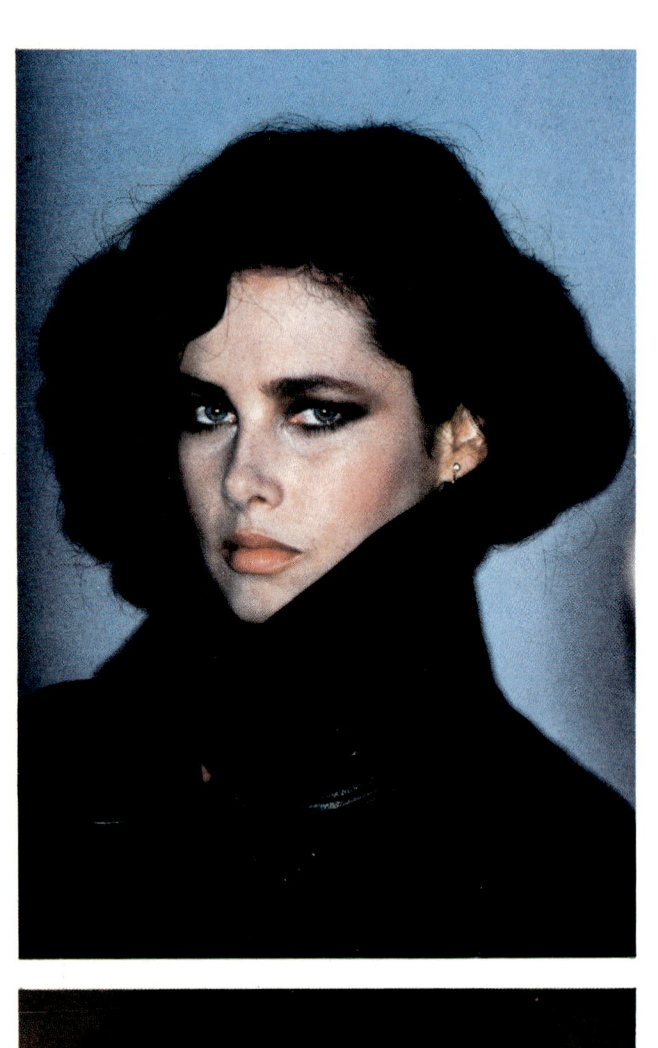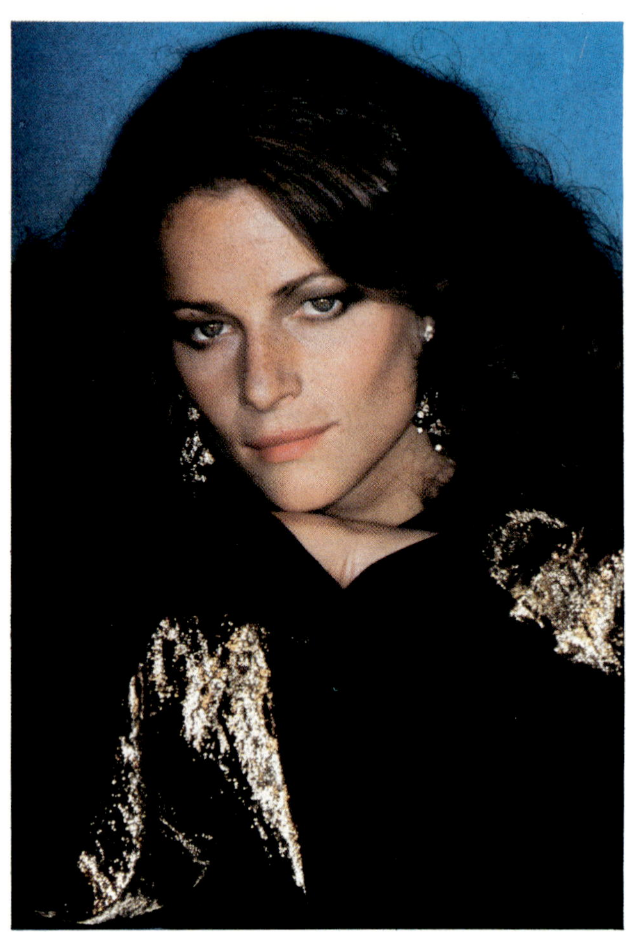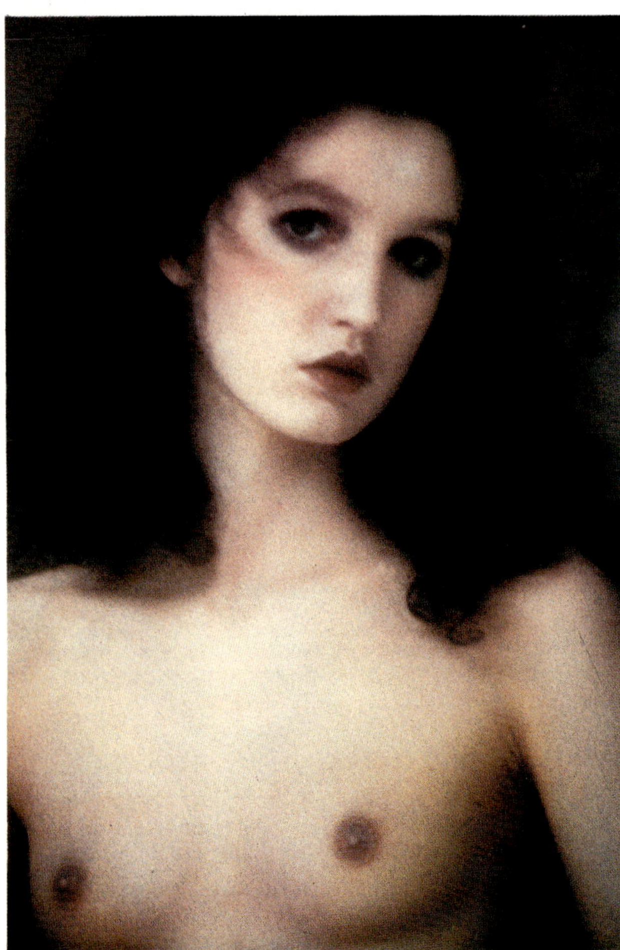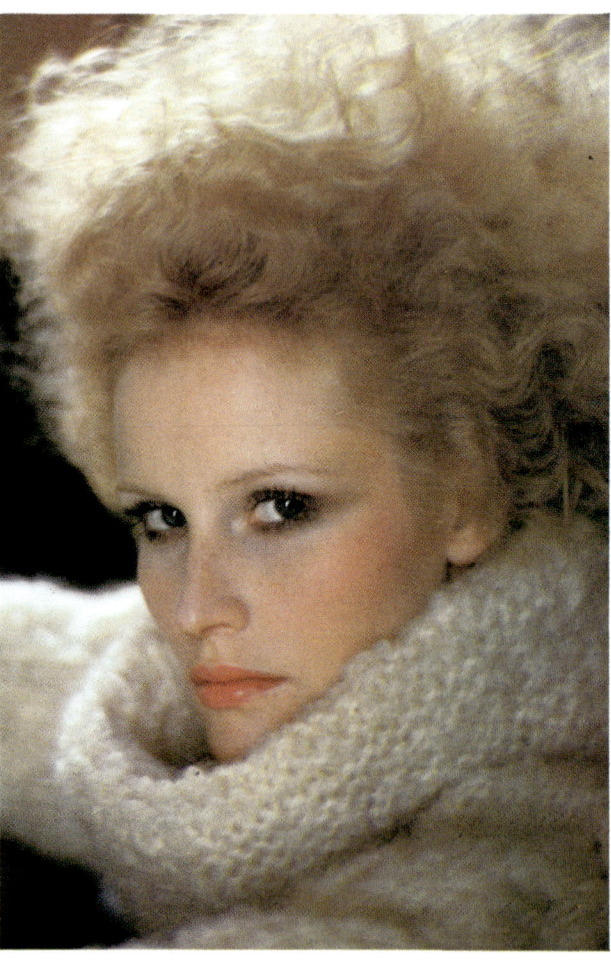

omic reasons, as well as the ever-growing shortage of well heeled customers with £5,000 to spend on an evening gown—and with no occasions at which to wear it.

When Sue Blair joined Nina Ricci's, she was only the fourteenth girl, but became the one whom the resident designer, Jules-François Crahay, used as a model for his designs. These days Crahay is the designer at Lanvin. American, Scandinavian, and German girls were more sought after in Paris than the French girls because they were more professional, and this has not changed today. The Americans move beautifully as far as fashion goes, because they tend to be less inhibited than their continental cousins. Models either have that vital inner sense of chic, or don't. Like star quality, it is intangible and cannot be taught. The French girls weren't particularly interested in the clothes; to them, modelling was a job, pure and simple—it paid the rent and provided fodder. However, for girls who cared little about the clothes, they usually managed to 'feel' the garments and show them to surprisingly good effect.

The models worked from nine to five, except for the two weeks before the day of the collection, when they worked into the night. Once the show started, they showed only three hours a day; one hour showing in the morning, and another two hours in the afternoons. For the rest of the day they idled away their time. 'We were treated like circus ponies', recalls Sue Blair, 'prancing around the ring, but once you sat down, you just sat around, *like* circus ponies, waiting for the next house. I never noticed so many girls before with such narcissistic complexes! They sat in front of the mirror all day long glaring at themselves, doing their make-up, and then re-doing it.' Sue used to knit.

Although the minimum height requirement for show models in stockinged feet in London is 5ft 8in, the average woman's height in Britain is 5ft 4in. The most important requirements in a model are to be able to move elegantly and to have a sense of clothes; short girls, with the best will in the world, simply cannot show clothes with the flair and style the taller girls have. A pretty face is not essential for show modelling, and although a boyish figure,

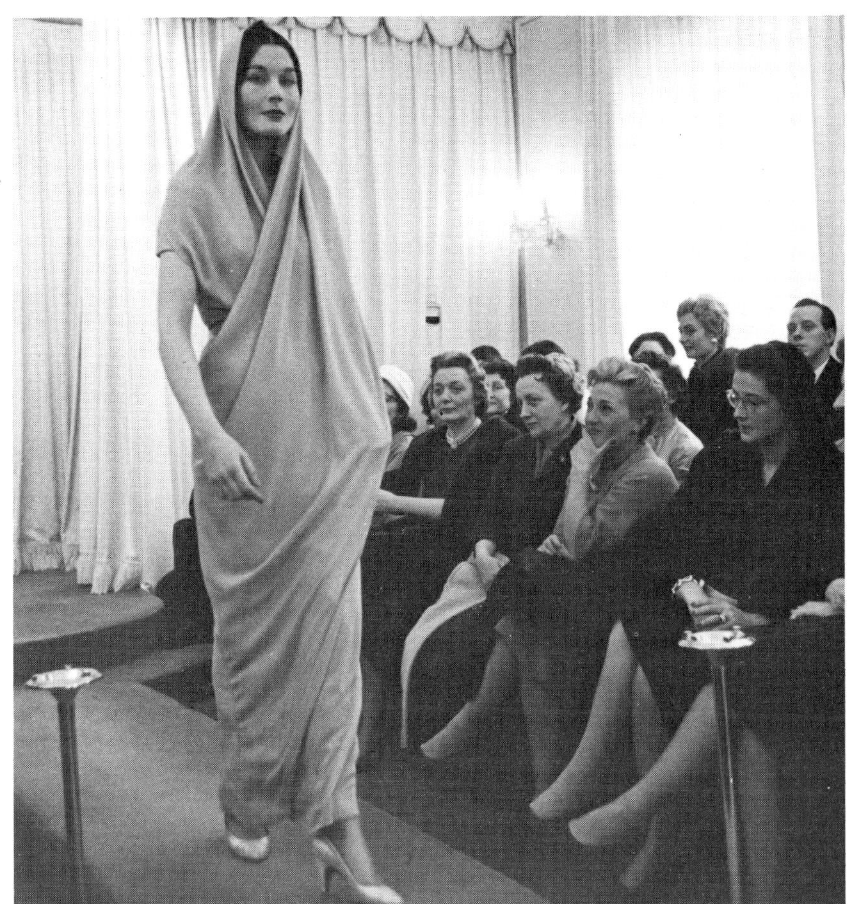

Above: Too tall to model in England, Bronwen Pugh became one of the leading Parisian show models

Opposite. Above left: Dayle Haddon by Helmut Newton—*Vogue* France

Above right: Charlotte Rampling by Helmut Newton—*Vogue* France

Below left: Anne B by Sarah Moon —*Vogue* France

Below right: Gunilla Lindblad by Hans Feurer—*Vogue* France

Cynthia Oberholzer, photographed by Alfred Crossberg

with slender hips and small bosoms, is preferred by some houses, others like a bit of bust and buttock. Sir Norman Hartnell admits that he has never known the actual measurements of his models; as the clothes are made specifically for them, they need not be stock sizes. He relies more upon the look and the style of the girl than her vital statistics.

Sir Norman, one of Britain's top couturiers, won the highest accolade of all British fashion designers when he was created a knight by Queen Elizabeth in her 1977 New Year's Honours List; he is the first designer of high fashion ever to be so honoured. Sir Norman, who opened his salon in 1935, has made clothes for the Queen and other members of the Royal Family for many years. His first models in the thirties were a beauty queen from Berlin named Fritzy, and an English girl, Patsy Quinn, who became Countess Lambert. Avril Anstruther was another of his good models at that time. His two current house-models, Mara, the smart, tall, dark girl, and a beautiful girl called Gillian, not only show the clothes, but train aspiring models in the Hartnell School of Deportment three nights a week. A six-week course costs £75, but, although they teach make-up, hair styling, movement, and general beauty care, they make no promises to convert students into models.

'I've had two ready-made girls, Dolores and Cynthia, who were simply model-girls by nature', says Sir Norman. 'They walked into the room and didn't need tuition at all.'

Dolores was the Queen Mother's favourite model girl at Hartnell's. The antithesis of the Queen Mother, she was tall, slender as a rake, and had a sort of Spanish vamp. She wore her black hair in a tight chignon, and had tremendous theatrical flair. An English girl from Sidcup, her real name was Dolly Stevenson. Probably about sixty years old today, she left Hartnell's to settle in South Africa, where she opened a model school, when Hartnell's new discovery from South Africa, Cynthia Oberholzer, arrived on the scene. 'If she stays, I go', threatened Dolores when she saw the new girl, and exercised her threat when Hartnell asked Cynthia to stay.

'Cynthia was chosen in a rain-storm in Johannesburg', recalls Sir Norman.

'I was on a tour and couldn't afford to take all my own girls, and so these gorgeous girls came in to meet me at a tea-party at Lady Oppenheimer's. There was one big girl in a squashed raspberry hat, very much made-up, who gave me a sort of old-fashioned wink. "Are you the head-girl?" I asked. "Yes, bossy", she replied, and she became my head-girl on tour right away. Then I brought her back to London to work for me.'

Cynthia, who was 5ft 11in, blonde, and terribly chic, with a lovely, wicked, arrogant twinkle about her, was Sir Norman's top model for many years. An attractive, amusing girl, she had a penchant for millionaires and the aristocracy. It was as though she aimed to be a rich dowager in her old age. She was wined, and dined, and much fêted by them, but the nearest she came to actually getting a millionaire to the altar was when her richest suitor called on her, believing her to be the innocent idol he had admired so much on the cat-walk in Hartnell's salon. In rather an ungentlemanly manner, he happened to flick through her diary in the next room whilst she was dressing. When she returned, he had disappeared, never to be seen again.

When Cynthia gave up modelling, she went to live in New York in search of true love, but her luck only changed when she adopted the title, *Baroness von Oberholzer*, since which time her social success in America has abounded and she has *almost* achieved her ambition.

'Given a reasonable garment, I'd back Cynthia against any other model girl, *ever*', Sir Norman adds as a fitting tribute to his South African discovery.

'We had one beautiful model girl here from Austria', Sir Norman continued. 'She was a lovely girl who turned out to be an international crook. She went *inside* for pinching one of our mink coats and some dresses specially made to fit her.'

The Austrian model had been fitted for some exquisite clothes to be shown in the new collection, but on the day of the show she was nowhere to be seen. The commentator announced to a waiting audience, 'We apologise, ladies and gentlemen. Mr Hartnell's head model-girl isn't here today. Her mother is terribly ill, and she had to fly off to Vienna to be by her bedside.'

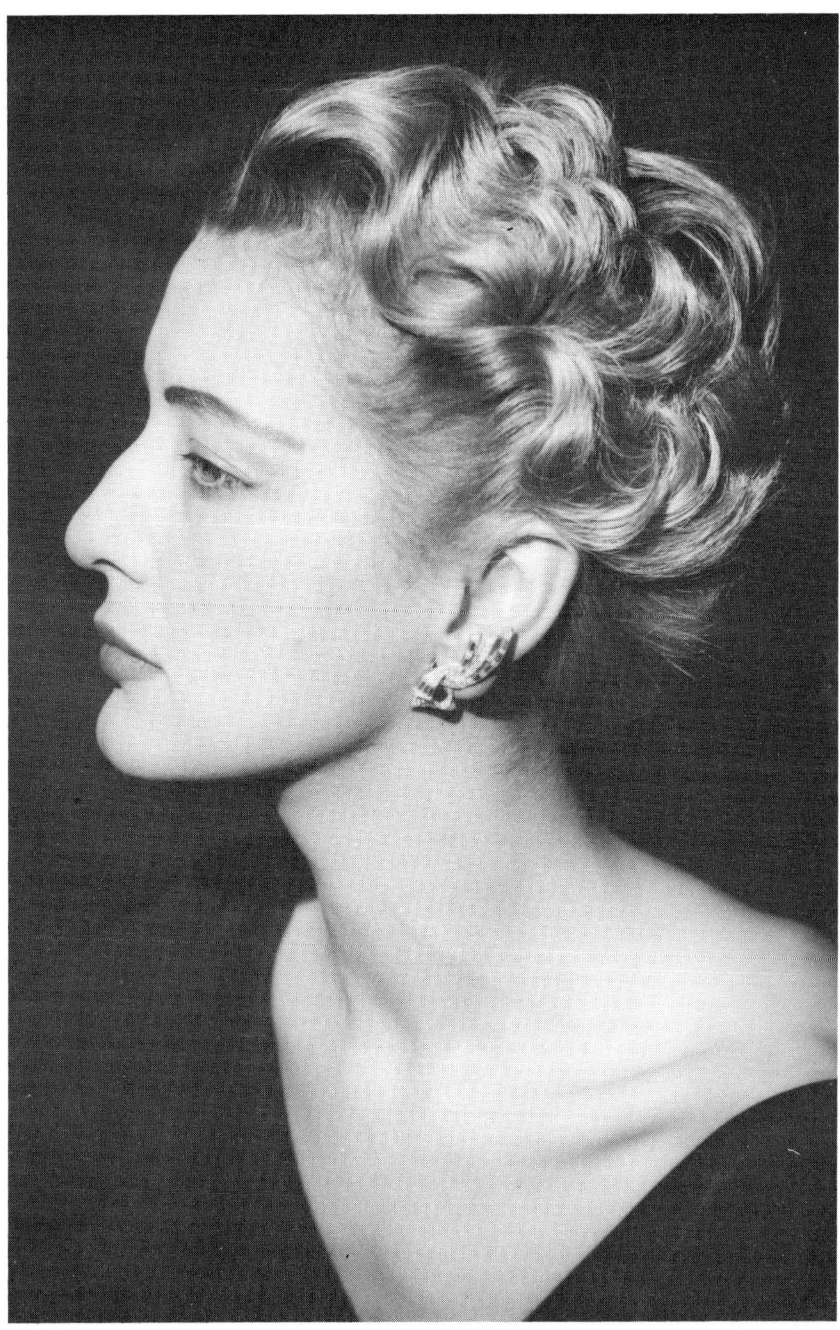

Models employed at these events are selected not only for their professional abilities, but show directors and choreographers like them to have a sense of humour, to bubble over, or be dramatic, depending on the mood of the dress they are showing.

The models, however, who work the hardest, both physically and mentally, to sell clothes to hardened buyers, are the girls employed by the wholesale houses. The showroom model is the most underrated of girls because she is the one who really has to sell the merchandise. She shows it at the fashion show, and then again, afterwards, to the department store or high-street dress-shop buyer who will all but pull the dress apart at the seams.

America has little to offer in the field of high fashion show modelling, and so, for the girl who wants to become a show model, Paris is the first port of call, where there are many houses from which to choose: Madame Grés, Jean-Louis Scherrer, Hubert de Givenchy, Yves Saint Laurent, Emanuel Ungaro, Lanvin (their designer is Jules-François Crahay), Dior (where Marc Bohan designs), Philippe Venet, Pierre Cardin, Louis Féraud, Ted Lapidus, Guy Laroche, André Courrèges, Patou (designer, Angelo Tarlazzi), Nina Ricci (Gérard Pipart), and Pierre Balmain. The Paris model agencies, Elite, Models International, Viva, Modelplanning, Pauline's, Christa Modelling and the many others, should be contacted in the first instance.

In London, the leading designers who regularly employ show models are Zandra Rhodes, Bill Gibb, Yuki, Jean Muir, Gina Fratini, Norman Hartnell, Hardy Amies, and, of course, the major dress manufacturers, the names of which can be secured by joining one of the top London model agencies.

Amongst the top fashion-show producers, commentators, and choreographers, the leaders in this field in London are Michael Whittaker, Patricia Laffan, Malcolm Goddard, Kenneth Partridge, and Leonard Pearcey. Peter Hope-Lumley, who, until recently, ran one of London's top model agencies, is the leading public relations authority on fashion and modelling, ever-knowing and helpful to both established and enthusiastic new aspirants.

'Don't be silly, dear,' one of the other models whispered in his ear, 'her lover's waiting in the car outside, and I've just seen her slip out of the back door with that new grey mink coat she was going to show today, over her arm.'

When the police picked her up she was found not only with the priceless grey mink and a carful of Hartnell's latest creations, but some diamonds from Cartier's as well.

In London, full-time show models employed by the high-fashion houses are paid about £50 for working a five-day week, with hours from nine to five-thirty. Freelance models are paid £60 a day for working an eight-hour day showing collections in hotels, but there are few of these occasions in the year. They are paid £20 a day for showing a couturier's new collection to a select, invited audience, and if they do shows in department stores, such as Harrods or Selfridges, they receive £15 a show, which may run an hour-and-a-half. They are paid £80 for a press show, which includes their photographic fee, plus £30 for rehearsals. Agents fees of 20 per cent are paid by freelance models. The girls who appear at industrial shows at large hotels, cinemas or theatres, are expected to dance, giving character to the new mod-clothes, or move in rhythm to the lively music.

Male Models

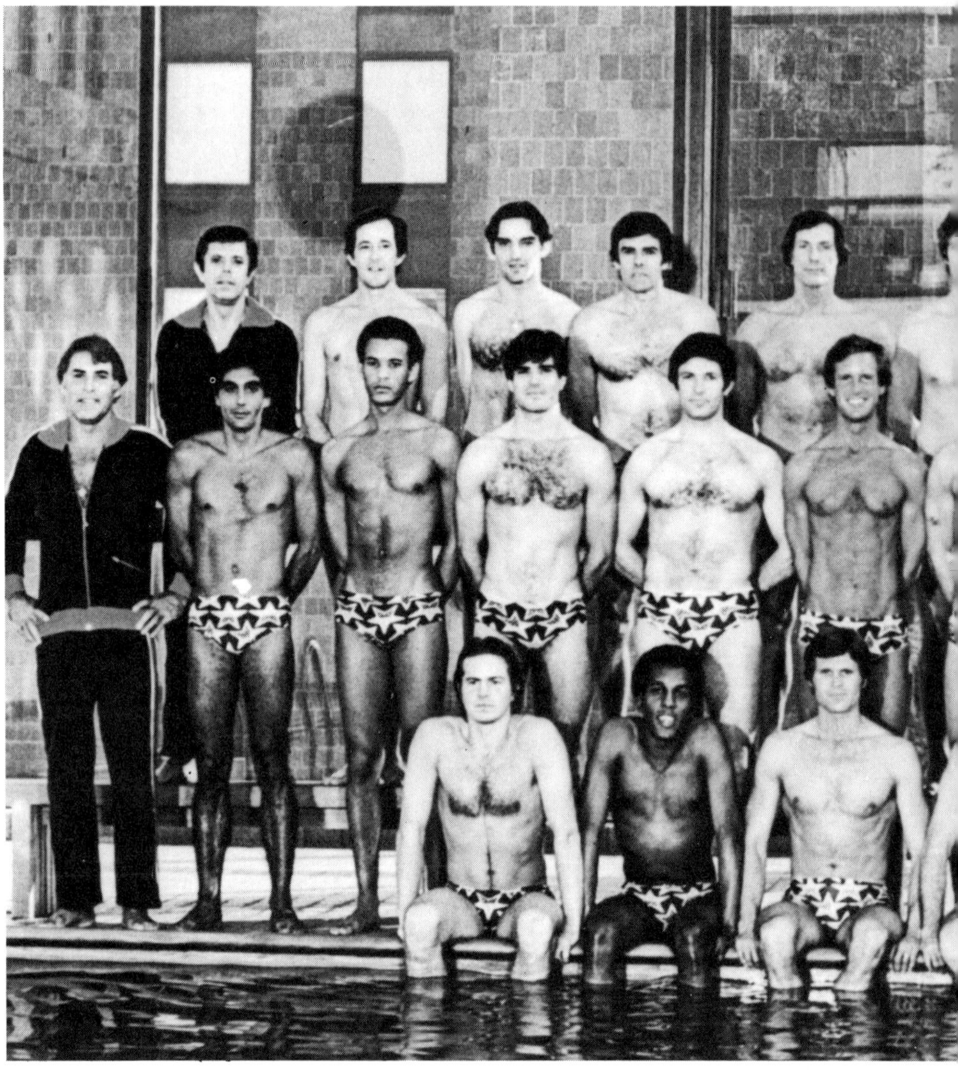

The advertising media is dominated by the female image, and so the male model is regarded as an accessory to the model girl. Because of this, in New York, a top girl earns up to $1,000 a day for cosmetic advertising and her male counterpart is lucky to receive half as much. However, in London, where equal rights prevail, a male photographic model's standard fee is £15 an hour, or £100 a day, the same as the model girl's fee. But the model girl trains harder, pays more for the initial outlay to launch herself with photographs and composites, fighting stronger competition from the thousands of other beautiful young things. A mere handful of male models dominate their exclusive market, unchallenged and uncompetitive.

The basic requirements for top male models are masculine good looks, a minimum height of 5ft 11in, broad shoulders, narrow hips, silm waist, and long, muscular legs. A serious, virile, and aggressively reliable image is what advertisers look for, and it is unlikely that men looking boyish, or younger than thirty, will make the top grade. Punctuality, grooming, and dependability are essential.

With one possible exception, male models have never reached the moviestar heights and gossip column fame achieved by their female counterparts. Husky Australian, George Lazenby, who made his reputation in England on television with the 'Big Fry' advertising campaign, is the exception. He became a movie star, playing James Bond in one Bond movie when Sean Connery abdicated the role, but has sunk into professional obscurity in the last few years.

Another manly Australian, Ted Dawson, is the reigning top male model in the world today. Operating from New York, where he belongs to the Ford's model agency, his daily rate is $500. The highest earning male model today, Ted Dawson is the most photographed

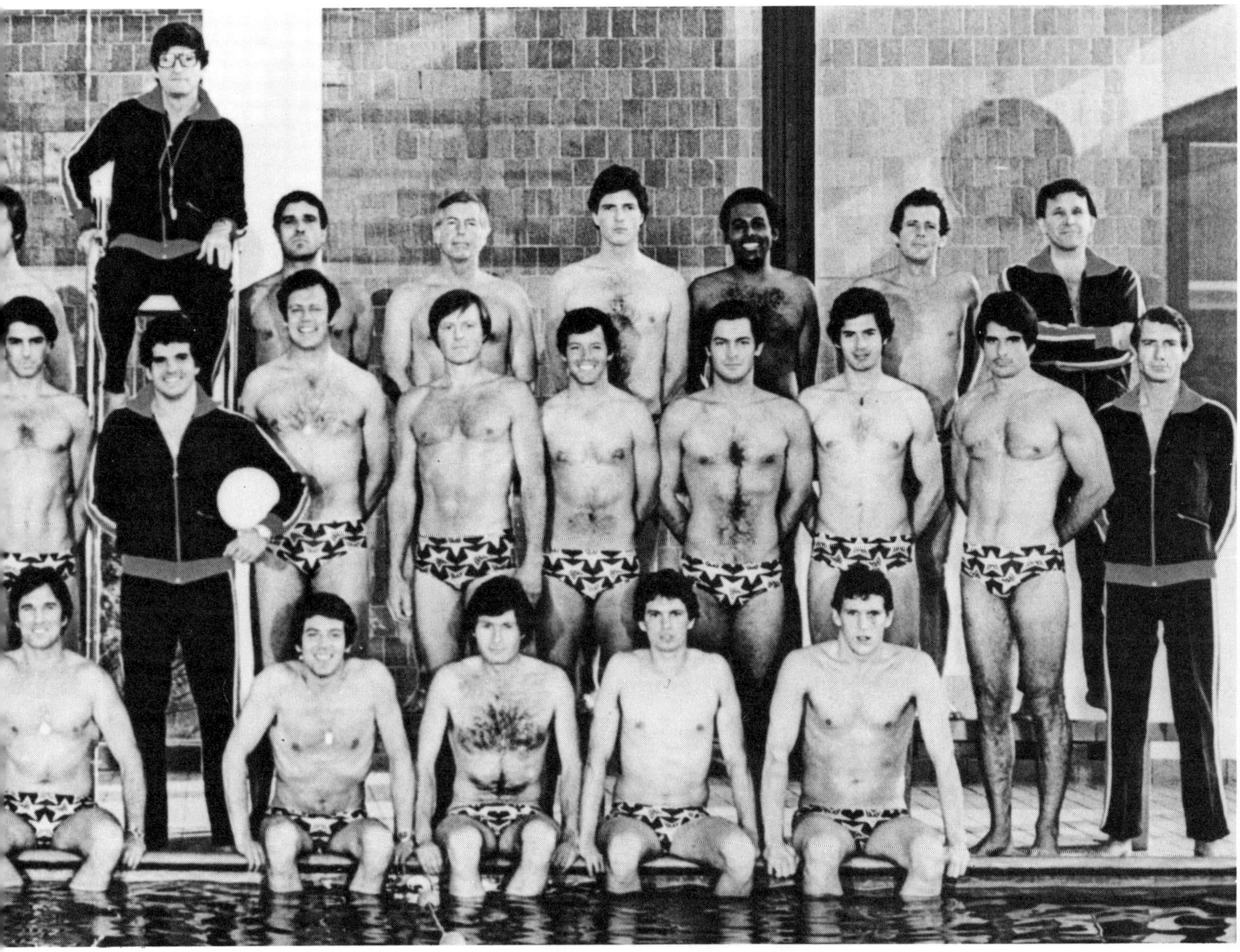

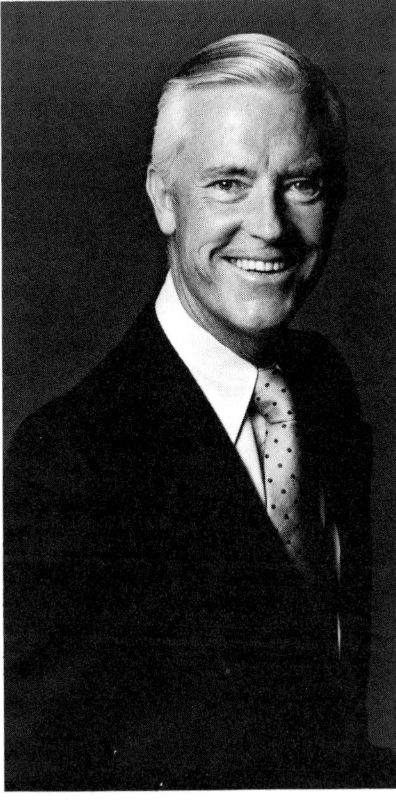

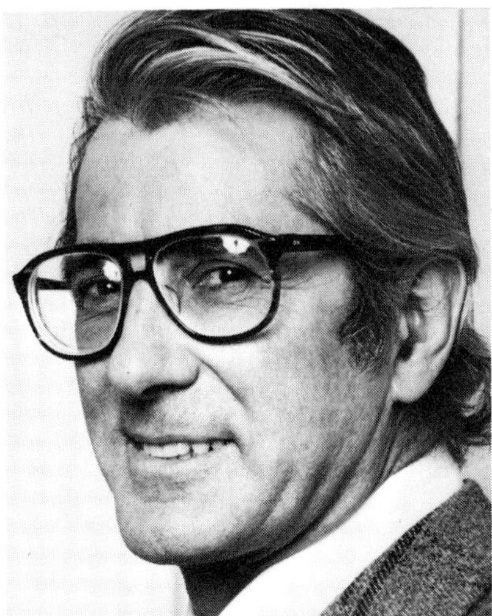

Above: Gene Barakat, by Stanley Rumbough

Right: Colin Leslie Fox, by Carl Saraishi

model in the world.

Australians seem to have cornered the market in manly models. Before Ted, another Australian, Gene Barakat, who, these days, runs the television and sports promotion side of the Ford's agency, was the world's leading male model. Gene came to London, where he became top boy after appearing in the 'Rolls Royce and Roses' advertising campaign. He progressed to New York, where he became the highest paid male model ever, achieving modelling fame. He is affectionately referred to as 'the daddy of them all' by women's liberationist Germaine Greer.

Although Jack Challenge is another male model to have had a long run—forty years to be exact—the first important male model in America was Colin Leslie Fox, who appeared in the Revlon adds in the forties and fifties with Suzy Parker. He retired from modelling for a short while, but has now resumed his career, appearing as the

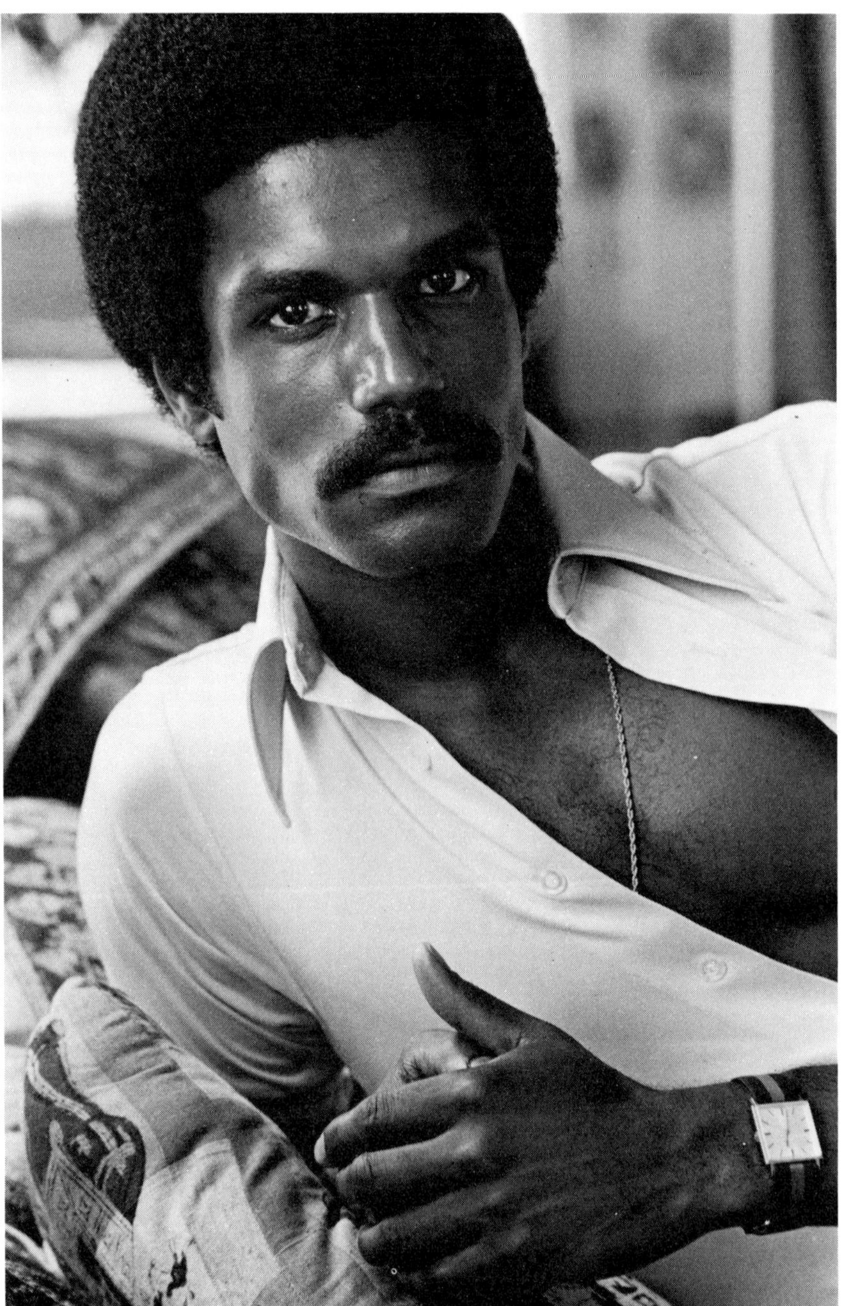

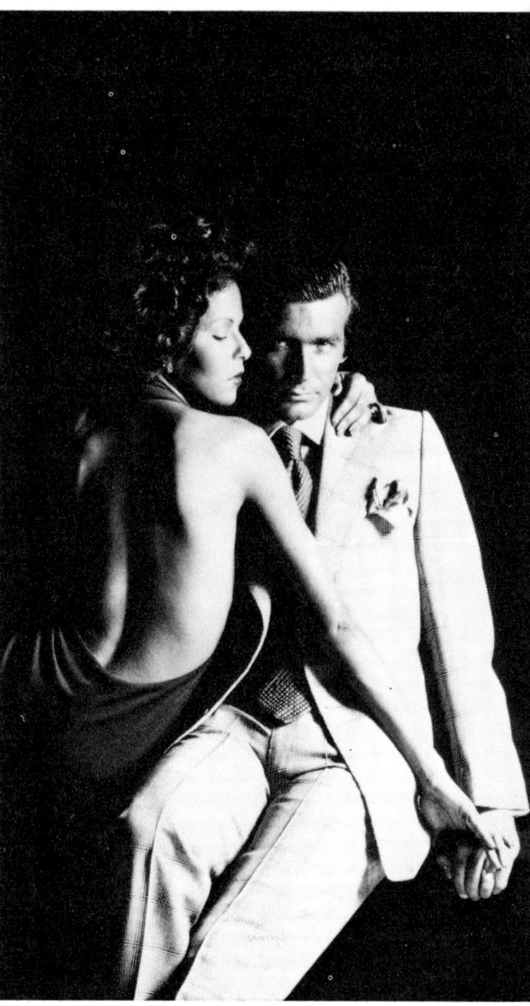

suave, greying businessman with Cary Grant good looks and charm.

Colin Leslie Fox is handled by the Zoli agency in New York, the closest rival to Ford's as far as male models go. Zoli's top black model in the US is Renauld White. In Britain there is not enough work available to keep a black male model fully employed because there simply isn't the market in Britain for a lucrative black consumer trade. Menswear manufacturers cannot see models such as David Clay, who is the top exotic black model in Britain today, identifying with the image associated with their goods. America has a colossal black community, and Renauld White appeals to the immense advertising campaigns aimed at this market.

Britain's first top male model in the fifties and sixties was Michael Bentley. His elegant, lean, good looks appeared in more advertisements for menswear than any other British male model. He continued his successful modelling career until he joined the Hardy Amies menswear division in London. Geoffrey Jones, another top male model of the same period, although a little younger, has become the men's fashion buyer for Bergdorf–Goodman. He travels the world selecting menswear and accessories for the exclusive New York fashion store.

The top male model agency in London is Nevs, run by former model Neville Gates, who manages most of the top males in London.

Graham Rogers, who models the famous Dormeuil fabric, is sent by Nevs to Chicago for the photographic sessions for the rather erotic advertisements, with a possessive-looking model girl holding onto her man—in his Dormeuil suit—ever protectively guarding her belongings.

Peter Benison is the other high ranking male model agency in London, followed closely by Gavin Robinson, who used to be a model boy himself. Gavin's is one of the top agencies for

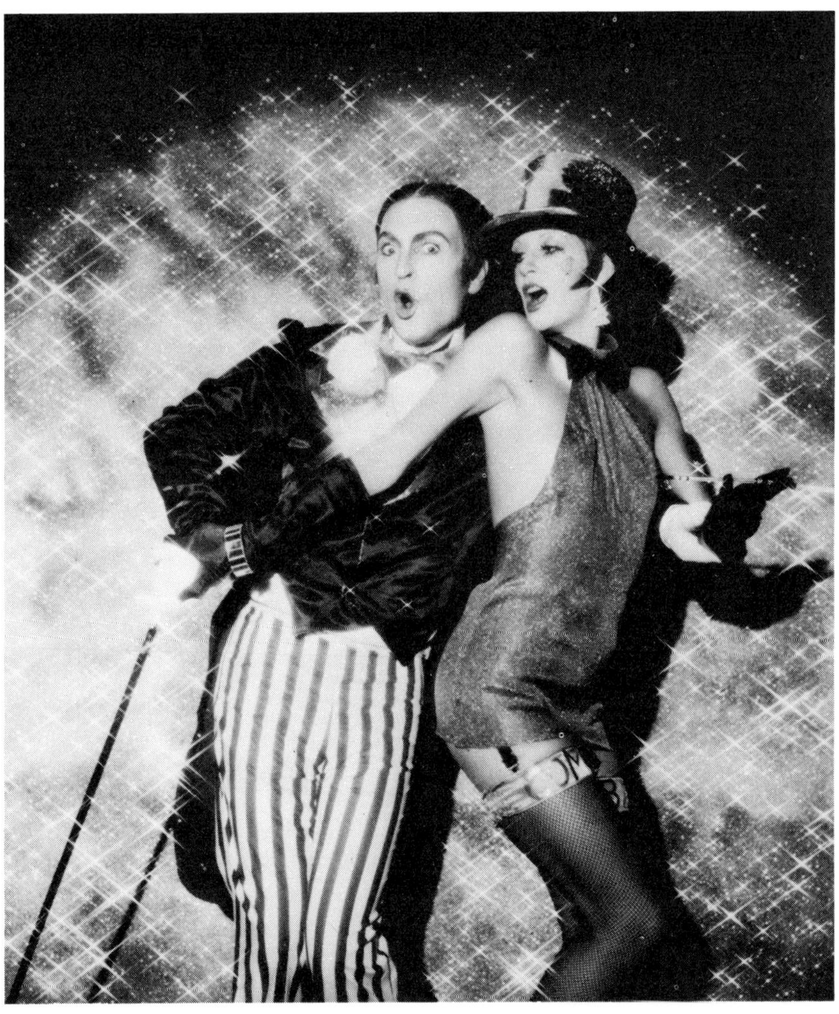

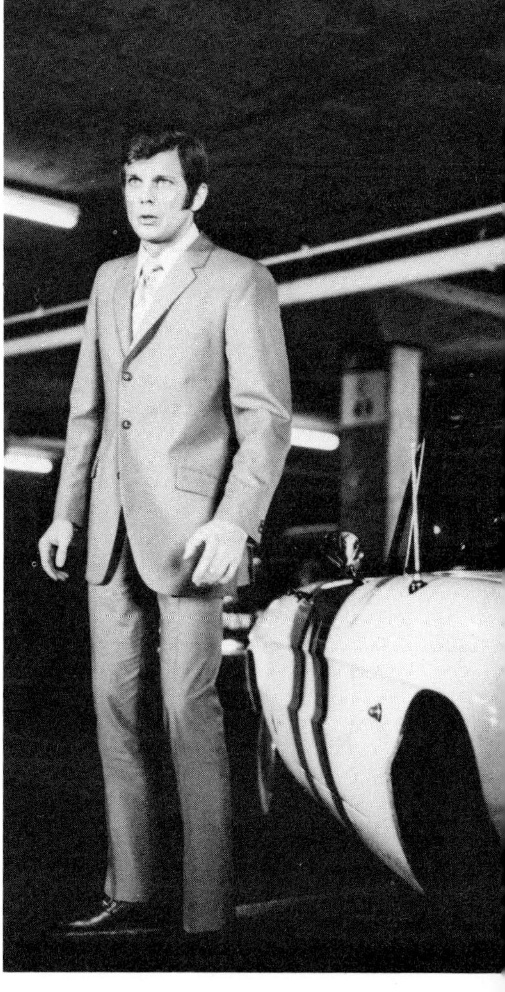

model girls as well. The male model side of Gavin's agency is run by another English top male model, Gil Barber, one of the most versatile of male models, who has appeared in every type of advertisement and a variety of fashion shows throughout Britain and Europe. Patrick Bashford, Tony Newton, and Derek Nesbitt are the current top male models in London. Tony Newton's masculine good looks are in demand in Europe as much as in London. He spends as much time travelling between Italy, France, and Germany for the top photographers and fashion houses as he does in Britain.

Although male modelling is not as competitive as the distaff side of the profession, the strongest threat to the model boy is the actor or movie star whose reputation and famous image is highly sought after by well known advertisers. American Karl Held is one of the top earning actors in the modelling field today. He gave up living in California, where he was under contract to Warner Brothers and NBC, appearing as guest star in many American television series, including *Perry Mason* and *FBI*, to settle in London with his actress wife Sarah Marshall. As well as appearing on British television, in films, and with the Royal Shakespeare Company, he is now under a life-time ex-clusive contract to appear in a well known series of television and film commercials in every European capital. He has signed one of those exclusive American-type contracts, normally reserved for the Lauren Huttons and Margaux Hemingways, agreeing to drink none other than their own world famous beverage in any form of advertising for the rest of his life! His gaunt masculinity and pale blue eyes guarantee him a record annual income.

Burt Reynolds, too, has appeared as a male model, but his contribution to *Cosmopolitan*'s centre-fold was more to delight readers with his physical attributes than to endorse a well known product!

The Calendar Girls

Although commercial calendars originated in Victorian times, the first calendar girl did not appear until 1912. She was an American girl, Julie Phillips, living in Paris, and was discovered in a Parisian café by the celebrated French artist Paul Chabas, who asked her to pose for him. He produced his painting *Matinée de Septembre* of Julie Phillips bathing in the morning mist of a French lake, and sent it on to New York where it shocked the Americans to learn that the subject depicted was the flower of American maidenhood.

This painting, which was copied and parodied by many artists throughout the United States, appeared on matchboxes, posters, and postcards as well, but it was not until the forties that the real commercial value of girls on calendars was realised. *Esquire* magazine's contract artist, Alberto Varga, had produced a considerable number of colour reproductions of oil paintings, but the technique was developed by several other artists who used live models as their subjects. The most notable artists were the Americans Rolf Armstrong, who produced cowgirls in pastel, Earl Moran, whose curvaceous beauties appeared on Brown and Bigelows calendars for over twenty-five years, and Zoë Mozert, herself a former model, whose typical American glamour girls smiled down from calendars for over thirty years. It was very much the period of inoffensive, wholesome beauties who bore broad smiles and buxom breasts. The models resembled the perfect Hollywood musical beauties of the fifties, emerging with wide-eyed, innocent looks, revealing stocking-tops and suspenders from skirts blown by lusty gusts of wind!

Gilette Elvgren, who rose to success with his illustrations of girls in early Coca-Cola advertisements, preferred to paint his girls from his own colour photographs. Across the Atlantic Ocean, his English counterpart, Archibald Dickens, chose a more elegant looking model, blonde, blue-eyed and innocent, with clean, wholesome lines.

Total nudity was never considered acceptable to advertisers, and this was confirmed by a slump in sales when their girlie calendars revealed a little too much. However, the look of calendars was revolutionised when the young

Golden Dreams, the classic calendar pin-up which helped to launch Marilyn Monroe in 1951

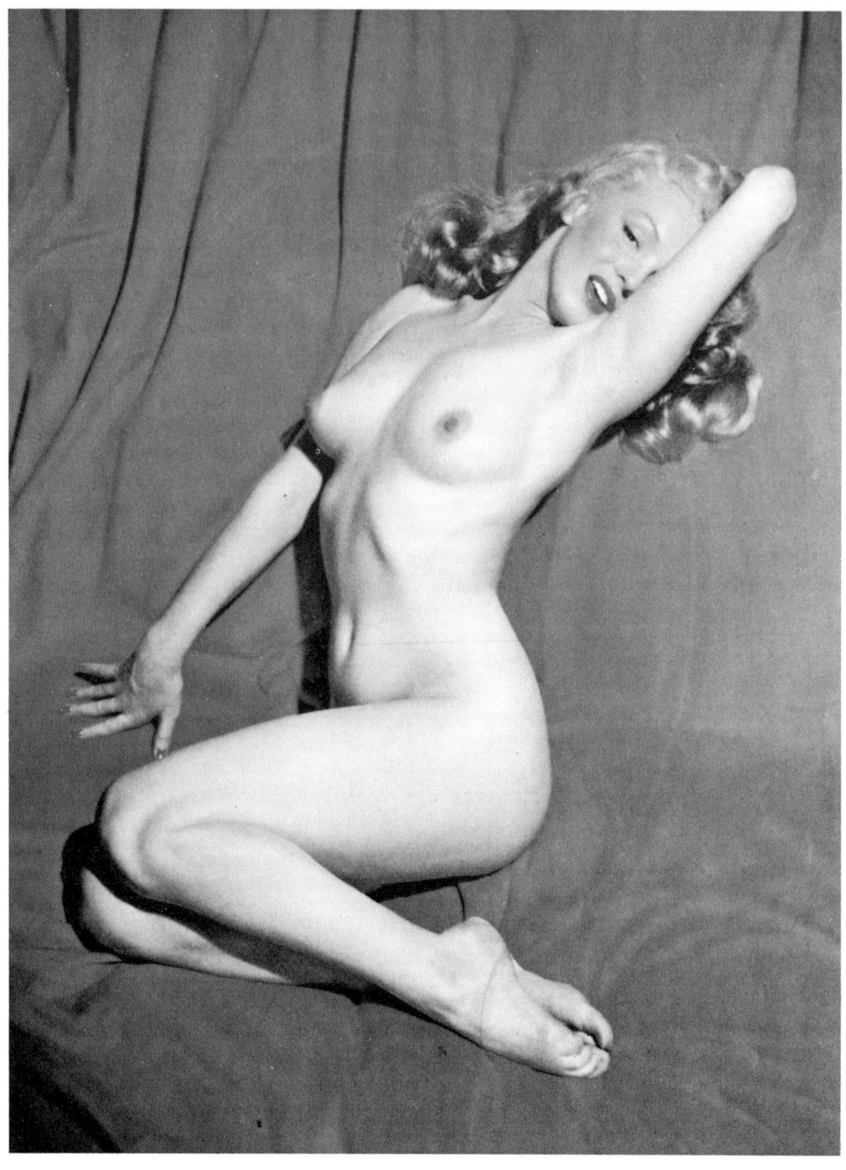

Californian photographer, Tom Kelley, produced the now famous nude photograph of Norma Jean Baker, the model who became better known as Marilyn Monroe, posed in her birthday-best against a vivid red background. The Golden Dreams calendar went on to sell eight million copies, and, despite many subsequent attempts by artists and models to recapture or copy this pose, it has never been equalled.

With the advent of the first photographic nude picture of Marilyn Monroe came the famous Petty girls who appeared in *Esquire* magazine. The artist Petty produced girls revealing sensual, sexy breasts and buttocks, voluptuous girls in sailor suits with firecrackers ready to explode. Today's calendar girls look almost nun-like by comparison. The Petty girls were certainly the fore-runners of the saucy seductresses seen much later in calendar form.

The sophisticated glamour of the Pirelli calendar became an art form, heralded by advertisers, photographers, and artists. Derek Forsyth was the first Pirelli calendar art director, and together with designer Derek Birdsall they produced the first 35,000 copies of the calendar for distribution in January 1964. They were clearly conscious of the importance of the selection of top photographers, and so chose Robert Freeman, who had worked with the Beatles, for the first series.

The models, throughout the ten-year Pirelli calendar run, were chosen from model agencies, and the majority, perhaps, from Lucie Clayton in London, which selected girls who, although reticent about appearing in fashion advertisements in underwear, were more courageous on beaches in swimwear. Although Frenchman Peter Knapp, *Elle's* leading fashion photographer, the third photographer chosen by Pirelli, produced the 1966 calendar, photographed in Morocco, their second-year choice was Brian Duffy. Duffy chose the South of France for his daring young beauties on the beaches, yet surprisingly enough, although Pirelli developed such an international reputation for its calendar girls, Duffy did not reveal *one* bare breast in the 1965 edition.

However, he did reveal a little more when he was invited to produce photographs for the 1973 edition. He chose a London art gallery for his background, and produced photographs of remarkable artistic merit. However, Duffy was put-out, to say the least, when he discovered what art director Allen Jones had done to his photographs with his

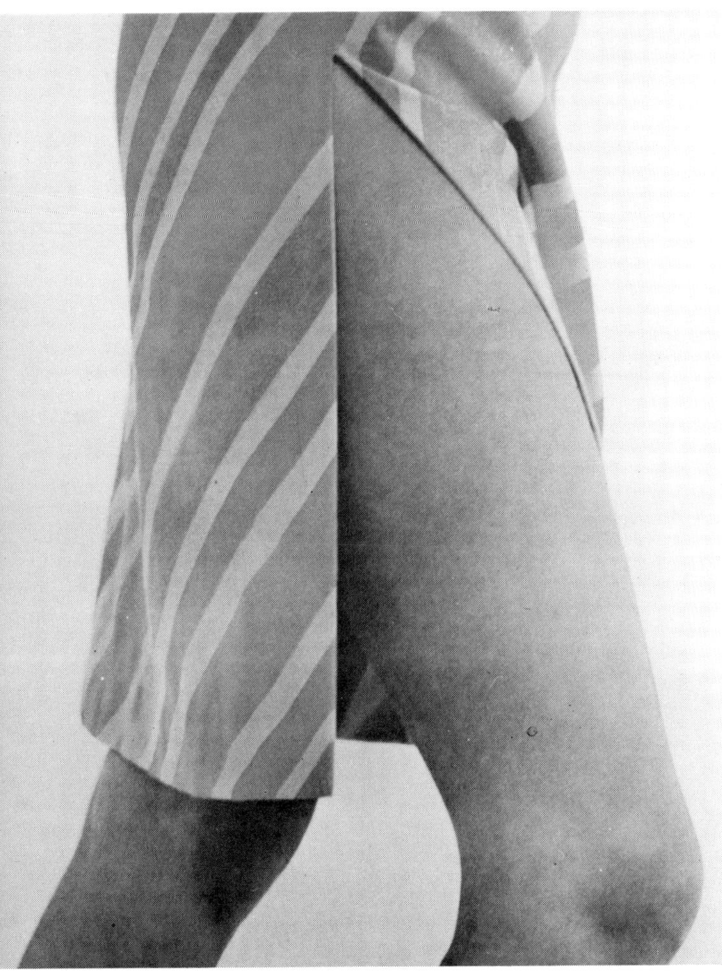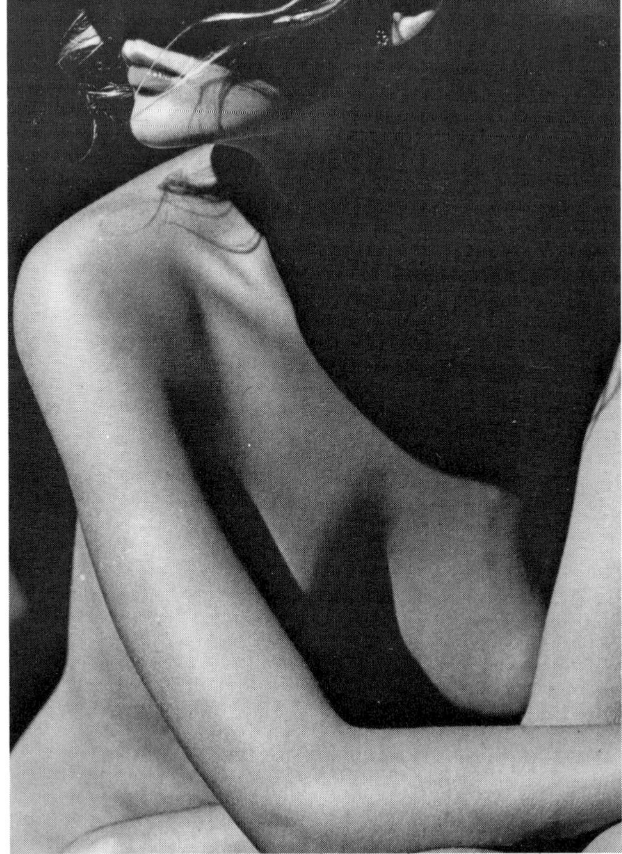

Shots from the first and last Pirelli calendars. This classic series, which appeared from 1964-74, elevated the calendar into an art form. Courtesy Pirelli (UK) Ltd

Right: Once Pirelli had shown the way, other manufacturers were quick to follow. Some, like this Avon calendar of 1971, tried to keep at least some link with their products! Courtesy Avon Tyre Co Ltd

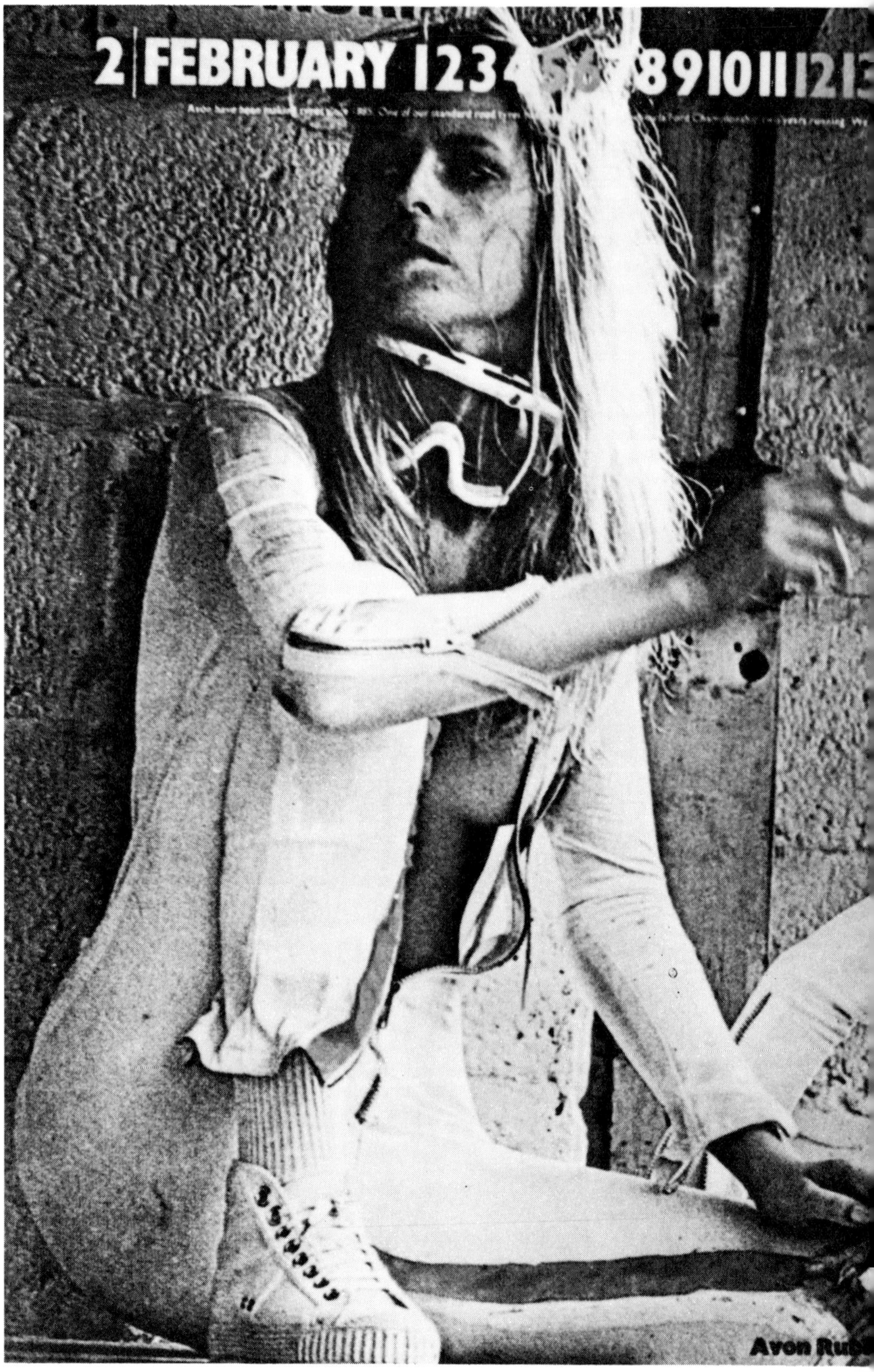

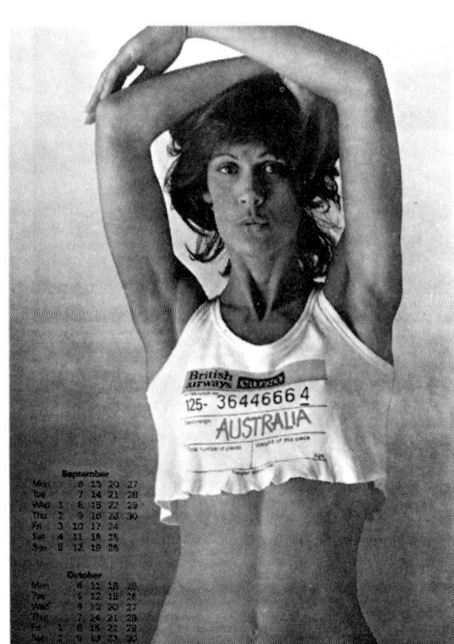

colour-brush and, rebelling against this interference with his work, refused to appear at the press conference.

What was intended as the sensual erotica in this penultimate edition of Pirelli calendars emerged as too arty for the press and critics who felt cheated out of visual titillation.

And so 1974 saw the last of the famous Pirelli calendars. The Swiss photographer, Hans Feurer, one of French *Vogue's* top fashion photographers, was chosen to fly to the Seychelles with his models, but for all that the photographs were produced in mid-shot or close-ups of heads and might just as well have been done in his Paris studio.

Pirelli had triumphed over its competitors. The other leading tyre manufacturers, like Firestone, Dunlop, Avon, and Motorway, had themsevles attempted to rise to the Pirelli heights but failed to get into its league. However, in explaining why his company had taken the step in ceasing publication of their famous calendars, Italian managing director Antonio Rosetti said: 'The enormous world-wide public interest which has developed in our calendar has reached far beyond the basic reason for its introduction ten years ago, that of promoting our name in all markets in which our products are sold.' A stronger

Below: A page from the calendar photographed by Tony Page for the Esso Petroleum Company

Opposite: A subtle combination of client's name and model by Sam Haskins for British Airways Cargo Division

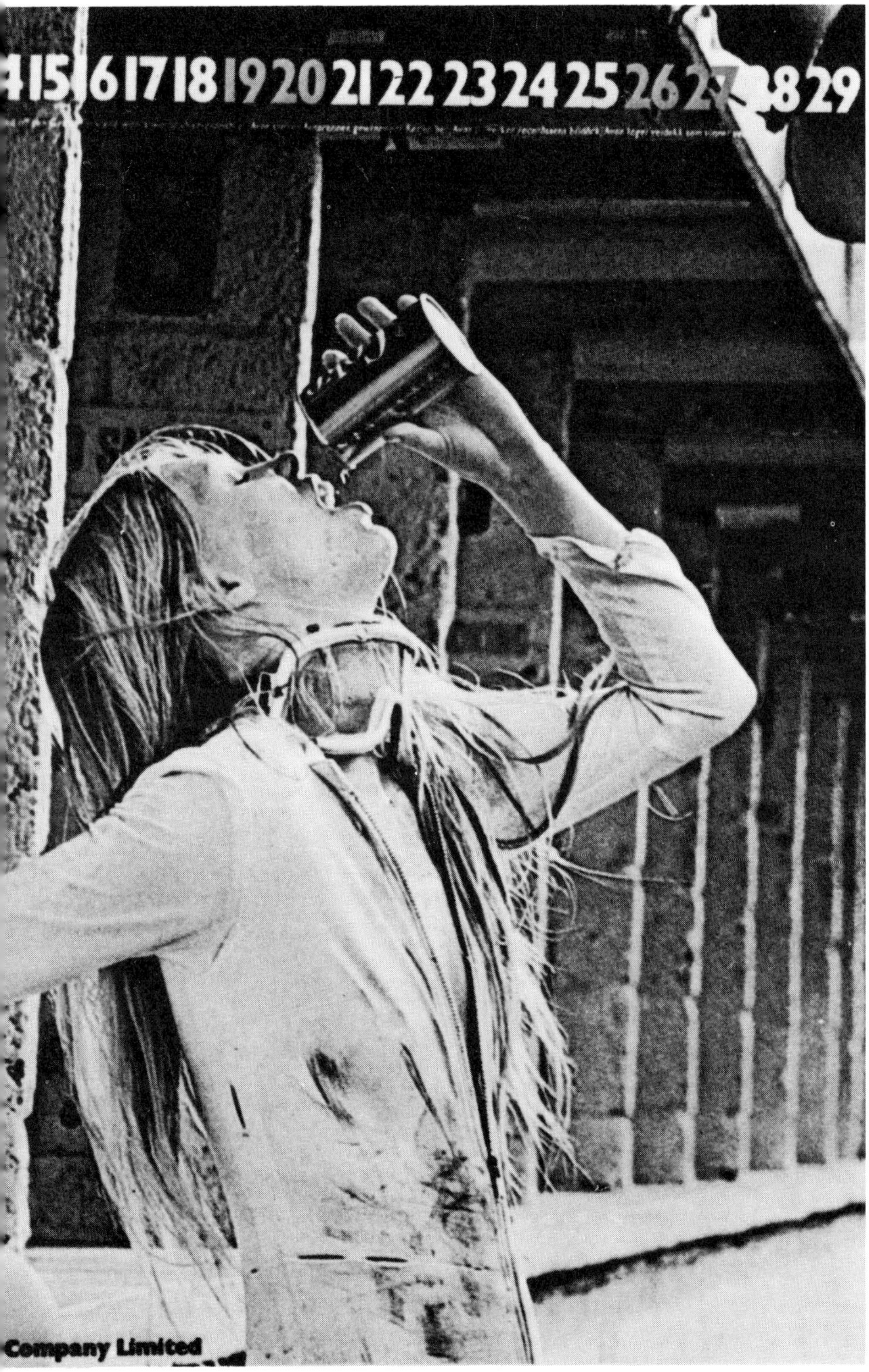

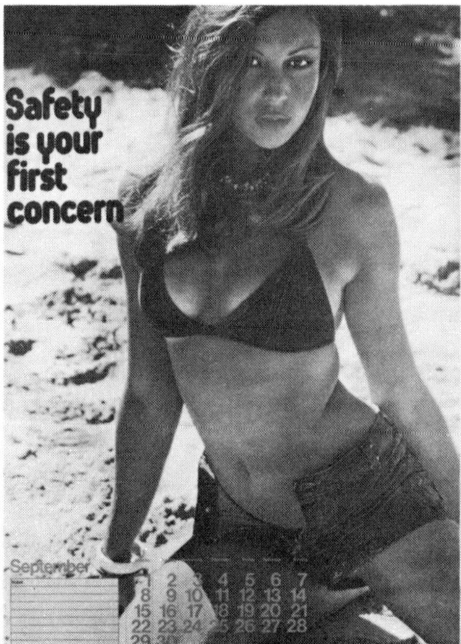

means of advertising was now sought by them, and although appreciating that from the public's point of view their calendar had become a phenomenon, they were withdrawing whilst they were still on top.

That year, Pirelli put up for sale a complete set of calendars at Christie's in London, where it was hoped at least £1,000 would be raised for charity. 'A collection', as Christie's catalogued the calendars, 'of pictures of not always the most beautiful women, but certainly the most interesting and desirable', fetched £504.

However, the story of the calendar girl does not end there. Lord Snowdon produced a calendar for ICI of remarkable aesthetic quality. He photographed ballet dancers, representative of various ballet roles, in the English countryside, introducing inventive and breathtaking imagery to the calendar art-form. Other big industrial names such as Esso, Castrol, Chrysler, Godfrey Davies, and Lambs Navy Rum continue to supply the demand for calendars. Year by year, calendars of smiling, buxomy sensual, and tantalising teasers are hung in offices, garages, pubs, and on any available hook or nail where discerning male eyes feel the urge for a little provocative fantasy.

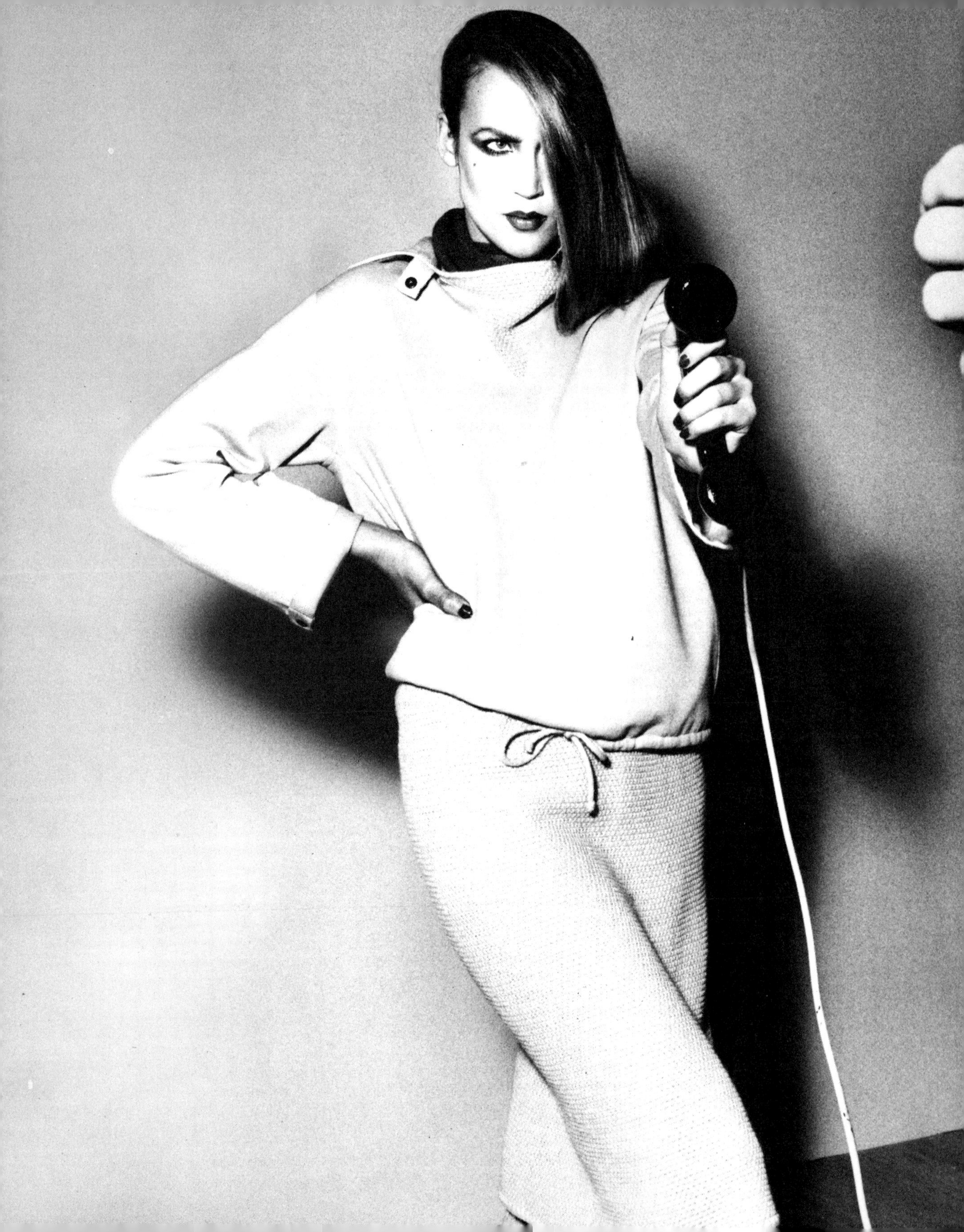

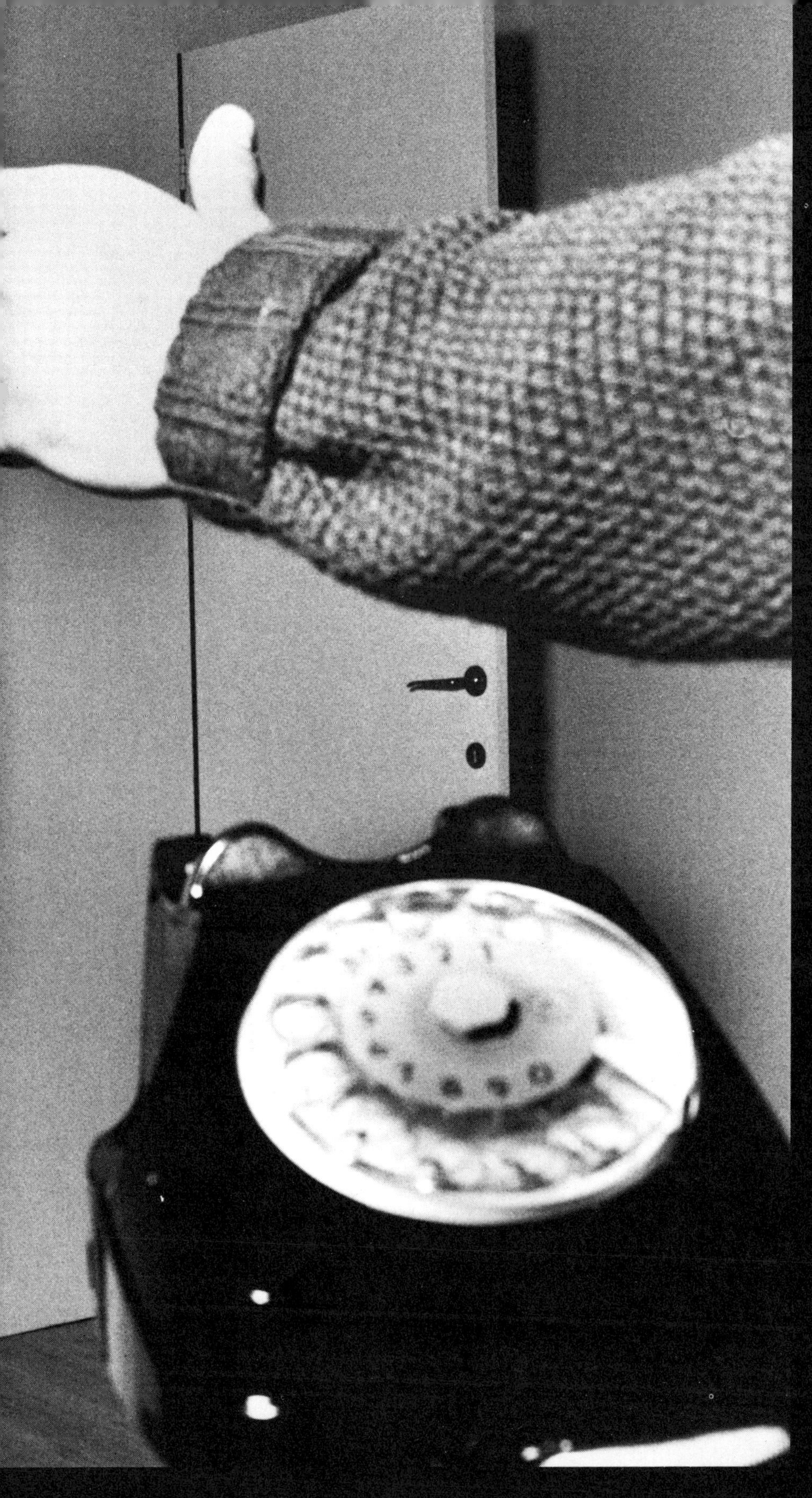

Creating
an Illusion

The model is 60 per cent of the photo-graph, and the photographer is the vita link between fashion and the media Fashion editors commission photog-raphers, hire the models after consulta-tion with the photographers, and choose the clothes and accessories. The photog-rapher often suggests his own choice o model and many top photographers wil refuse to work with models they don' like. They have a powerful role. ' usually work with friends', says Davic Bailey candidly. 'They don't give trouble. I don't work with difficul models; if they give me trouble, that' the last time they work for me.'

The list of top fashion photographers in the last fifty years is impressive Edward Steichen was the first to photo-graph a live model for publication ir Paris in 1913, and became the highes paid member of *Vogue's* staff until he was succeeded as top photographer fo Condé Nast Publications by Baror Gayne de Meyer.

Adolf de Meyer's camera defined the beauty and elegance of the 1920s. He helped to set the taste of an era, and ir the course of so doing, established a new genre—fashion photography. This ha never, to this day, ceased to show hi influence with his remarkable style o back-lighting his subjects, giving them an almost three-dimensional effect. O. unknown origin, but generally though to be German, de Meyer was an eccen-tric, the *poseur* or *boulevardier* incarnat —and the embodiment of the *belle epoque* that saw him rise from obscurity marry a great beauty, acquire a title through a whim of King Edward VII and achieve a formidable reputation as a gentleman photographer. He worked for *Vogue* and later for *Harpers Bazaa* for over a decade, and his style was sc entirely distinctive that his bold signature on his many photographs of exquisite women and famous men was hardly necessary. A photographic pioneer and authentic genius of the camera, he betrayed his own art-form by refusing to acknowledge his craft when he moved into the higher echelons of society, becoming a frightful snob in the process.

Russian-born George Hoyningen-Huene was one of the great photographers in the twenties and thirties, de Meyer's natural successor. He was a superlative portrait photographer, and his fashion photography too has the style and depth of great works of art. He turned to film-lighting when he went to Hollywood, where he joined veteran movie director George Cukor as his adviser on many movies of great distinction.

Hoyningen-Huene's great protégé, Horst, who inherited the Russian's remarkable photographic archives, succeeded him in the thirties, working for *Vogue* as fashion photographer until the war. He rejoined *Vogue* after serving in the US army and became the first to photograph many of the great models in New York in the late forties and fifties.

While Man Ray did venture into fashion work, his inventive, avant-garde photography with shapes and irregular dimensions, dominated any fashion work he might have undertaken. Although Man Ray was born in America, he lived most of his adult life in France, except during the war years. He was a central figure in the Surrealist and Dadaist movements and a close friend and collaborator of Duchamp, Picabia, Ernst, Breton, and Eluard. He has stood at the centre of European and American modernism since about 1911, as a painter, conjurer of magical and poetic objects, inventor, and photographer. Few contemporary artists have played such a vital role in the creation of imaginative visual realities.

The artist who has achieved more than any other living photographer is Sir Cecil Beaton, who was a great innovator in Paris in the twenties and thirties. After the war he worked consistently for *Vogue* in New York. He goes down in history as one of the great figures of our time, his contributions to fashion and the theatre as photographer

and designer, as well as author of many works on the great periods of fashion, being some of his finest achievements in the fine and applied arts.

Of the Americans, Louise Dahl Wolf was one of the forerunners, followed by Richard Avedon, Irving Penn, Erwin Blumenfeld, Clifford Coffin, and John Rawlings, as the exceptional photographers of fashion. 'The greatest fashion photographer, I think, is Irving Penn', says Lord Snowdon, formerly Tony Armstrong-Jones, whose own contribution to the applied arts as a photographer is of the highest order in Britain. 'Penn has got impeccable clarity. He influenced me tremendously. I love him as a person, and respect his work enormously. He is a quiet, humble, sweet man.'

Penn, however, has a distinct dislike of models, even though his wife, Lisa Fonsagrieves, was perhaps one of the

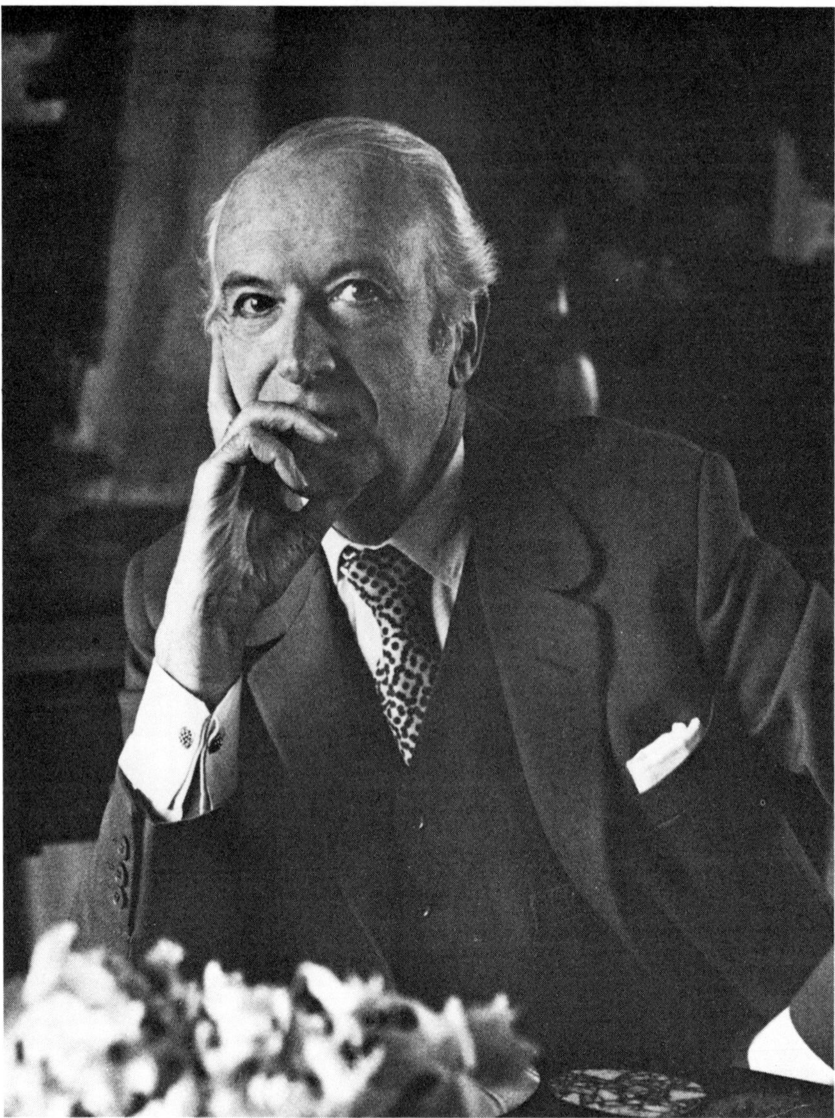

Above: Sir Cecil Beaton, the great theatrical designer and fashion photographer whose work has spanned five decades. Photograph by Louanne Richards

Opposite: A photograph of Dovima characteristic of Cecil Beaton's eye for imagery and composition

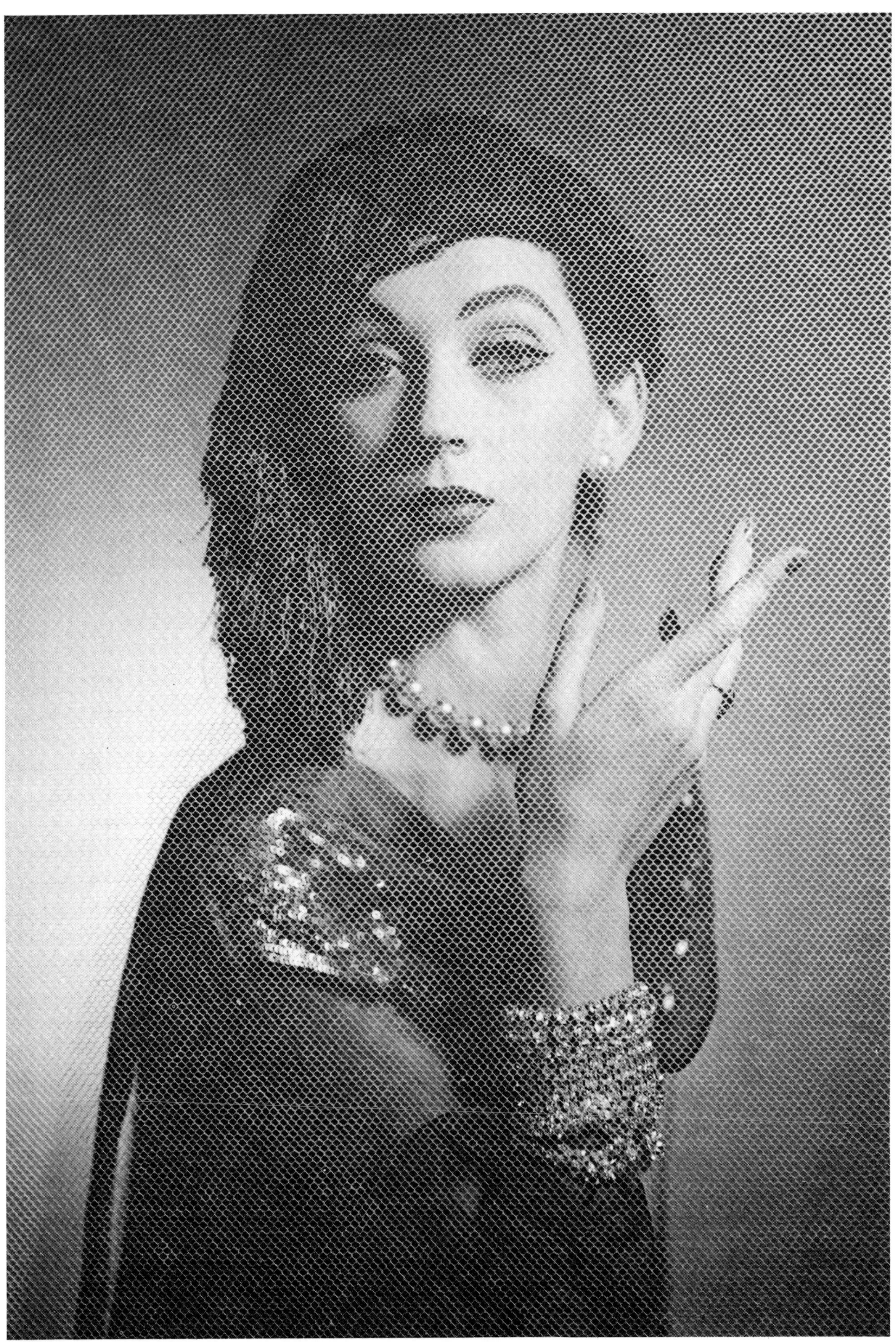

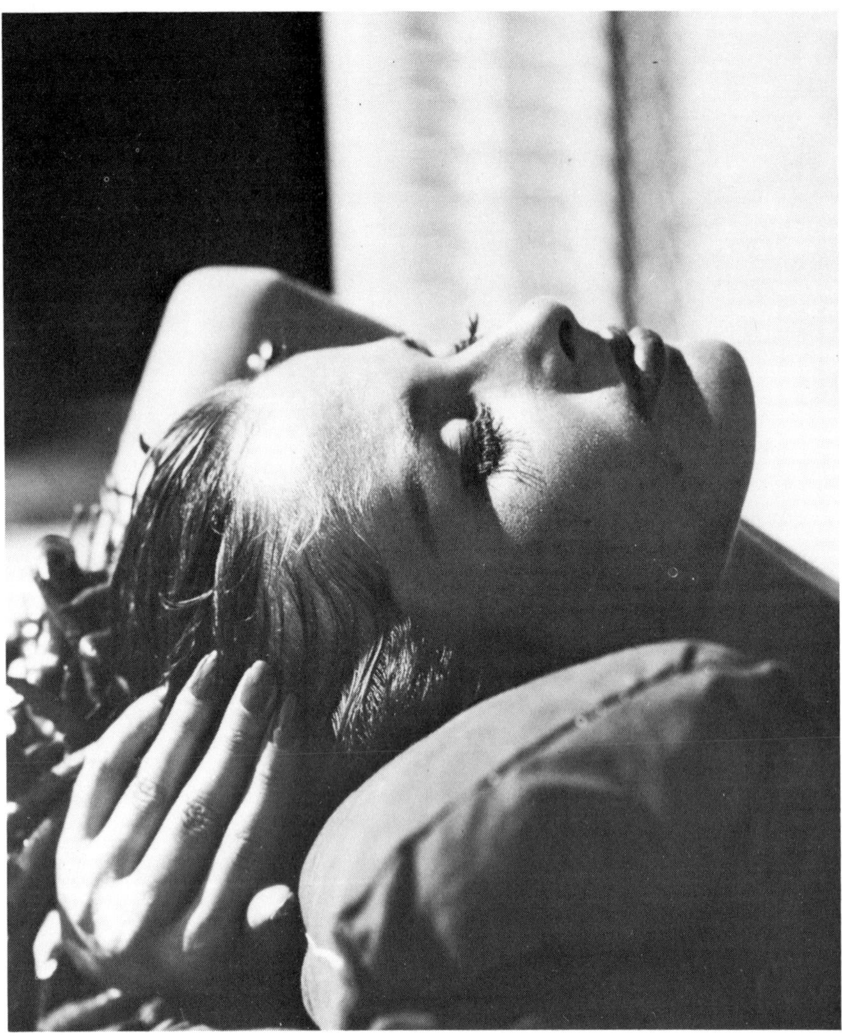

Above: The Finnish model Tamara, photographed by Henry Clarke

best models of all time, reigning in Paris in the thirties and New York in the forties and fifties. Models find it impossible to communicate with this great advocate of models in terms of imagery, and he refuses to discuss them for fear of being disparaging. 'I do not want to talk about models', he says. 'To photograph them is enough.'

The only models Penn worked with were lady-like; he has an intense dislike of vulgarity and will have no association with models he suspects of promiscuity. Jean Patchett was one of his ideals as a model, not only because of her exquisite looks, but because of her unquestionable private and professional behaviour. Another top model who worked with him practically every day for six years complains that he never once thanked her or said he was happy with her work at the end of the day. 'However, he did give me a kiss one Christmas because I returned from Chicago three times for a retake', she laughs. 'I thought the secretary and assistant would pass out.

That's how removed he wants to stay from models. He can't stand them. If he were to discuss models he would hate himself afterwards for telling the truth. Penn does not lie!'

Blumenfeld and Coffin, although being superlative fashion photographers, lasted only a short while. Blumenfeld had a row with American *Vogue's* editor, Alex Lieberman, bringing to an end his brilliant career, and Coffin became unpopular with models and fashion editors alike. Wilhelmina recalls that Clifford Coffin was the first photographer she ever worked with in New York—because all the other models refused to work with him. He had genius, though, and was a master when it came to creating lighting. 'He was a wierd, wild man', Wilhelmina adds. 'He used to throw the editors down the staircase.' You were afraid to disagree with him, and you never let him get close to you under any circumstances, because, as he was so creative with make-up, you weren't going to walk out of his studio looking the way you came in. He thought only of the picture he was going to take, and when it came out it was sensational. You looked like a different girl, but he ruined you for three weeks; nobody else bought you from what they saw in that picture, and nor would he. The following week he wouldn't want you that way. Having plucked all your eyebrows out, and drawn strange and wonderful images on your face, he would say, "Who plucked those eyebrows out!"'

In America top photographers come and go. John Rawlings made a model feel that there was nobody in the world like her. But if it was Bert Stern, the models pretended that the camera itself was human because he was so impersonal. Hiro, Sokolsky, Derujinski, Scavullo, Bill King, James Moore, Rico Pullman, Chris von Wangenheim, Debbie Turbeville, William Connors, Arthur Elgort, Steve Horan—the list of good American photographers is impressive.

The rapport between model and photographer is vital. Contact, and the ability to work together, is reflected in the finished photograph. In photographic modelling, the eyes are of utmost importance. Eyes are the means of communication; they are the first contact one has with people in life as well as

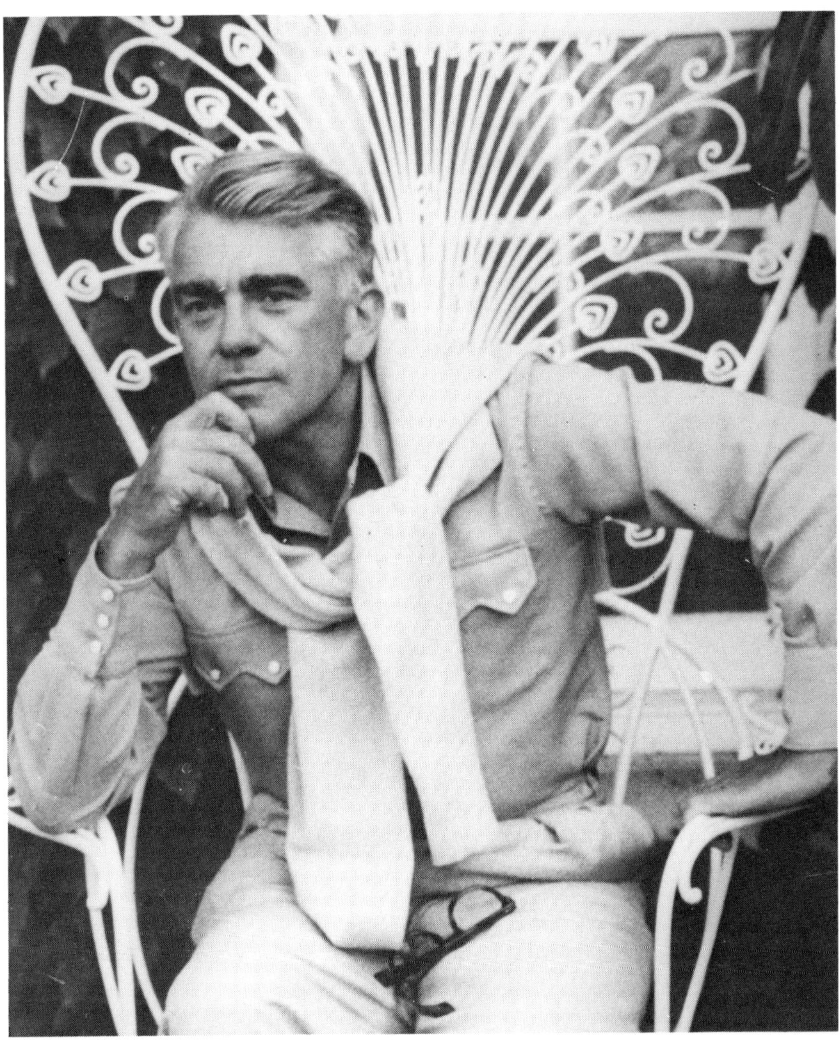

Left: The great German photographer, Horst, taken by Ian Graham

in photography. 'The camera is somebody that you pretend is there', says Wilhelmina. 'It's the wonderful attitude of flirting with the camera that works, but it's not easy.'

German-born Horst is one of the most powerful and long-lasting photographers in New York today. He studied applied art in Hamburg and architecture in Paris in the early thirties before moving into photography. Today he is the most well known and valued member of *Vogue*'s photographic staff. His photographs have appeared not only in English, French, American, and Italian *Vogue* and in *House and Garden*, but also in many other European and American magazines. He was the first to photograph Dorian Leigh, Suzy Parker, Sunny Harnett, Lauren Hutton, Veruschka, and many others.

Born Horst Boormann, he changed his name to Horst P. Horst when Hitler's notorious henchman of the same name came into prominence in the thirties. Horst, who was George Hoyningen-

Huene's protégé, began photography by chance. They were lunching in Paris one day, and were joined by Erich, a great artist who used to do fashion drawings of the collections for *Vogue*. He suggested Horst try photography, but as Horst had neither a camera, experience, knowledge about fashion nor acquaintanceships with fashionable women, he was reluctant. However, he went to a studio three times a week, and, with the help of an assistant who handled the technicalities, he tried his luck. His guinea pig was the model Agnetta Fisher, and when he succeeded in selling his first and subsequent fashion photographs, he launched himself into this new-found career, under Hoyningen-Huene's critical and helpful guidance.

Horst photographs by instinct and imagination. 'Sometimes you have a vision, when travelling, for instance. You see a painting or a statue, and then start dreaming about it. When you come to photograph a model, you try to re-

produce that image.' When he met Chanel, he had never seen her before. She arrived at his studio in Paris to be photographed, but she was displeased with the result. 'It's a very good photograph, but the dress is nothing to do with me', she complained. And so she asked Horst to dinner, so that he could discover how she lived and how she moved. He was then able to arrive at the right photograph for her, capturing her mood. It became her favourite photograph.

'You have to start off with an idea', Horst advises. 'I feel myself into the person and the situation, and that goes for fashion too. I feel what the dress is supposed to mean, what possibility that dress has pictorially.' He relies on lighting for mood and effect, managing to bring out the qualities of both model and garment alike. Whereas Irving Penn manages to hide a woman's sexuality, or Richard Avedon reveals her bi-sexuality, Horst conveys her femininity.

Next to Horst, Irving Penn, and Richard Avedon, Francesco Scavullo is the top fashion photographer in New York today. His apprenticeship was spent as Horst's assistant in 1948, and he branched out on his own to photograph for *Seventeen* magazine. The teenage models he photographed were unknown, but he worked consistently for magazines, catalogues, and advertising. Jackie Michelle, Sandy Brown, Anne Murray, and Pat Gehagen were the models who worked with Scavullo at the time. He went on to work for *Today's Woman*, *McCall's*, and *Ladies Home Journal*, with his ex-wife, Carol Macausen, as his favourite model, and progressed to *Harpers Bazaar*, on the *Junior Bazaar* side, working with Iris Bianchi, Sandy Brown, Sandra Peterson—and Dolores Hawkins, who was one of the top models in the fifties. He then worked for *Harpers* proper, with his favourite model in the sixties, Agnetta Darren.

'A good model is like a thoroughbred horse', Scavullo defines. 'But a thoroughbred has got to have a good rider. And a good model has to have a good photographer.' His ideal model has to have big eyes, full lips, and good hair. She has to have good proportions and it is best if she's between 5ft 8in and 5ft 10in. 'It's difficult for small girls to do fashion. I don't mind if she has pimples', he continues, explaining that they can be retouched, but he prefers to have beautiful skin to photograph. Scavullo finds that girls between eighteen and twenty-five are the best to photograph. 'I love them when they're twenty-one!' But he prefers black models. 'They've got more style, more energy, more zoom.

'I like models to have an attitude; a sense of drama in front of the camera. And they need a sense of humour with the clothes the editors put on them these days. You've got to have a very good sense of humour to be a photographer, too!

'I like working for a good magazine and a good editor. If you've got that, and a good model with a good hairdresser and a good make-up man, you're as good as the team you're working for. At that point, the dress becomes unimportant, particularly when you consider the clothes they give you from Seventh Avenue to photograph. They're all uniforms!'

New Yorker Melvin Sokolsky began fashion photography because he felt the pictures he saw in magazines lacked individuality. His own first photographs were considered vulgar because he included articles such as an egg or a rubber band in the picture. *Harpers Bazaar* editors felt he was trying to make a rude comment. 'But that wasn't what I was trying to say', protests Sokolsky. 'It was purely because the shape interested me, and I was working in a purely visual level; there was no message I was trying to put over. Most of my pictures take place in my head, and I try to put what I see in my mind into the camera.

'What I look for in a model is something that's pure. Psychologically pure. Somebody that hasn't been broken by a bad childhood, or, if she has, someone who can overcome that and can arouse my feelings.

'Illusion is the relationship you get with somebody when they are prepared to show you something of themselves; the aspects of how they think or feel; whereas another person would photograph that girl and find that she's withdrawn and can't move. It's creating a kind of work/love affair.'

Sokolsky finds photographic lighting fascinating and regrets the fixed, mechanical lighting system used nowadays. 'I always changed lights and used them to find a place in reality. It was always creating new ways of lighting and seeing people in new ways with different kinds of light that interested me. When the sixties ended people began to get uptight and began to show things in less of an illusionary manner, and started taking pictures straight on with strobe lights. Then there was a cycle for the editors as well as for the models where they didn't want to be repressed that way either; there was a whole new world in the sixties of what I call children models', with Twiggy leading the field.

Sokolsky believes that ten years as a fashion photographer ought to be enough, otherwise it becomes destructive. 'I don't think that in the last ten years Dick Avedon has said anything in his work', he claims. 'I think that the years before that, some of the best fashion photographs ever done came

Donna Mitchell, by Melvin Sokolsky

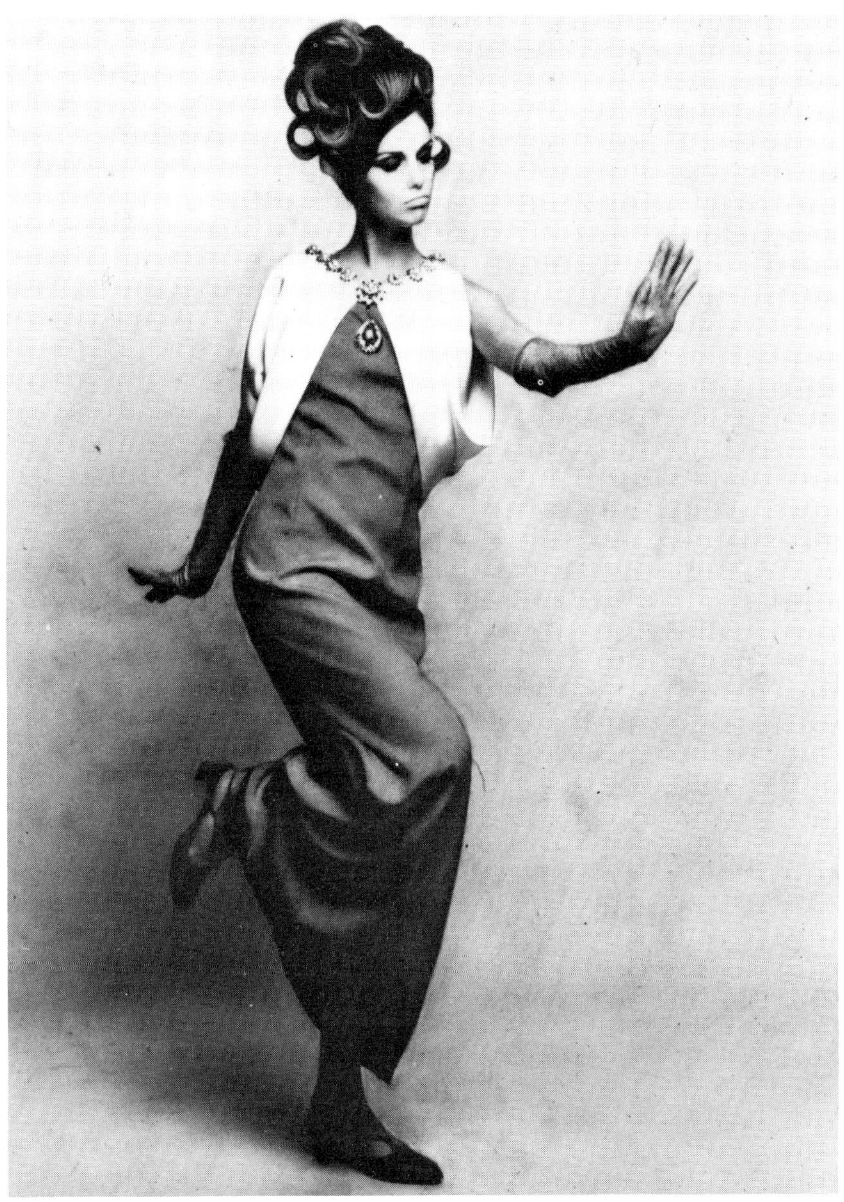

from Avedon and I believe that he has become jaded by repeating the same thing.

'It is the learning process that brings in new ideas, and when one settles down from that learning process, it tapers off, and that's why I moved off. But when I go back to it periodically, I enjoy it, because there's a relationship that you have with a model when you're working together that you can't have in a real life relationship.'

Sokolsky finally gave up fashion photography when, in the late sixties, he felt trapped by the magazine editors' policies and opinions. 'Do that picture again. It's too strange', they would say. 'Do that one again', and they gave other reasons for finding fault in his work. He returned to *Vogue* briefly when he found another model, called Ushi, who he

thought was 'fabulous'. She was a German girl who had sent Richard Avedon a picture of herself a year earlier. Avedon replied saying that he would like to see her when she got to America. But when she got there, she went to see Sokolsky instead, who booked her for a week. 'Avedon, my censor, called up to say that he wanted to photograph her first. I explained that I had a studio full of people and was about to begin working with the girl. He threatened *Vogue* that either I left or he would go. They would have to choose. Naturally, they chose him. So he took one picture of her, and left her to stay at her hotel for ten days. Having exercised his prerogative, he wasn't interested in her anymore.'

Sokolsky gave up fashion photography for a new career in Los Angeles, as a television commercials director, but

after ten years away from the fashion industry he has a yen to return to photograph the new girls of the seventies.

Whereas Horst, Penn, Avedon, Blumenfeld, Coffin, Rawlings, and Louise Dahl Wolf were the star fashion photographers in America in the fifties and sixties, Norman Parkinson, John French, and Richard Dormer reigned in Britain. Parkinson stands alone with his individual style and presentation, taking full advantage of the breathtaking settings he finds throughout the world, hues of pinks, reds, and oranges often dominating his work. But although he is one of the best, few people know about him. 'I'm the *best* unknown photographer', he admits.

The late John French began fashion photography because he could not make a living as an artist. Before he took up photography he used to do illustrations. His first work for the *Daily Express* was a series in 1937. During the war he was in the army in Italy and the Middle East, but he never seriously considered doing anything but photography when the war ended. His most famous model was Barbara Goalen, with whom his name has been linked since they first started working together in 1948. 'At one time, I would only be photographed by John French', admits Barbara Goalen. 'I loved him dearly. I found him terribly easy to work with and he always did such attractive photographs of people. He was a very sweet, gentle man. He had a good sense of humour and was totally meticulous. He was frightfully neat and beautifully dressed. He always looked fabulous—the exact opposite of the way photographers look these days!'

Richard Dormer was another product of the fifties and has worked in high-

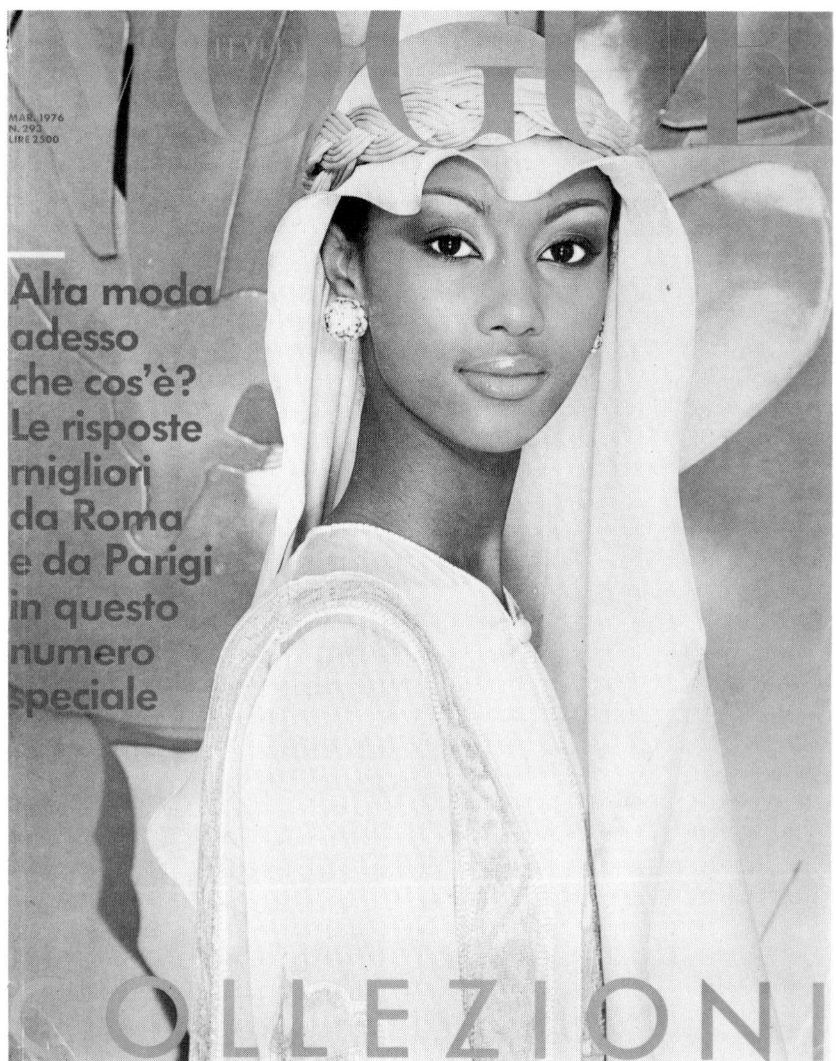

Above: Imen, by the renowned English photographer, Norman Parkinson. Perhaps one of the greatest fashion photographers of all. Courtesy *Vogue*/Italy

Opposite above: John French with his leading models over twenty-five years, photographed by Terence Donovan for the *Daily Express*.

Back row: Joy Weston; Sandra Paul; Mrs Edward Pickering (Rosemary Whitton); Mrs Charles Parnell (Shelagh Wilson); Lady Royle (Shirley Worthington); Princess George Galitzine (Jean Dawnay); Jennifer Hocking; Rosalind Watkins.

Centre row: Mrs Robert Nesbitt (Iris Lockwood) and, in front of her, Mrs R. McAlpine (Rosemary Chance); Mrs Nigel Campbell (Barbara Goalen); Celia Hammond; Mrs Somerset de Chair (Sylvia Shelley); Mrs Sportoletti-Baduel who as Marla Landi starred in many films; Mrs Harold Bamberg (June Clarke); Tania Mallet; Evelyn Spilsbury.
Front row: Patti Boyd; Mrs Rachel Severne; Lady Hastings (Katie Hinton); Mrs John Heine (Jackie Cahill); Mrs Laurence Harvey (Paulene Stone)

Opposite below: John French in 1957. Photograph/Snowdon

fashion photography for the past twenty-five years. London-born, he went to Paris after the war and began taking hand-cut photographs for the Paris couture houses. Maxine and Alan de la Farge, who ran a public relations company, took him on and he undertook public relations photography for them.

Ernestine Carter, then the fashion editor of English *Harpers Bazaar*, saw his work and invited him to London to work for *Harpers*. As *Harpers* and *Vogue* had recently closed down their photographic studios, Dormer paid John French a commission for the use of his studio and dark-room facilities on a freelance basis. Barbara Goalen was the model who helped Dormer to reach international recognition as a photographer.

Richard Dormer maintains that a model is 60 per cent of a photograph, and that she helps to establish the photographer's reputation. 'You cannot work with a bad model, no matter how good you are; you can't get anything out of her. The good model is a vital factor in your work, and you have to have sympathy together, otherwise you can't work together.'

Dormer finds that models are underestimated as a profession, and that photographers are divided into two or three categories. He is not a creator of models and never likes to work with new or unprofessional ones. He prefers girls who know their job, so that together they can produce good work. 'Somebody like Norman Parkinson has created many models', Dormer says. 'He likes absolutely raw clay. There are a number of girls who "Parks" really has discovered. Seeing them selling cosmetics in Selfridges he selects them and produces them. Richard Avedon is somebody like myself, who only likes working with professional people.'

In America, a girl is not sent on the road until she knows her business. Eileen Ford, one of the world's top model agents, does not take on a raw model. She sees their photographs, and, if she thinks they will make the grade, grooms them and pushes them around the good studios to get them going.

Just as John French and Barbara Goalen 'clicked', so did Richard Dormer and Anne Gunning, producing their best work together. Anne was sent to

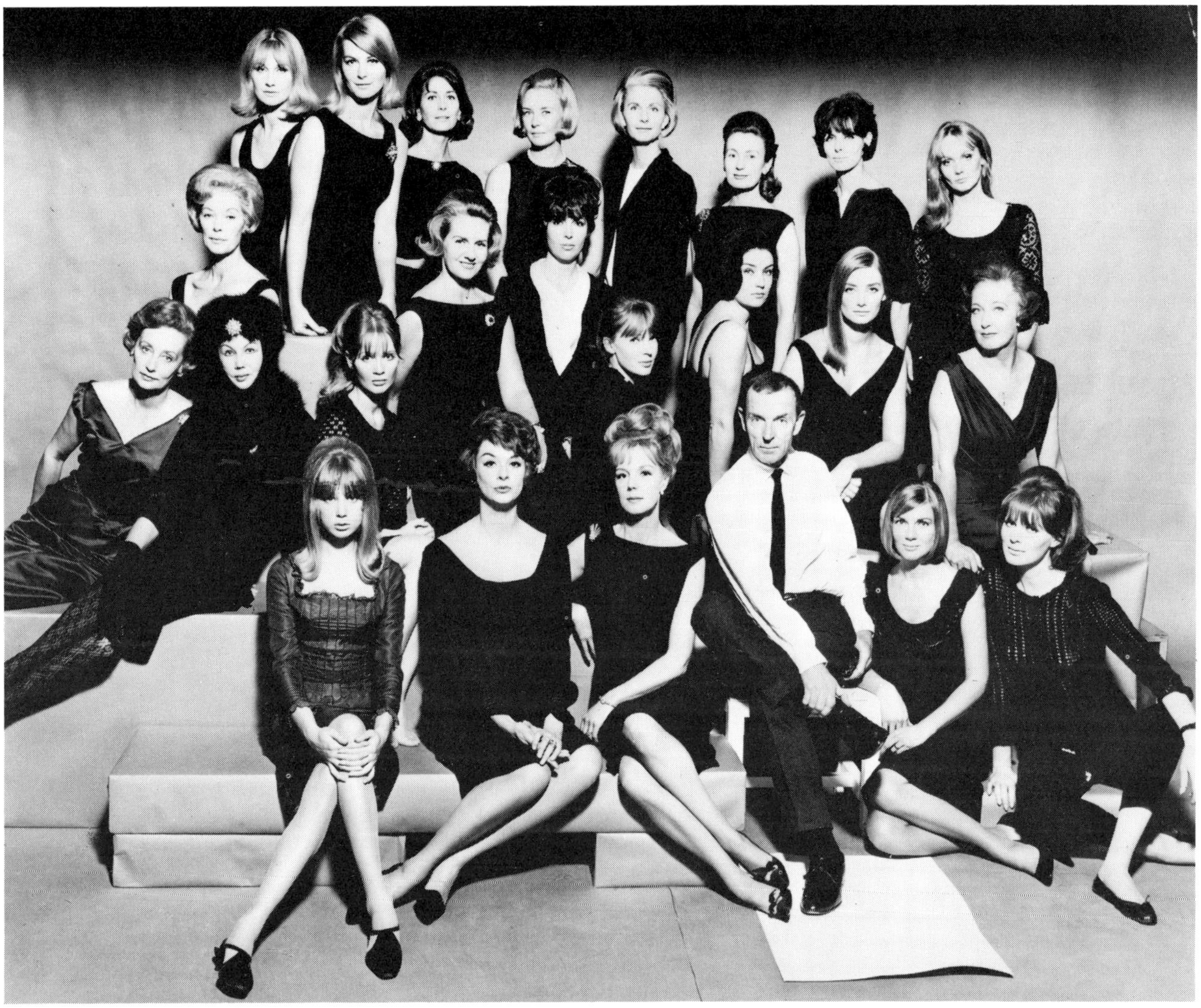

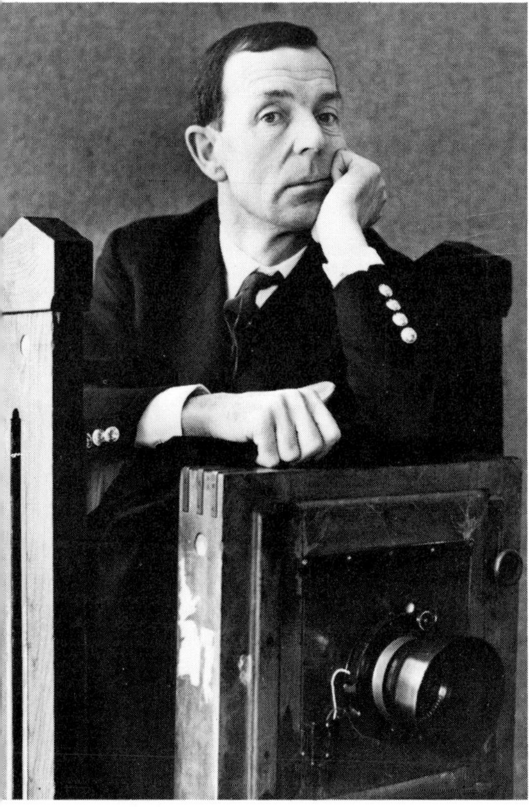

Dormer by John French's wife, Vere, who believed that Anne had the makings of a top model. She had been a Rank starlet, but had done nothing. Dormer photographed her for an advertisement, and found her absolutely terrified. He managed to calm her down, and they began working together. It was luck with Anne Gunning, who became one of Britain's best models in the fifties and worked successfully for many years. But Dormer, equally lucky to have found a good model, dreads the bad ones.

'To have a bad model forced on you against your will is the worst thing that can happen to a photographer. This only really happens in commercial work, when somebody insists you have the girl, either because it's the girl-friend, or for some other unprofessional reason. I can spend the whole morning coaxing them, but I never lose my temper. Some people start shouting and screaming at them and make them cry. I don't do that. I warm them up because I hate rows. I can't work with disharmony. I don't think I worry about the clothes half so much. You can be given the most monstrous thing to photograph, but if you've got the right girl wearing it, the camera and you can make something of it.'

As a tribute to the working relationship between photographer and model, Anne Gunning recalls a difficult trip they did together, for *Harpers Bazaar*. They travelled to India, Bangkok, and Australia, but difficulties arose when it was decided to make a television film of the model and photographer at work. Whereas Dormer wanted soft light—his style is gentle, soft focus—the film cameraman wanted hard light. This required a heavier make-up for the model. And so each shot had to be done twice, once for Dormer, and once for the television film camera. As a consequence, they began getting behind schedule, which, not unnaturally, agi-

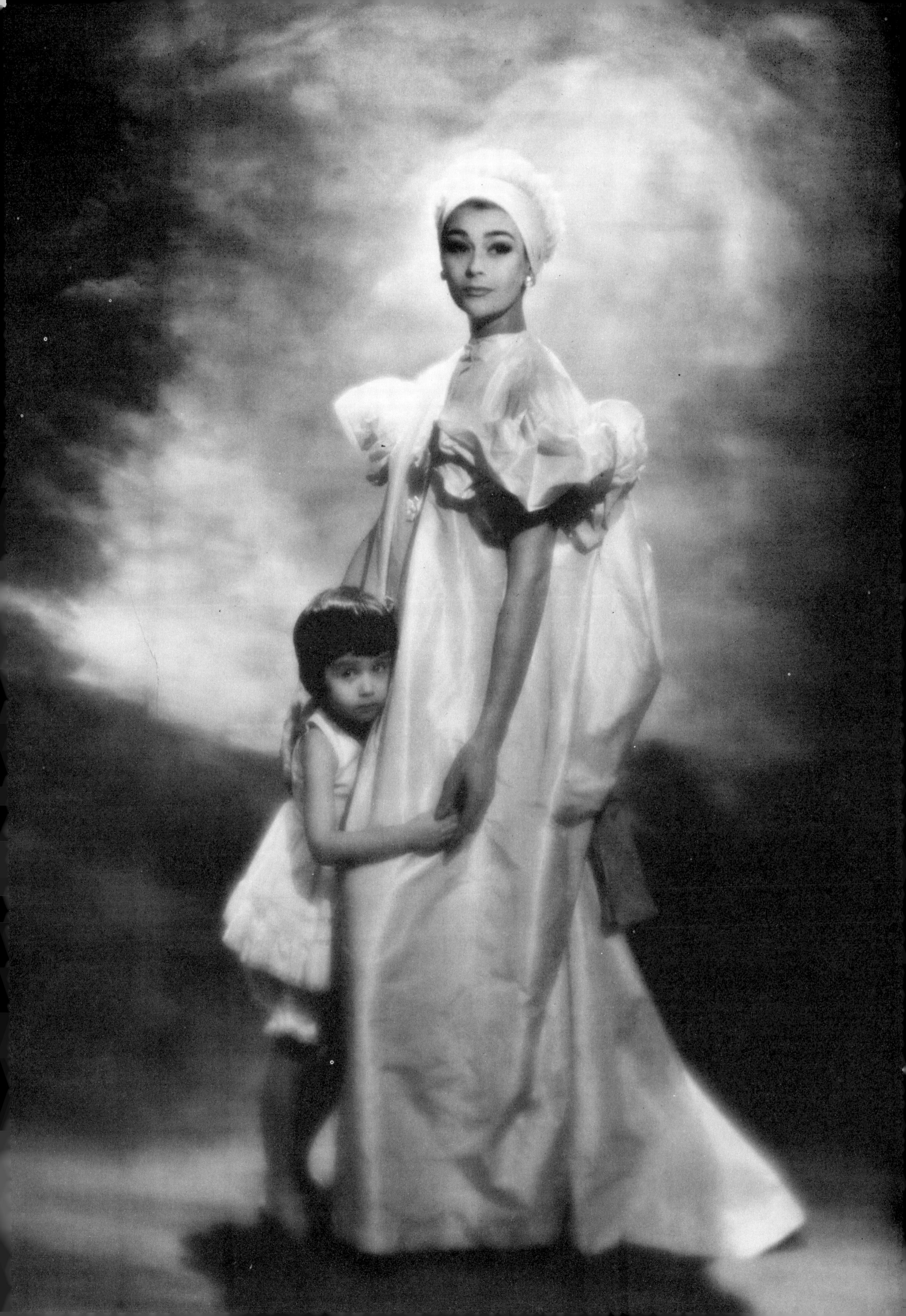

tated Dormer who had a rigorous six-week schedule. The editor didn't help matters; although a sweet woman, she was a ditherer, undecided about which accessory should go with which garment, and so she too asked for retakes. 'So Dick got into a nervous, ratty state', Anne Gunning recalls, 'and the obvious person to take it out on was *me*. I suppose he knew I'd understand, really. However, we had a filthy row, and as a consequence we worked for a solid week in Bangkok without speaking to one another. But to prove the rapport that we had established together, it was not necessary for Dick to say, "Do this", or, "Do that", or anything else at all. We simply continued working in dead silence and produced wonderful results. Needless to say, it made no difference to our friendship.'

Some of the finest fashion photographs of Suzy Parker were produced by Richard Avedon and Henry Clarke. American-born Henry Clarke has lived in Paris since the fifties, working not only there, but in London, New York, and all corners of the globe. His work for French *Vogue* is in stylish contrast to the more avante-garde photographers of the seventies, but Clarke's work provides sophistication and 'class' of the 'old school'. Born in California, he began working as a buyer for I. Magnin and Company in San Francisco.

Feeling the need for change, he took six-month's sabbatical in New York, and there found that *Vogue* needed a prop-boy as holiday-relief for two weeks in their photographic studios. He began making decorations for decor for photographers, and one day saw the then top model in New York, Suzy Parker's older sister, Dorian Leigh, being photographed by Cecil Beaton. 'It was total magic watching them work together', Henry Clarke enthuses. 'Dorian was modelling a suit—and I was knocked between the eyes. I knew there and then that I wanted to be a fashion photographer.' However, he had yet to learn his craft and went along to the New School of Photography, which was run by Alexi Brodevitch, also the art director of *Harpers Bazaar*, where he studied photography by night. He gave up his job in San Francisco, deciding to stay on in New York where, still with *Vogue*, he bought, hired, or

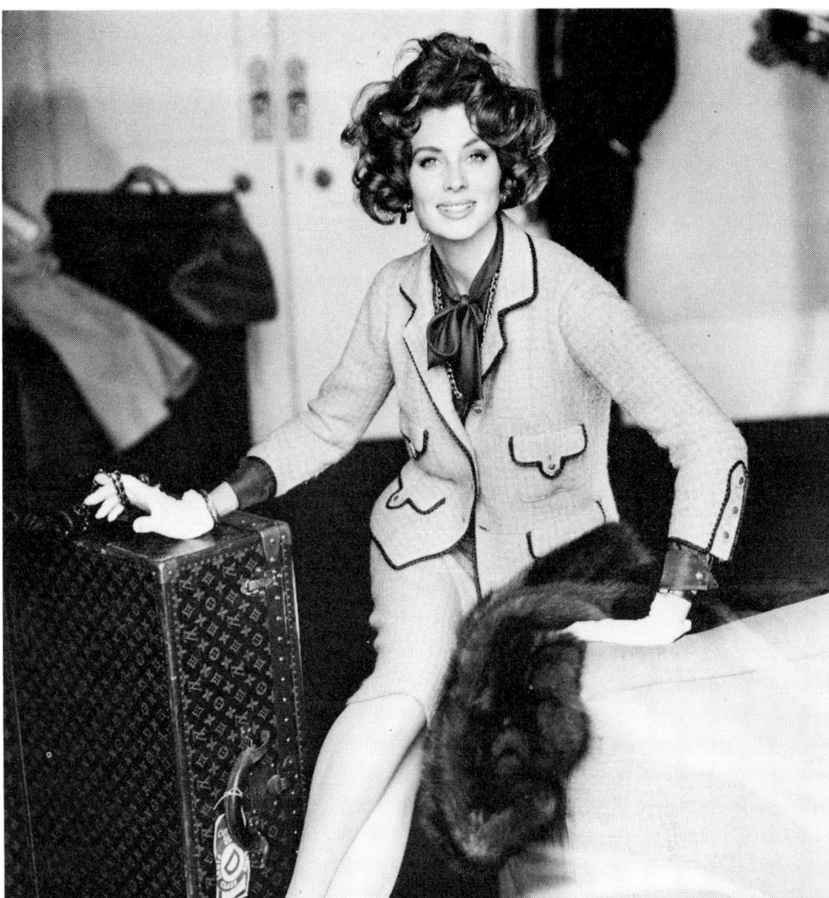

Above: Suzy Parker, photographed by Henry Clarke

made props for Beaton, Horst, Irving Penn—and every other photographer who was commissioned by the magazine.

Clarke spent his weekends learning his craft, and met a new young model called Chérie Martinelli. He photographed her in his spare time, but, as *Vogue* weren't interested in the pictures, he hawked them around until he was taken up by a new magazine who agreed to employ him as a photographer. However, after three months the magazine went bankrupt, owing him $2,500. He lunched with Horst who suggested he try his luck in Paris, and, taking the photographer's advice, he left on the next boat.

He had been given letters of introduction to Molyneux, Dior, and Jacques Fath by Horst and, on meeting Fath in Paris, was asked to photograph his new collection after showing him his portfolio of photographs. Fath was impressed with Clarke's work and showed his photographs to Comtesse Toulouse Lautrec (a descendant of the artist), who was the editor of the fashion magazine *Femina*. Clarke was asked to work for *Femina*, and within the same week

Opposite: The exquisite Anne Gunning, by her favourite photographer Richard Dormer

Opposite: One of Helmut Newton's fashion photographs with characteristic overtones of eroticism—*Vogue* France

Overleaf, left-hand page. Above: Ingrid Boulting, photographed for *Elle* by Barry Lategan Below left: Maudie James by Barry Lategan (By kind permission of Condé Nast Publications) Below right: Cathee Dahmen by Barry Lategan (By kind permission of Condé Nast Publications) Overleaf, right-hand page: Twiggy, photographed for *Vogue* by Barry Lategan (By kind permission of Condé Nast Publications)

photographed Molyneux's new collection as well. The following week he photographed the Jean Dessés collection and, shortly after, left *Femina* to work for the better-class fashion magazine *Album du Figaro*. Thereafter, he was asked by the London editor of *Harpers Bazaar*, Anne Scott James, to work under exclusive contract for *Harpers*, whose fashion editor was Eileen Dickson. After working for *Town and Country* and *Look* magazines in New York (under Fleur Cowles with the latter), he returned to Paris where he was taken up by *Vogue*, working under contract at the same time to the three *Vogue's*, English, French, and American, travelling between the three countries.

'I don't think my style has changed much since the fifties', says Henry Clarke, 'because I have always been after the maximum in beauty, or seduction, or allure. I'm a romantic photographer. I want things to swoon about. I want the impossible, in romance.

'I look for heroines in my models. I want people with character, but that is hard to find today. There are no great faces anymore. The models today are very, very pretty, but they're not individual. There is one girl in Paris I like, Vibéké, who is very beautiful. She has a face. I took her first good photographs. They were published in French *Vogue*!'

But now, in the sixties, a new, young and exciting look emerged through the lens of the *enfant-terrible* of English fashion, David Bailey, with Terence Donovan and Brian Duffy following close in his footsteps; all three were from the East End of London. Another top British photographer to reach international heights was Barry Lategan. Although, like Norman Parkinson, his name has never really become known to the general public, he was the first to photograph Twiggy.

Between them, Bailey, Donovan, and Duffy earned more than £100,000 a year. They were usually accompanied by some of the most beautiful women in the world. At thirty, Duffy was the star photographer for *Elle* magazine. With a quick, nervous intelligence, he is the only one of the three with an art school training.

Large and affable, Terence Donovan reached the top of his profession as a photographer by the time he was twenty-seven. Like David Bailey, he had learnt his craft as an assistant to John French.

While David Bailey was working as John French's assistant, French introduced him to Harold Keeble, who was the assistant editor on the *Daily Express*. Keeble 'discovered' Bailey, and commissioned him to do half-pages every Thursday. Bailey then worked for Tom Wolseley on *Town*, before *Vogue* (who claim to have discovered him) came into his life; he has worked for *Vogue* ever since. The first pictures Bailey took that were really noticed were of Paulene Stone for the *Daily Express*.

Bailey prefers black and white photography because he finds colour is reproduced so badly in Britain: 'Black and white is harder to do than colour because you're dealing in tones. If you've got a red dress and a green background, you've got a picture; if you turn it into black and white, it's reproduced as grey against grey.'

Had Bailey not been the first to photograph several new models, they might possibly never have become top models. He was among the first to photograph Veruschka in America, the first to photograph Jane Birkin, who has become a sex symbol in France, and the first to photograph Marisa Berenson before she became a top model and rocketed to film stardom. Apart from Jean Shrimpton, the other models he was first to photograph and discover include Sue Murray, Moyra Swan, and his present wife, Marie Helvin (his former wife was Catherine Deneuve).

'The key to taking fashion pictures is to make the girl look beautiful', says Bailey, 'because if the girl doesn't look fantastic and you can't see the clothes, then there's no point in taking the picture. It might be a beautiful picture, but it's not going to sell the frock.'

Bailey finds it difficult to find good models. 'But I'm a bit more flexible than most photographers, because I try and work around the girl as much as I try to make her look the way I want her to look.' He changes his style all the time, but does not change the way he works with models. 'It's all that jumping about that I'm glad is over. It's such a relief', he says, referring to the period between 1968 and 1971, when over-made-up doll-like models danced about

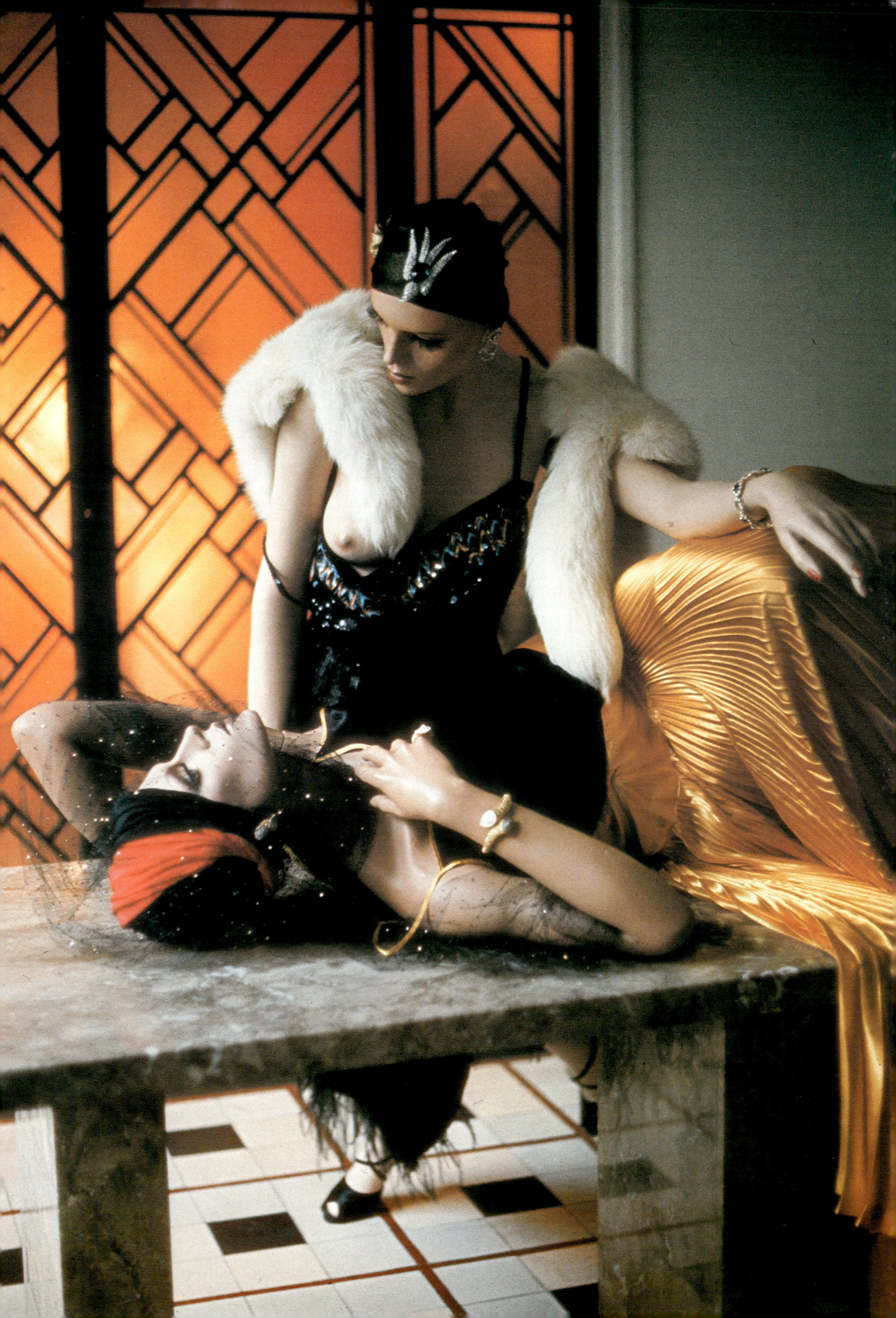

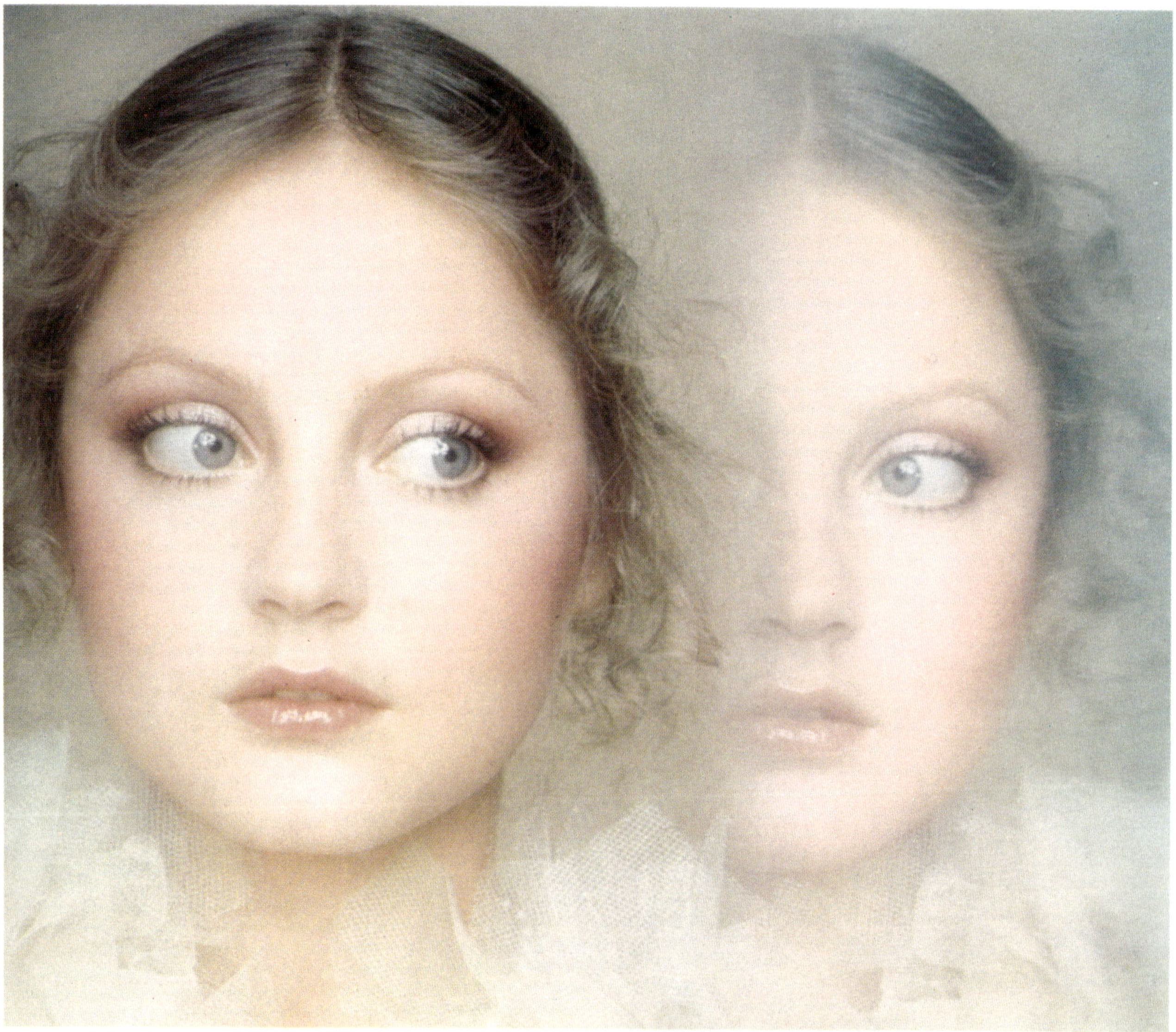

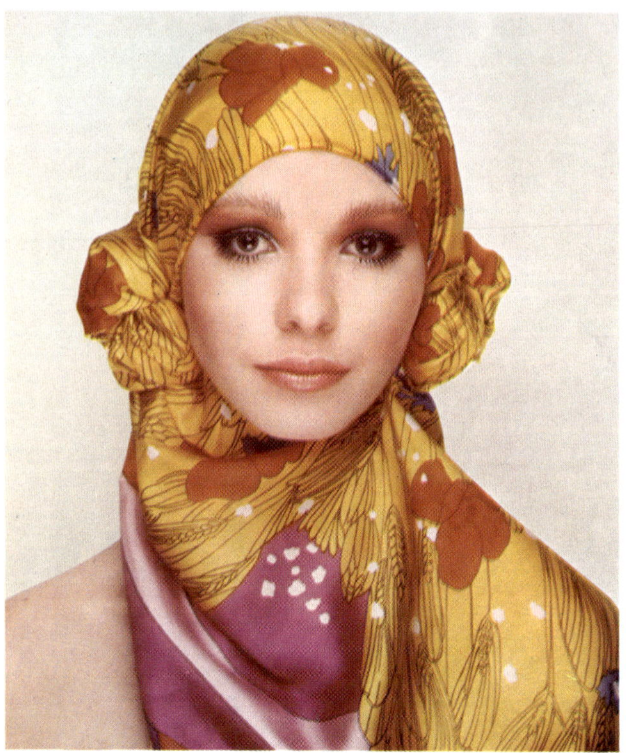
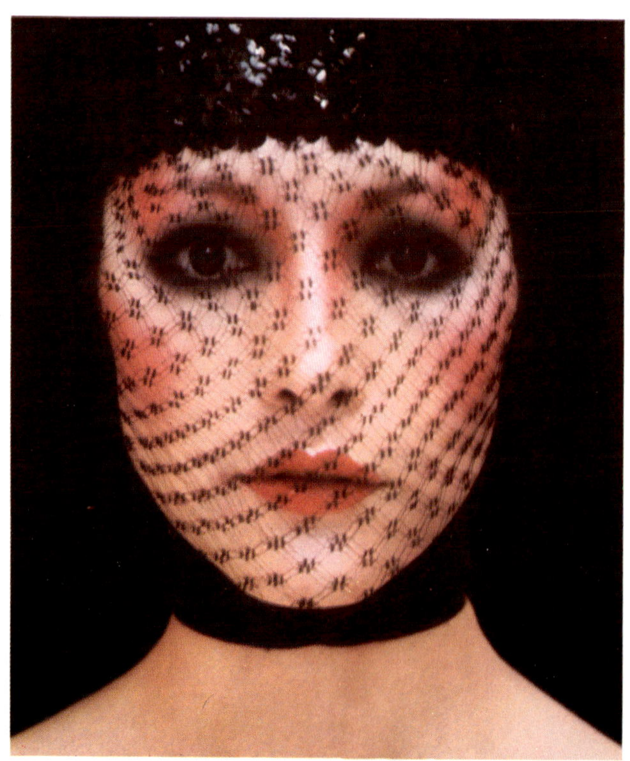

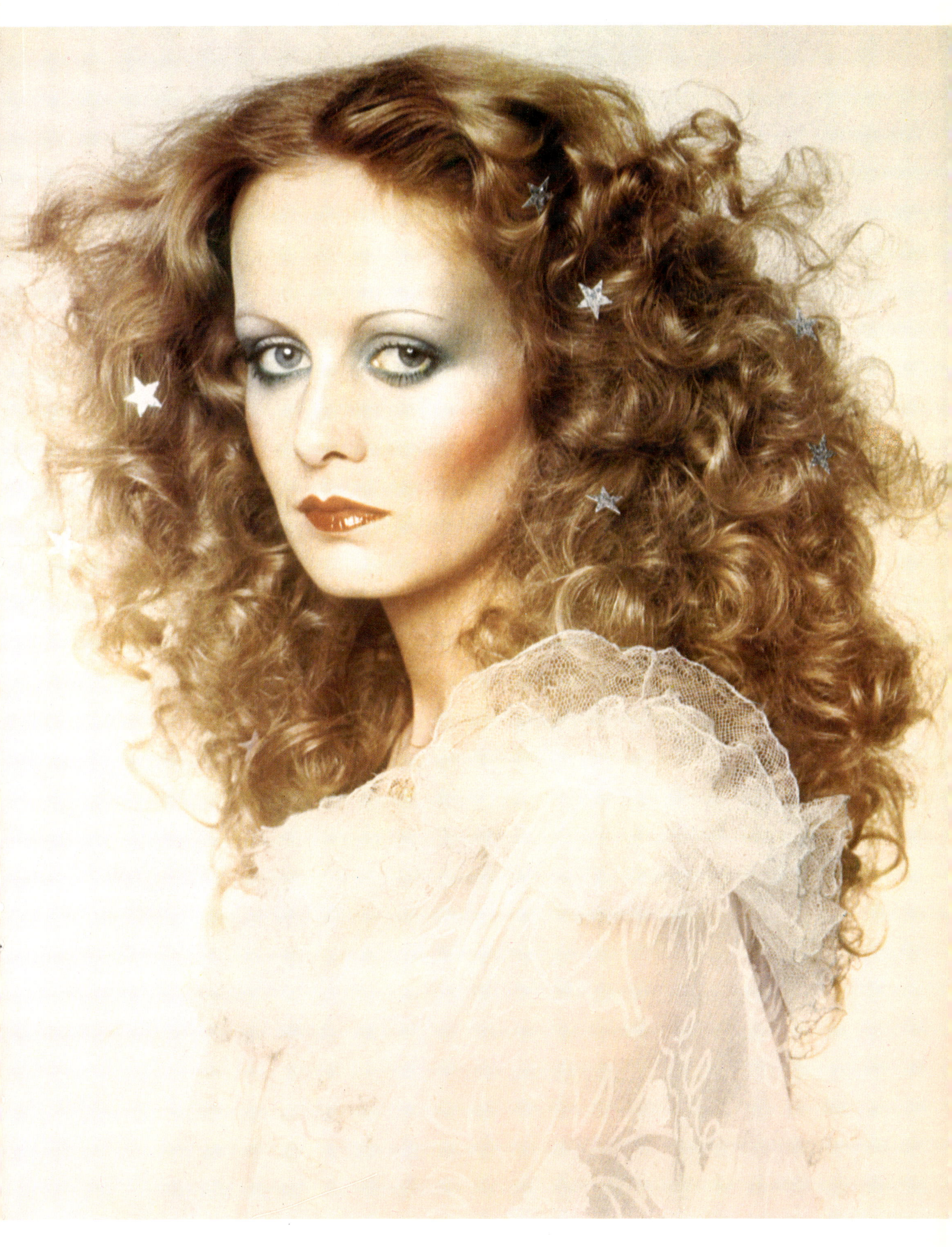

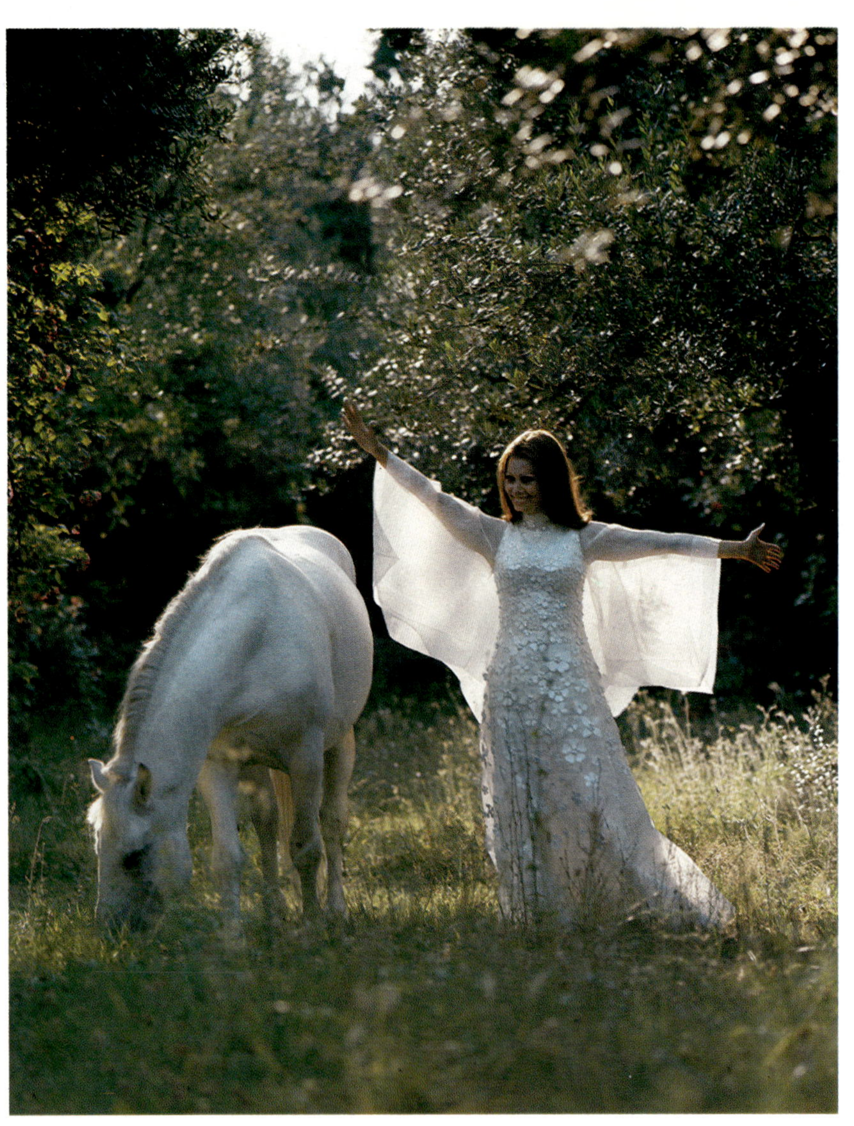

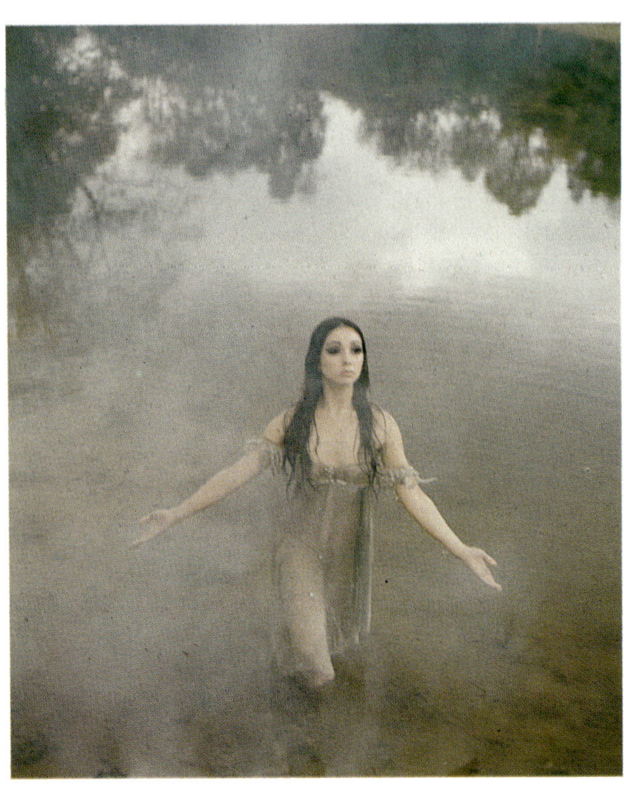

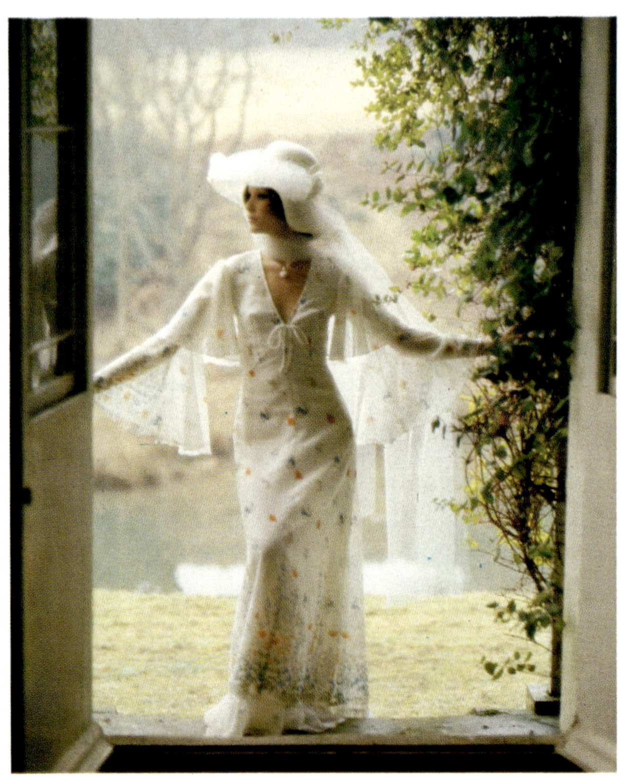

the studio in front of the camera to psychedelic music.

'I think Bailey's a great photographer', chimes top American model Jerry Hall, whose face regularly appears on English *Vogue* covers. 'I like the way he brings you down to earth. He says, "Look, baby, I know what sort of girl you are", and for a moment you're afraid to get into your "thing," and then you do it, looking *at* him. He's done so much for photography, and I think he's changed a lot. But it's a shame he's in England because they don't pay photographers of his calibre enough money. There's not enough work in England either. There are hardly any top models there. The trouble with Bailey is that he didn't move to America when he should have. He was very important in America, and they begged him to go there permanently in the sixties. They're still begging him, but he won't leave England.' He is, perhaps, too patriotic to give up his country for money.

'You've got to make money in this business', adds Jerry Hall with finality, giving little thought to artistic and creative achievement and satisfaction. 'You've got to have success and money That's very important', especially in America. She earns $1,000 a day doing cosmetic-advertising modelling in New York, and so she should know.

Once married to American model Lyn Kohlman, Britain's top cosmetic photographer, Barry Lategan, is a slender, casually clad, gently spoken forty-two year old, with neatly-trimmed, thinning black hair, beard, and moustache. 'I don't like the idea of a photographer being projected before his work', he says modestly, explaining why he has shied away from publicity for so many years. He lives and works in an immaculately laid-out studio in Chelsea.

Born in Natal, Barry Lategan started as a clerk on the South African Railways, ending up in Johannesburg, where his interest in amateur dramatics led him to join the National Theatre, touring with Leonard Schach. He joined the Bristol Old Vic School in England, but was soon conscripted into the RAF and was posted to Germany. He saw a notice pinned up in the NAAFI canteen encouraging members to join the RAF photographic club, and so he was introduced to the magic of the darkroom, where his interest has remained. After completing his national service, he returned to South Africa where he became employed as a photographer's assistant in Cape Town, but after two years he returned to England to branch out as a freelance photographer in London.

He developed a reputation for photographing girls for beauty and hair products and was introduced to Twiggy by a working colleague, hairdresser Leonard, who had cut her hair. Lategan was the first to photograph Twiggy, and when his pictures of her appeared in the *Daily Express*, heralding her as 'The Face of 1966', Lategan's reputation was made alongside hers. He began working for *Vogue*, and with Barbara Daly, an expert make-up artist, evolved new ideas in cosmetic photography.

He acquired a reputation for being able to extract more from young models at the beginning of their careers than from experienced models. 'It's because, in the beginning, girls don't really know what they should look like', he explains, 'and so they present themselves in a nice open way to the camera. Obviously, they are manipulated by me. I find it harder to work with them after a time when they have seen the success of a photograph, examined it, and then parody what they see. It's a kind of narcissistic repetition and then I can no longer extend them. And so, sadly, as fashion goes on, I move on to another girl.'

The illusions he creates are images of suspended, dream-like beauty. In cosmetic photography he looks for nicely lidded eyes, beautifully formed lips, and a sense of projection rather than perfect features. 'I try to make a very strong contact with the model. I get

Opposite. Above: Sophia Loren, photographed in her own garden in Italy by Snowdon (Courtesy *Vogue*, copyright © 1970 by The Condé Nast Publications Inc)

Below left: An impression of the ballet *Ondine*. Photographed by Snowdon at Nymans, the home of his mother, the Countess of Rosse in Sussex.

Below right: Michaela, photographed for *Brides* by Snowdon (By kind permission of Condé Nast Publications)

Right: The American model Maura McGaghey by Barry Lategan

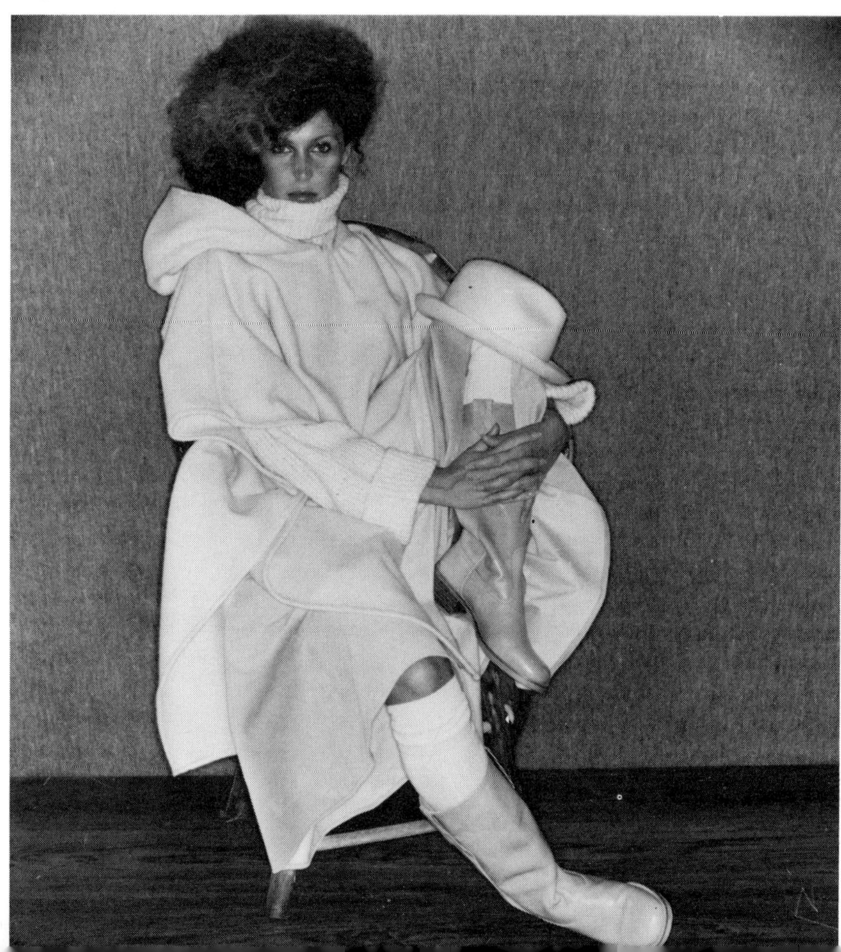

Snowdon, by Tim Jenkins

close to her. I talk to her, and coerce her. I take lots of photographs.

'I show her the polaroids before we do the actual shots, and draw her into the atmosphere. I never use noisy music. It excites them too much. I create a sense of dreamlike euphoria. If the model is edgy, I change the music. I sit down and talk to her in the dressing room, and create an atmosphere of intimacy before she appears in front of the camera, and get to know about her.

'Even the most experienced girls don't want five people around when she works, so I put screens around them, and that helps to create a feeling of intimacy.'

Tony Armstrong-Jones was one of the most inventive photographers in the fifties and sixties. He was a top photographer of people, personalities, and places, and was to be seen at every social and theatrical event of significance.

He was the innovator of many exciting, lively fashion advertisements, but says candidly that he has never much cared for fashion photography: 'I was forced into it by Audrey Withers, who was editor of *Vogue*. She came to have breakfast with me in my basement in Pimlico and said, "Tony dear, John Parsons [*Vogue's* art director] and I wondered whether you'd photograph Dior for us and we want you to find some way of covering every facet of his life and work."' In one photograph! He visualised pinning up stockings behind Dior, and dressing the photographs with bottles of scent and lengths of cloth, but they insisted that he visit Dior in the South of France to photograph him against an absolutely plain white background, which he did.

His interest in photography began in a chemist's shop in Eton, during the war, because there were neither photographic societies nor film available. 'I used to work with an old horizontal enlarger, a great big mahogany thing, at Oldhams. I used to go down there, when I was fourteen, to develop and print other people's snaps. Then I started the photographic society at school in a tiny little room.'

When he left school he planned to join the Massachussets Institute of Technology to read engineering, but instead went to Cambridge to read natural sciences. 'But I loathed that. I did it for ten days, and then changed to architecture, which I loved doing, but failed after two years.' However, he used his experience later when he designed the remarkable aviary at the London Zoo.

His photographic interest continued at Cambridge as a hobby, and he submitted work to the *Cambridge Daily News*. When he came down, he lived with his father in the Albany in London for two months, looking for work. His mother, the beautiful Anne Messel, had remarried, and become the Countess of Rosse; her brother, Oliver, became a noted theatrical designer.

Tony was offered a job with the family firm of Messel's, the stockbrokers, but he had no wish to work in the city and, instead, became photographer Baron's assistant for six months, at a princely £2 a week. He then joined another photographer, David Sim, in a basement in Shaftesbury Avenue.

He found an ironmonger's shop in Pimlico, which he converted into living accommodation and a studio. It was here that he evolved a completely new form of imagery in portraiture, for which he became well known and much sought after. Although he was working hard as a photographer by now, he did little fashion. 'I did *some* fashion for *Tatler*, which was frightfully bad', he adds disarmingly. 'I just wasn't good at it, besides, fashion wasn't good those days, either.'

He had published a book of his photographs of London, and designed a collection of women's ski-clothes in 1958, which his own tailor made up for him. 'They were knickerbockers with balloon-type smock-tops. They were long before their time; and if you're long before your time fashion-wise, you're just extremely stupid. It's not clever to be ahead of your time, because that's the wrong time!' His collection had a grand opening but the press gave it a poor reception. 'When people went into the shop after the collection, the assistant said, "No. I wouldn't buy that. It's funny. We've got some very nice Norwegian sweaters here, dear."'

At this time he designed the sets for John Cranko's revue, *Keep Your Hair On*, in which Rachel Roberts appeared, but it closed in the West End after three weeks.

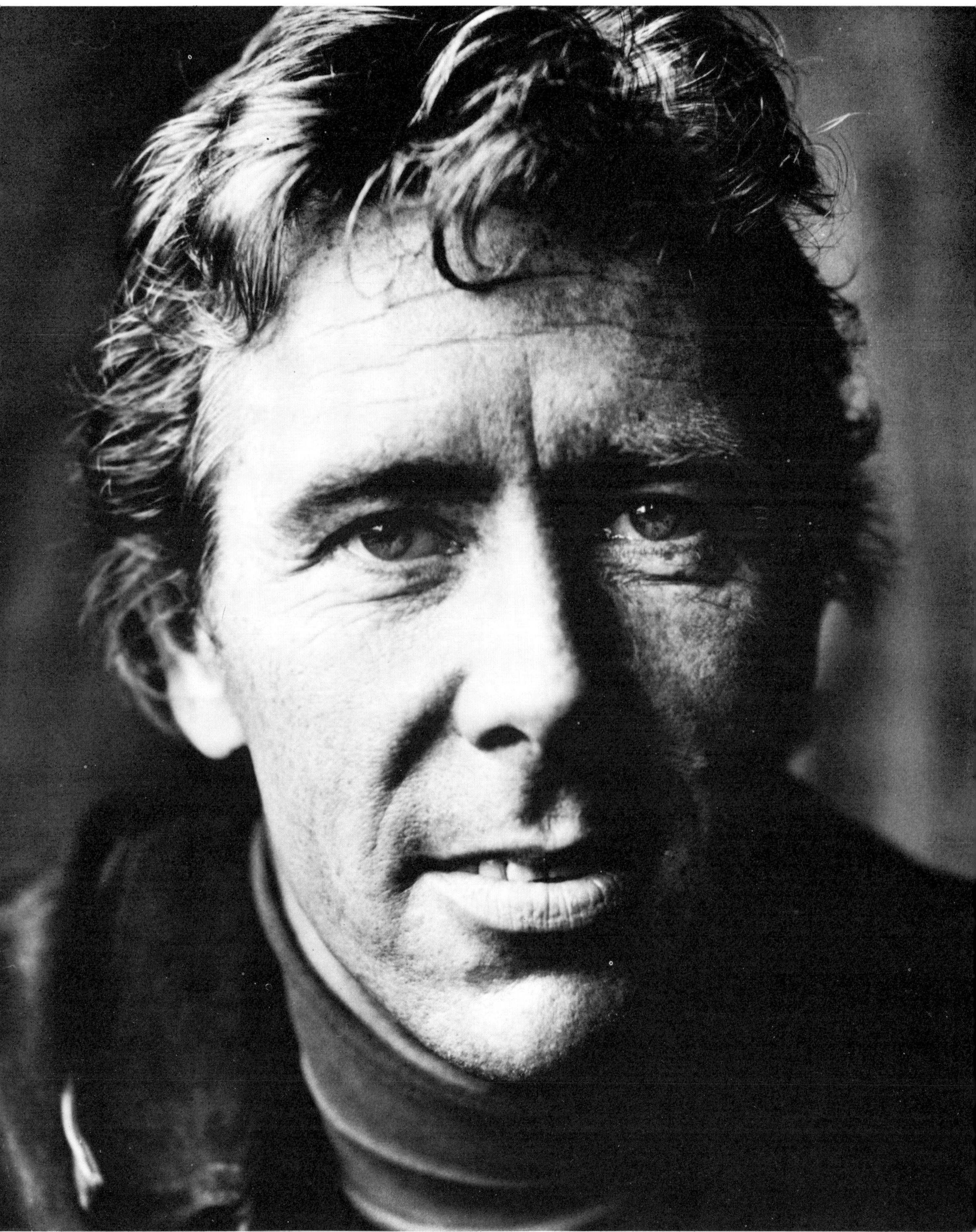

The *Daily Express* started using Tony Armstrong-Jones to photograph theatrical events, and he worked with John Barber, who was theatre critic for the newspaper. He ventured into fashion photography under the assistant editor, Harold Keeble's, influence.

He did a considerable amount of fashion photography in the late fifties, both editorially for *Vogue*, as well as photographic advertising for Acrilan and Michael Sekers' fabrics. His lively, inventive photography had models flying through the air, or being blown over sideways, with umbrellas turned inside out, by wind and rain. He devised a method of photographing champagne bottles and glasses tumbling down, luggage floating down to the street below from a balcony window, and model Anne Gunning playing cards with male model Robin Tattersall, making card-houses and blowing them down.

'As I had no flash-gun, I sellotaped the cards together and hung them with wires so that I could put every card exactly where I wanted it.'

After his marriage to Princess Margaret, he was created Earl of Snowdon and official duties afforded less and less time for the pursuit of his career as a photographer. However, he did develop as a serious photographer, and drifted farther and farther away from fashion. 'The only time I do anything remotely connected with fashion is when I'm escaping from having done a rather long social-problem feature documentary on cruelty, old-age, or loneliness, for *The Sunday Times*, which I find a lot more fulfilling because one helps, I hope, to make for more understanding over those problems, which is what I use the camera for. Then I need to go to *Vogue* afterwards, as a form of escapism.

'Fashion must be romantic escapism, I hate hard-edge fashion and I don't like treating it with enormous reverence. It's how people wear the clothes that matters; I think people should wear the clothes that suit them and just go on from there; they should not be affected by fashion that changes all the time. I've always tried to break models down to make them real, to make them look like part of a documentary, so each photograph looks like a *vignette* in a film.'

In 1976, Snowdon's fashion assignment for French *Vogue* featured Dayle Haddon in different scenes with top fashion designers, wearing a garment designed by each specific designer. The designers chosen included Madame Grés, Hubert de Givenchy, Yves Saint Laurent, Pierre Cardin, Ted Lapidus, Guy Laroche, Andre Courrèges, and Pierre Balmain. He had, however, to find a theme for the photographs, and with only five days in which to photograph sixteen designers, during the frantic Paris fashion collections, his task was daunting. 'It was on the way between the airport and arriving in Paris that I had this idea of the designers falling in love with Dayle, and I tried to make them fall in love with her in the mood of the garment and the location.

'Dayle was marvellous, quick and professional, but when I gave the direction, "You're alone. You've met for the first time, you're having *supper-a-deux* and you're in love", although Dayle, as an actress as well as a model, achieved the mood without any problems, it was difficult to get a shy fashion designer to relax to that extent and pretend they were alone, when, in fact, they were in a restaurant packed with people at the surrounding tables, out of shot.

'When I did the shot of Gerard Pipart (for Nina Ricci) and Dayle, they were supposed to be having a romantic picnic under a tree, but he sat there, rather formal and withdrawn. I took some shots, and said, "OK Finished. Lovely." Then I whispered to Dayle, "Pull off his tie." He thought I'd stopped photographing, and so he was relaxed. She tickled him and pulled off his tie, and he fell backwards, laughing, with Dayle leaning over him, and I got this lovely, natural shot.'

When working in a studio, Snowdon prefers the atmosphere to be calm. 'I can't bear all that music and noise in studios. I like absolute silence, and if I do work with an assistant, which I do with *Vogue*, I want them to look away, and not catch the model's eye-line. There is a very important relationship between you and the person you're photographing, and you have to preserve it.'

His eye for imagery and ability to create illusion is illustrated by his photograph of a ballet dancer in the role of *Ondine* for a calendar for ICI. 'The girl was in the lake, surrounded by pale, pale blue and she was just coming out of the water.' He photographed her in the lake at his mother's house, Nymans, in Sussex, one freezing April morning. 'I let off smoke bombs, but they didn't work, so I lit some leaves to make blue smoke. I thought the poor girl would freeze to death, so I filled one of those thermos buckets with hot water, and put it just below water-level, and she stood in the hot water—in gum-boots; but you wouldn't know it, because she was standing in the blue-lit haze.

'I believe that photographs should be simple technically, and easy to look at. I never want to put my stamp on anything. I want my photographs to be totally anonymous and change with the mood or the situation of the subject.' Although Snowdon protests that if he had an identifiable style and somebody recognised a photograph of his, he would count that as his failing, his work *has* individuality, mood, and a documentary-like sense, which is so easily attributable to him. His books, *London*, *Private View*, *Assignments*, and *Venice* are evidence of his essential worth as a photographer with a unique eye for observation.

His photography and film documentaries have gained momentum over the years as he continues his search for new subjects, using his camera to reflect and record social problems of our times.

American models fly over to London to get good photographs at reasonable prices for their portfolios, and then return home or travel to Paris to earn their keep in fashion and advertising modelling. Many of the best photographers these days are in Europe. Whereas in the fifties and the early sixties American photographers dominated the fashion scene, and London took over in the mid-sixties for a short while, it is Paris, in the seventies, that has the most imaginative photographers.

In Paris, the top photographers are selective about the magazines for which they will work, and the advertisement campaigns they will undertake. The models seen in French *Vogue*, for instance, are the creation of the Paris photographer who will devise the look, the make-up, hair-style, the mood, deciding for himself the latest trend in fashion. His influence on fashion, as portrayed by *Vogue*, is immense.

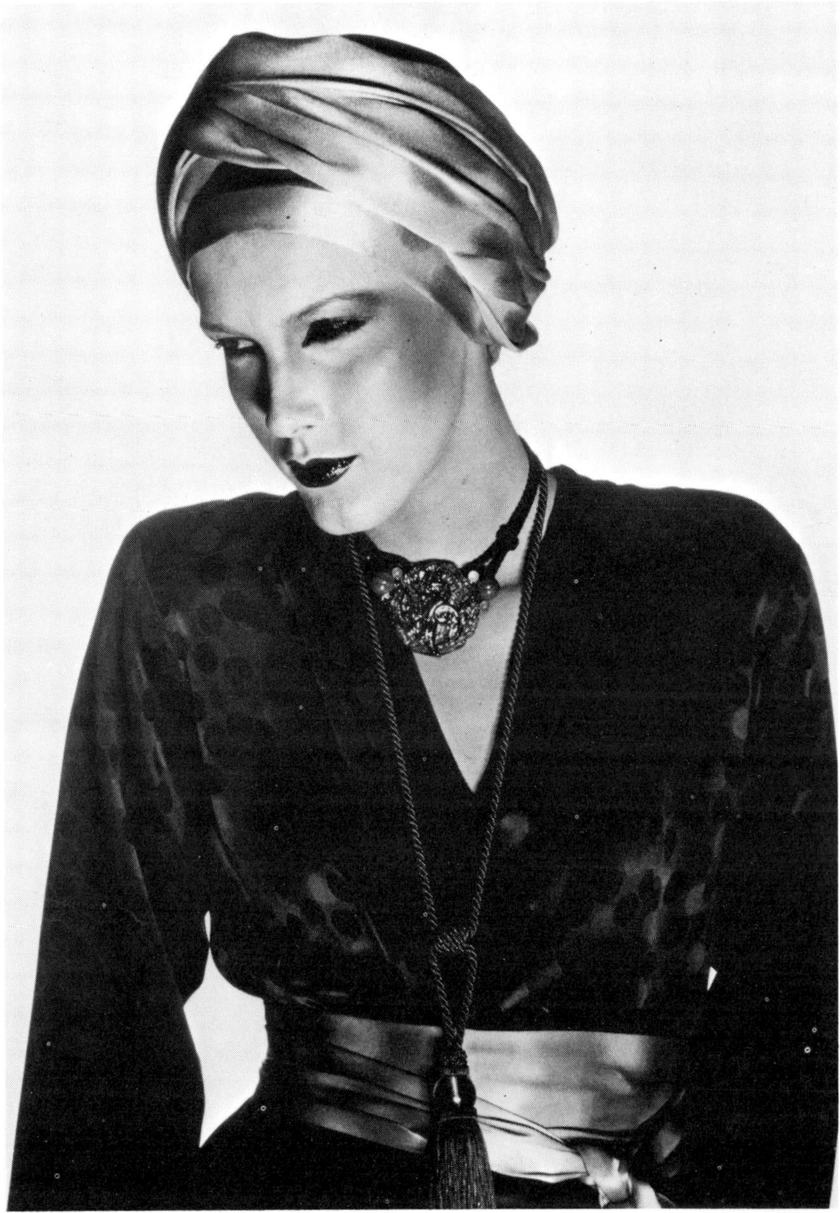

Carrie, photographed by Guy Bourdin. Courtesy *Vogue* France

Leaders in the field for French *Vogue* are cosmopolitan. Guy Bourdin is French; Helmut Newton, German; Hans Feurer, Swiss; Sarah Moon, British; Barbieri, Italian; and Henry Clarke, the daddy of them all, American. *Elle* and *Marie-Claire* have their own prized photographers. The magazines jealously guard both model and photographer, preferring them to remain exclusive to their publications. For a model to appear on the cover of *Vogue* and its rival *Elle* simultaneously is a catastrophe in the glossy magazine world, and fashion editors do their utmost to prevent this from happening.

Guy Bourdin and Helmut Newton are the tops, as far as French *Vogue* readers are concerned, and they like working there because *Vogue* allows them to experiment. They are encouraged to try out new ideas. A shy man with a boyish face, baby teeth, and an adolescent-sounding voice, Guy Bourdin started photography in the fifties. He began as an artist and was brought into French *Vogue* by Edmond Charoux. He became Charoux's protégé. His first photographs were barely acceptable, but he has developed an individual style which is easily identifiable.

Guy Bourdin's models have a definite 'Bourdin' look about them. He uses the same artists, Heidi for make-up, and Valentine for the frizzed-out hair styles, on all his models, who emerge looking identical. A catalogue he did for Bloomingdale in New York caused a controversy, and the editor who commissioned him was fired. One tends to look at his photographs as a whole, rather than at the clothes. The models, who not only all look alike, look miserable. It used to be that a girl dressed because she wanted to catch a man— Bourdin's girls look as though they have just lost their man. His style has a stark, avant-garde look about it.

Helmut Newton's models tend to look like German whores of the thirties, while Bourdin's models tend to vary— blonde, brunette, tall girls or fat girls, mostly unknown models; Newton prefers the tall, blonde, rather big and blue-eyed types. There is an almost pornographic connotation to his work. In French *Vogue*, his models might be photographed with one breast protruding from a priceless ranch mink coat—

or else heaving up a Nina Ricci creation to the navel in order to adjust a suspender. It is unlikely that the editorial photography Newton has published in French *Vogue* would ever see the light of day in either English or American *Vogue*, for the advertisers, most certainly, would not pay for the lurid look which has become his trademark. When he did a spread for American *Vogue*, readers protested, threatening to cancel their subscriptions. He does, however, earn considerable money and prestige from top advertising campaigns, but, out of necessity for the advertiser and consumer, waters down the suggestiveness of his poses. His work can be great and imaginative, but models of considerable standing, such as American Shelley Smith, have reservations about working for him. 'I don't think I would like to do some of his pictures', she admits. 'I think I would be embarrassed to be noticed having done them. I don't mind the toughness of the imagery, but I'm not crazy about the dykey whorish bit.'

'He photographed me with a steak on my eye', laughs American model, Jerry Hall. 'I had to pretend that I had a black eye. I had the blood dripping down from the steak. He loves doing lesbian things —with two models practically making love.'

The greatest of present-day Italian photographers, Gian-Paolo Barbieri, was born in Milan. His father lost everything when, as the result of an unfortunate business deal, he was forced into bankruptcy. At the age of eighteen, Barbieri set off to try his luck as a photographer in Rome, but, after failing, travelled on to Paris where he literally lived on beans. He used to photograph by the light of a small candle, as the light from the weak lamp in his small hotel room wasn't strong enough. He became assistant to Kublin, the Hungarian photographer, and worked with him on the collections in London and Paris before branching out on his own in Milan in 1962. His first break was working for *Town and Country* in New York, and, after a few assignments with American *Vogue*, he returned to Italy where he works largely for Italian and French *Vogue*. His most important clients are Yves Saint Laurent in Paris, and Valentino in Italy. He prefers

photographing advertisements for fur— mink especially—and *prêt-à-porter* because he considers haute couture to be dead.

'I go for reality in my photography,' Barbieri says, 'but I always ask myself whether what I do has simplicity. I always try to make the girls beautiful because fashion needs that in order to maintain quality. There are many aspects involved; sophistication, elegance, graphic sense of style—all of which have to be composed in one picture. If you put an unattractive dress on a beautiful woman, the dress must look beautiful too, because you want to sell it to the girl in the street as well as to a princess.'

Barbieri is the only fashion photographer of any significance in Italy today. His rival was Franco Rubartelli, who gave up his brief career as fashion photographer when his model girlfriend, Veruschka, left him for pastures new. Rubartelli learnt all he knew about photography from Veruschka, who gave him his first Nikon and taught him how to use it—on her. She thereafter refused modelling work unless Rubartelli was employed as her photographer, but unfortunately, Rubartelli's work was not as highly regarded as the top model herself, and they soon both lost work, seriously damaging Veruschka's remarkable career as an international model. There is severe criticism of photographers who tie models to them, rendering it impossible for fashion editors to use the model without employing her boyfriend or husband, the photographer. Editors eventually tire of this, and it can mean death to both model and photographer, unless, as in the case of David Bailey, the model is changed periodically for a new face with a different style, keeping abreast of fashions and the times.

'I love being photographed by Barbieri', enthuses Jerry Hall. 'His style is very dramatic, very Italian. He likes the model to play the role of a movie star. In one photograph I had to pose, shocked to find my lover with another girl. The picture was composed of another model on the couch with her Italian lover, and me standing at the door looking shocked. And we were modelling fashion!'

Barbieri prefers working with ex-

perienced models because he finds the job difficult enough for a photographer, without adding additional anxieties about the model's capabilities for the job. He does, however, try out new models as he is always looking for the models of the future.

The majority of creative, artistic fashion photography is in Europe nowadays. Whether it is Italy or France, the look is different from the American approach. 'Many years ago I looked to America for their technical achievements,' Barbieri admits, 'but they lack creativity. I agree that Guy Boudin is one of the best photographers in the world because he is creative. He understands and he learns all the time.' For his own part, Barbieri, too, continues to learn all the time. He spends his money on books and visiting exhibitions, learning and observing. He tries to understand people who achieve success in a world of everchanging art—painters, graphic artists, photographers.

Barbieri leads a private existence in Milan. He keeps away from restaurants frequented by models and fashion folk, but he is aware of their attraction to him, all the same. 'Perhaps they work for me because they know I make them more beautiful', he adds. 'It's a big problem getting top models for someone like me who works outside the big fashion centres. Fashion only really got started in Italy about ten years ago. But fashion in Italy is fantastic. For me, French and Italian fashion are the best and the most exciting!'

Opposite: Swedish-born Ann Anderson, rated as one of the top models in Europe in the seventies. Photograph by Barbieri

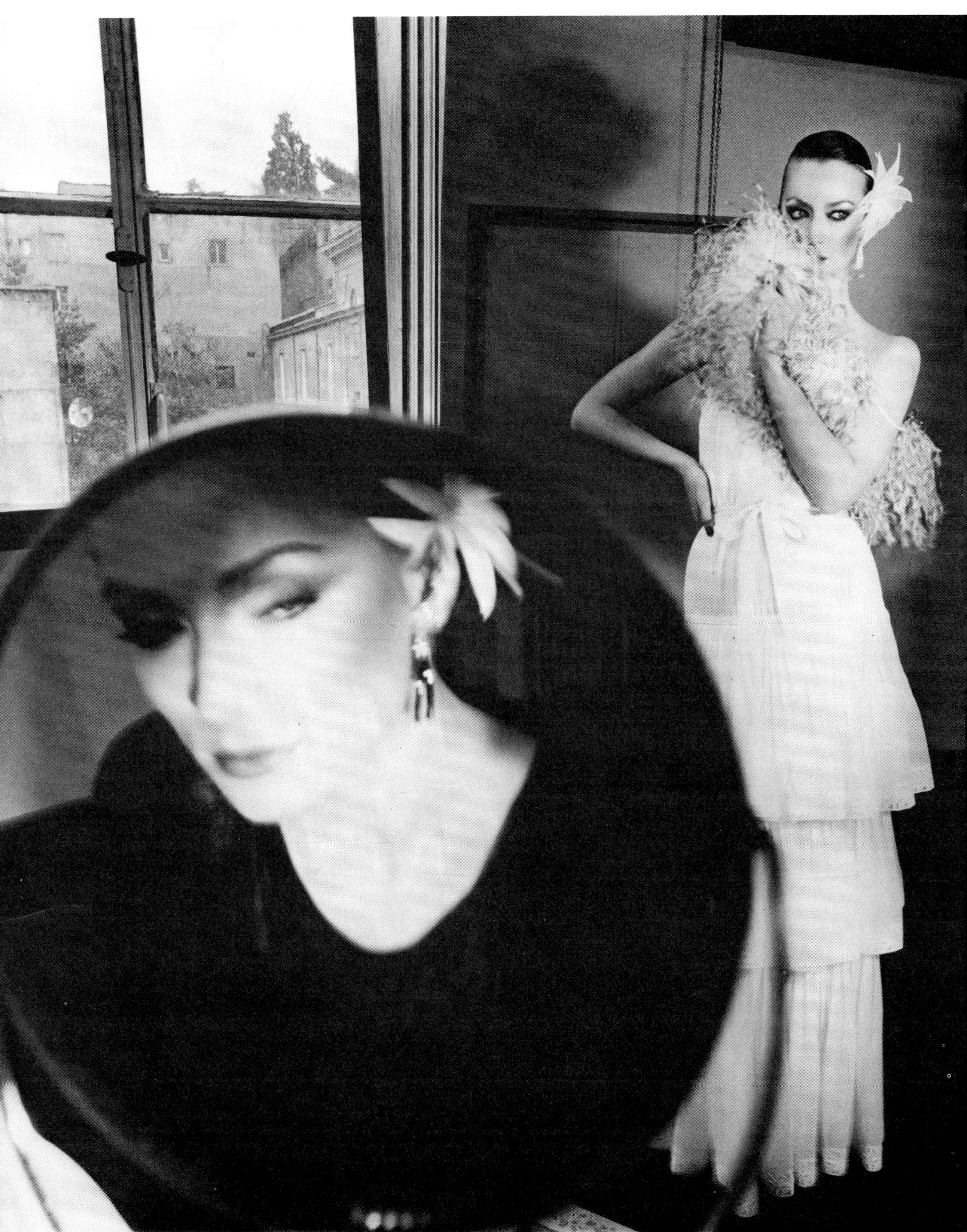

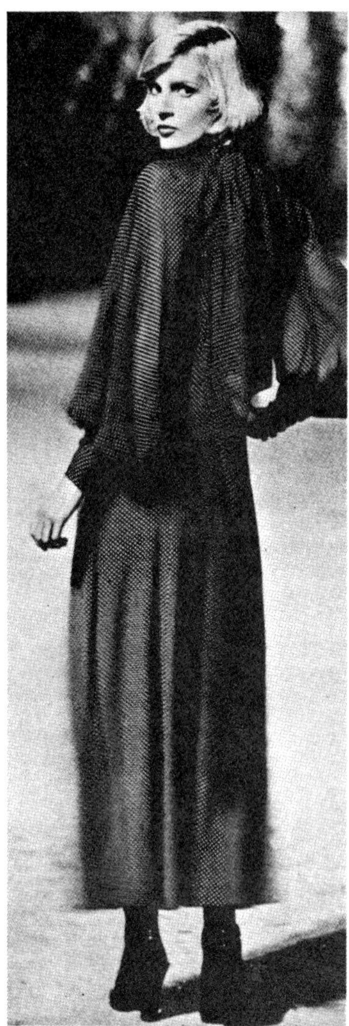

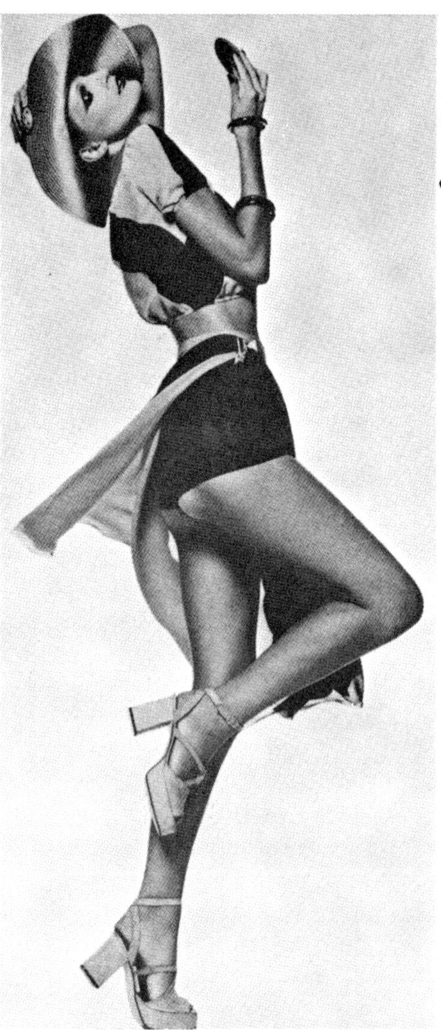

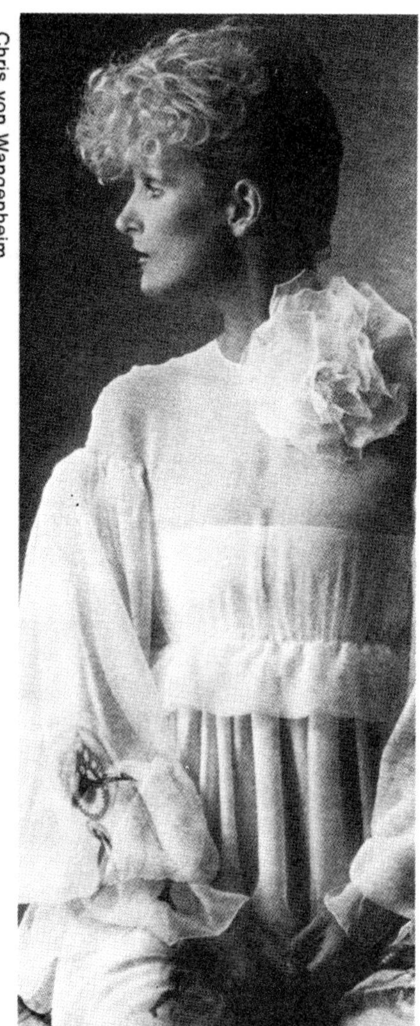

New York apartment can cost over $400 a month, which would mean $200 each. Then there's the telephone bill and electricity, and $50 a week for running around and eating. She needs at least $400 a month to keep going. She might get one booking for $75 an hour, or a three-hour booking, and that would help, but many new models take jobs as part-time waitresses, especially where alcohol is served and people are more generous with tips. A model can 'take off' within a period of two weeks, like Patti Hansen, the top model in America today. Other girls, like Shaun Casey, took well over a year to get off the ground.

Girls should, however, come with a background of training in speech, acting, or drama which might have been taken in school. As many dancing classes as possible should be taken, but ballet must be avoided because it is too stylised. It ruins a model for natural poses, because it gives a certain stance that cannot be undone. It is the one type of dance that will ruin a potential model.

Model agencies in New York, London, and Paris differ in what they can do for a new girl on their books. In London the agency will do no more than find her jobs, negotiate adequate fees, arrange transport and accommodation, and periodically advance money if the girl has waited too long for her fees from the client (clients can take up to four to six months to pay). For this the agency receives a commission which varies from company to company.

In New York the model signs a three-year contract with an agency if it believes she has potential. It will then do all it can to help develop and foster that girl's career. The agencies charge 15 per cent commission and they advance the model 70 per cent of the fee received for her services. The other 15 per cent of the fee is put in a reserve fund for the model, which is a hedge against future advances given to the girl until such time as the client pays. Commissions at some of the top New York agencies rise as high as 20 per cent for

their services, for their expenses can be enormous—telephone bills of $1,000 a month; total running costs, a million dollars a year.

If models choose the 20 per cent commission scale, the agency advances them the full 80 per cent the week after they have done the work. The agency guarantees the fee, and bears the loss if the client doesn't pay, or if there are bad debts.

In Paris, the model agency system differs from America or Britain. In Paris the model is considered to be employed by the agency, whereas in America or Britain the model is employed by the client and the agent represents the model on a commission basis. If the client doesn't pay, the model loses. The Paris agent pays all the social charges for the girls' travelling and living accommodation, and invoices the client accordingly. The model pays the French agent a 20 per cent commission.

Top New York models earn more than any other models in the world. There are a handful of them who earn $200,000 a year, but a great number of them earn between $90,000–$125,000 a year. The top model in Paris who works every day and night, every Saturday and Sunday, couldn't earn more than $50,000 a year and, in London, the top model can earn considerably less. Fees these days are higher than they've ever been—photographic modelling in New York pays $600 a day; while for beauty advertising, it's $1,000 a day. The hourly rate is between $75–$100 an hour, depending on the model's popularity.

In Paris, they earn 1,500 francs a day for advertising, but editorials pay considerably less. For *Vogue*, the models get 300 francs a day. At *Elle* and *Marie-Claire*, they get $400 a day. These fees apply to new models, perhaps on their first job, as well as to the established girls who work throughout the world.

London pays less than New York or Paris and it is perhaps for this reason that there are very few top international models in London. Marie Helvin lives in London (she is married to photographer David Bailey), but works all over the world; she is London's top model. American Jerry Hall, one of the top ten in the world, lives in London, not because of the money she earns there but because she is engaged to be married to pop singer Bryan Ferry. Cathee Dahmen, Sue Purdy, Maudie James, and Maura, who are other top London models, command a maximum of £20 an hour (£12 an hour for editorials), or £100 a day for photographic modelling. £200 a day is the highest for advertising. Many agencies impose a minimum booking, however, of, say, two or three hours, otherwise it simply is not worth the girl rushing across London in a taxi for £20—less commission.

Although New York is where the model can earn the most, her craft should be learnt and applied in Paris, where the creative photographic work is done today. There is considerably more work available to girls in Paris because of the amount of fashion magazines, and their tremendous fashion output. In Paris or London the model can build up her portfolio and working reputation, and move on to New York where she will earn top money. Models in Paris are, however, particularly unprofessional, and so are many of the

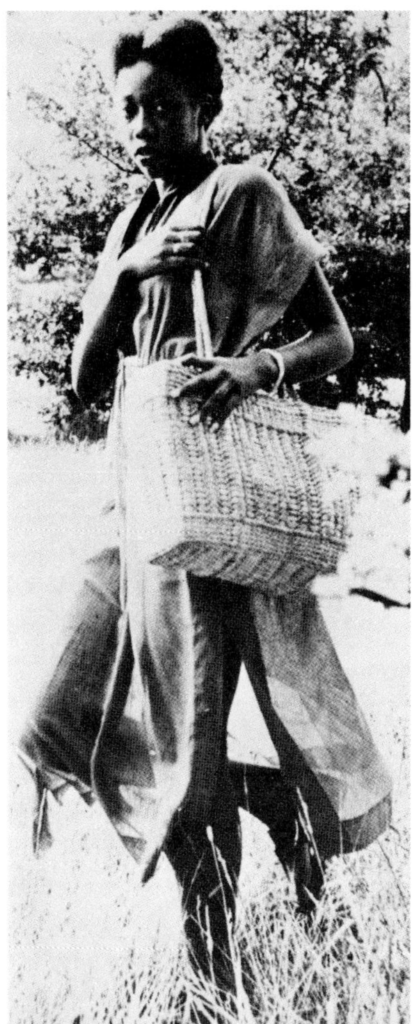

Opposite: Flip side of the composite card of one of Europe's top models, Jeanette Christjansen

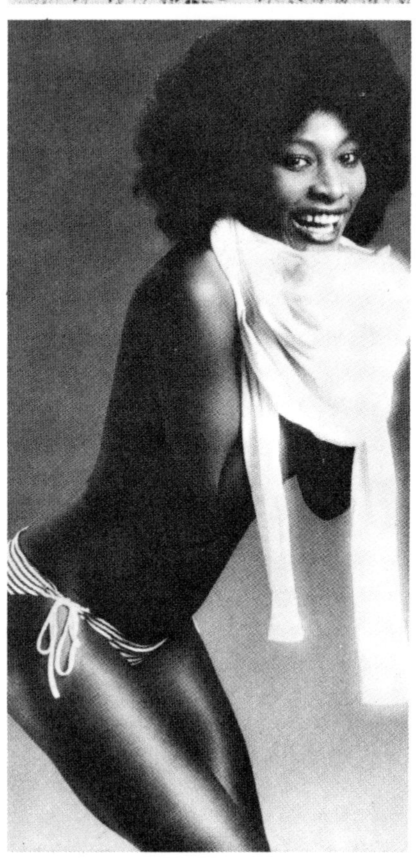

Right: Details from the cards of two young British models, Sandra Boyd (above) and Normaline (below)

photographers—unlike their New York cousins who have the reputation of being the most professional in the world. In New York you work by the hour. It's a nine to five job. You're expected to be absolutely prompt, and if you're five minutes late, you're expected to work five minutes longer; they want a full hour's worth out of you. You have to arrive ready in New York. You walk through the door and they virtually hand you the garment to put on, whereas in Paris it is extremely lax. The booking in Paris is normally for half a day, or a full day. When the girls arrive in Paris there is usually a hairdresser, and generally a make-up artist. Hours are spent waiting, but it's calmer and friendlier.

A top agent in Paris complains that American girls who arrive in Paris with a nine o'clock booking telephone her to say, 'Listen, you've given me the wrong address. There's no-one here'. She reminds them that they're in Paris, suggests they go down the road for some coffee, and return in an hour or so. No-

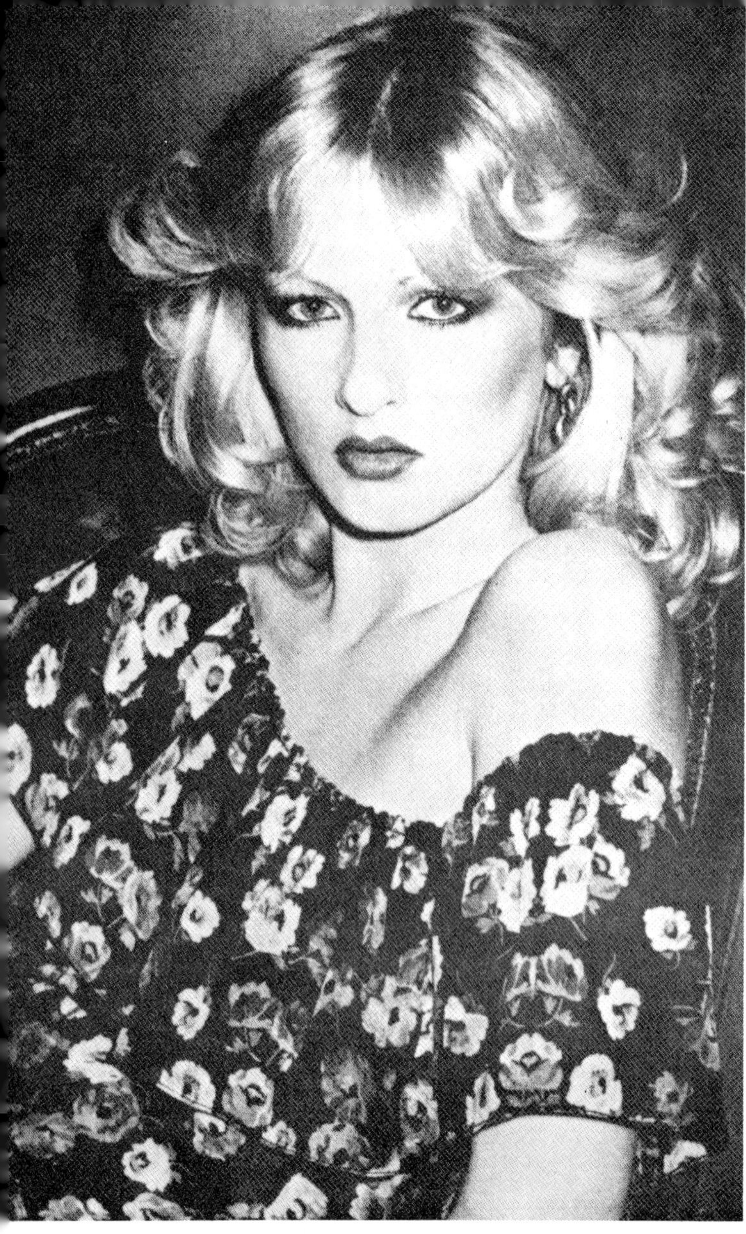

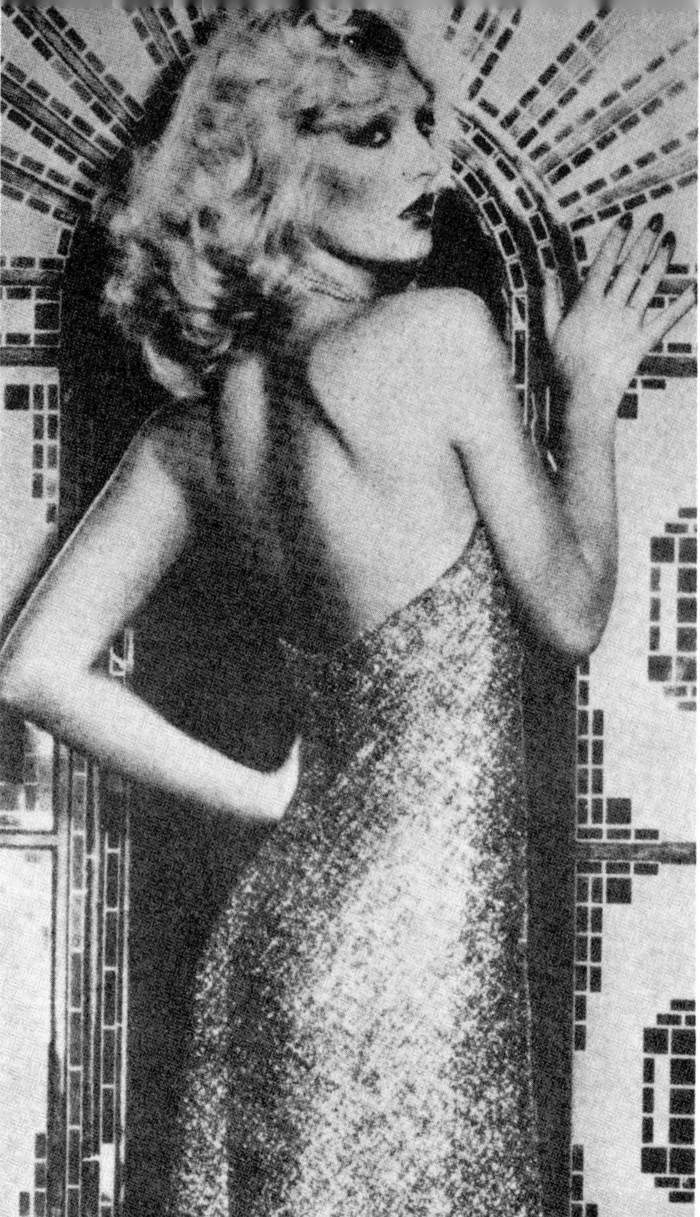

body arrives until at least an hour and a half after the appointment, and by the time hair and make-up are done, it is lunch-time. Work begins after lunch, but it might continue until nine or ten at night because there are no time limits. In New York, models are paid time-and-a-half for working late. Not in Paris. Modelling becomes a way of life in Paris.

In New York, models arrive for work with their accessories—jewellery, shoes, bras, different-coloured stockings; in Paris, the girls who earn 1,500 francs a day very often have not a pair of shoes to their name. One girl who had a booking in Germany needed accessories and shoes. The agent advanced her some cash to buy shoes, but when she returned to Paris she told the agent she needn't have bothered, because 'one of the other models had shoes and accessories, so I borrowed what I needed from her'. A top photographer in Paris complains that quite often the European models can't even stand up in shoes with heels, and that on one occasion he waited an hour for one to learn how to do so!

Models need to work for the glossy magazines. It is essential for them to do the editorials because it is their shop-window. Once they hit the glossies the work starts coming in. Advertisers want models who have appeared in the glossies, because they are considered to have reached the top of their careers once they are taken up by *Vogue* or *Harpers Bazaar*. Achieving the cover can change her career. It is the pinnacle of a model's career to appear on the covers of *Vogue* and *Harpers Bazaar*.

A photographic model's career can start at sixteen, but will end at, say, thirty. Anyone over thirty is unusual, but there have been exceptions. In couture, or show modelling, girls go on for considerably longer.

Top New York photographer Scavul-lo finds that models are best to photograph when they're between eighteen and twenty-five. 'I love them when they're twenty-one', he confesses. 'I look for good hair and big eyes in a model', he says. 'I like full lips. If a girl has thin lips, I can't be bothered. If she has small eyes, I can't be bothered either. I like her to have an attitude in front of the camera; a sense of drama or a sense of humour. And the girl has to have length; proportion of the body. I prefer models between 5ft 8in and 5ft 10in. It is difficult for small girls to do fashion.'

If a model is determined to succeed, the best advice she can have is to keep her sense of humour and not to believe her own publicity. That, however, is difficult to tell girls of seventeen and eighteen years old who can earn $100,000 a year. No matter how 'on top' a model is, physically, she can be her worst enemy if she does not take

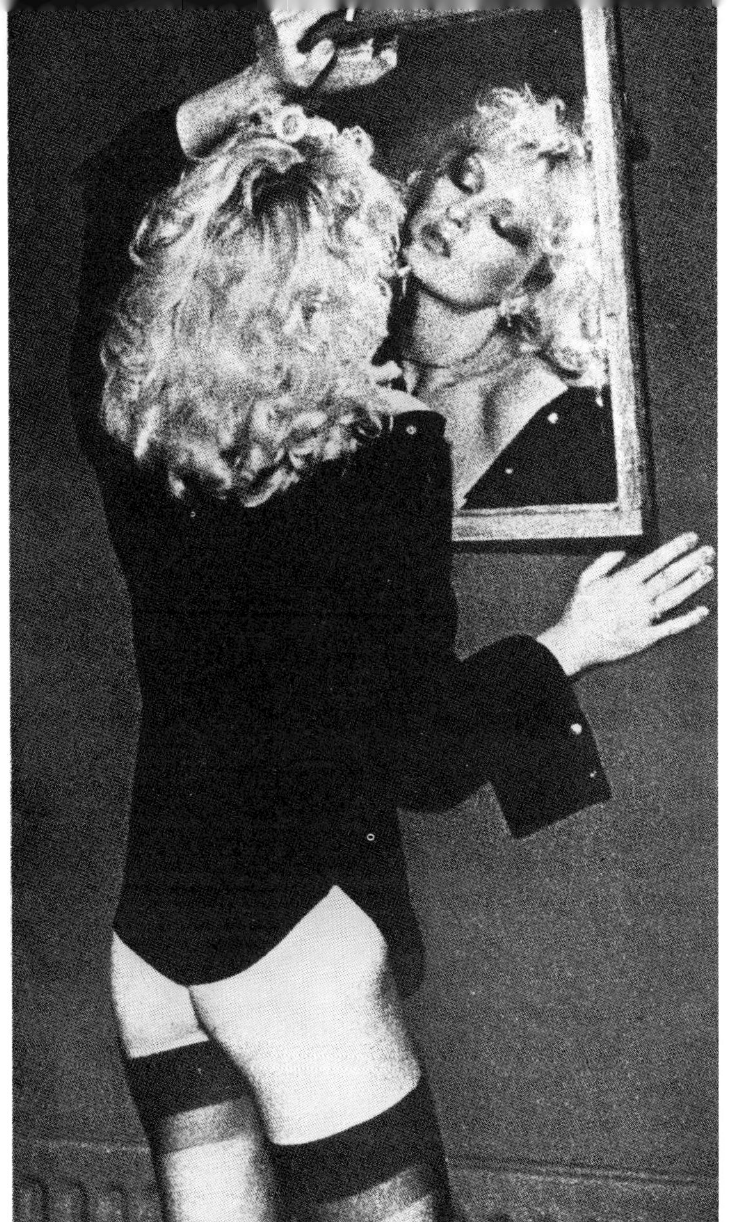

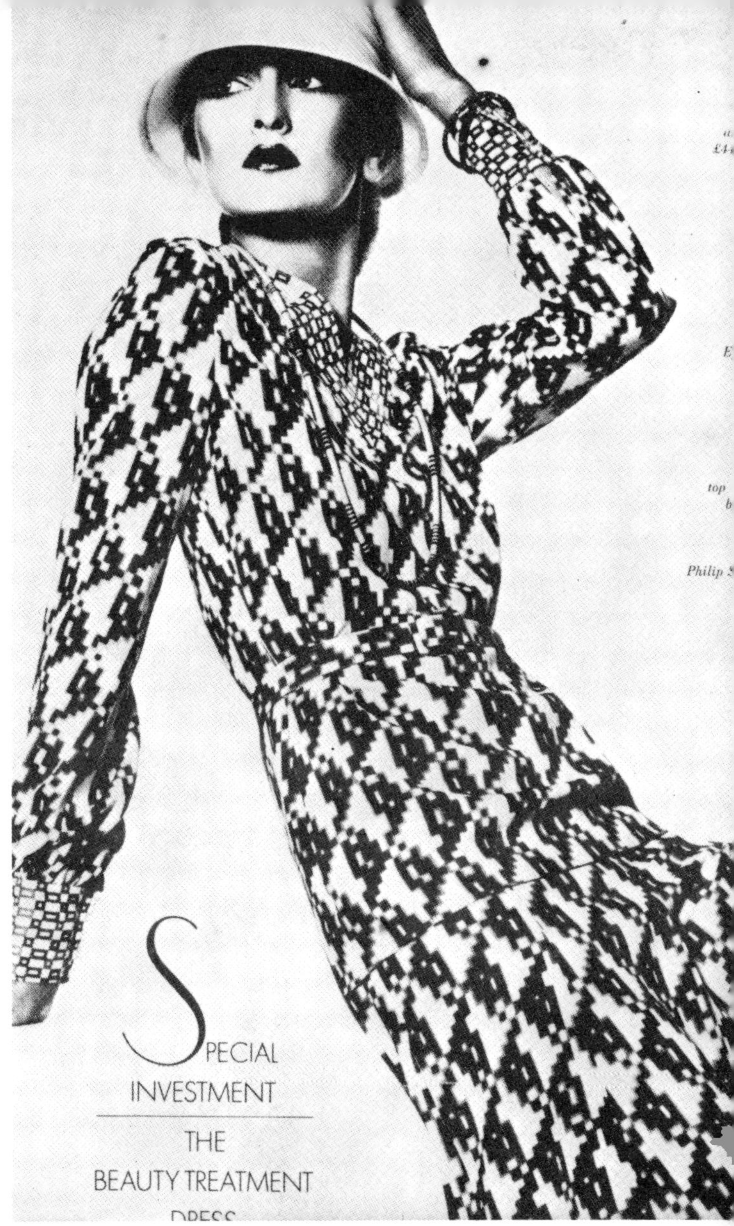

care of herself, and of the friends she has made. If she steps on her friends, or the people who have helped to mould her career, as much as they helped her on the way up, they can slap her on the way down.

But before a girl becomes a top model she would be well advised to consider a college education. The more intelligent she is, the better model she becomes; beauty is skin deep. Beautiful girls can stand in front of a camera, but only for a certain length of time; to have a college education and a background to fall back on when they've reached thirty and the money stops coming in is to be fore-warned.

'What is the greatest caution a young girl coming into the industry should heed?' I asked a top New York model.

'Don't spend all your money', came the reply. 'And don't think it's going to last forever. Moreover, find a rich husband very quickly!'

Above: A variety of poses from the card of Jane Goddard

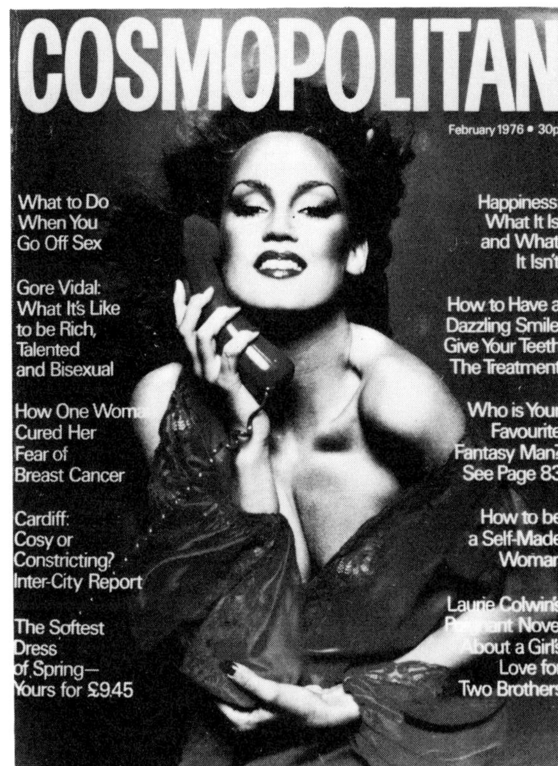

Left: The top American model, Jerry Hall, on one of her many covers. Photograph by Bill King. Courtesy *Cosmopolitan*/**UK**

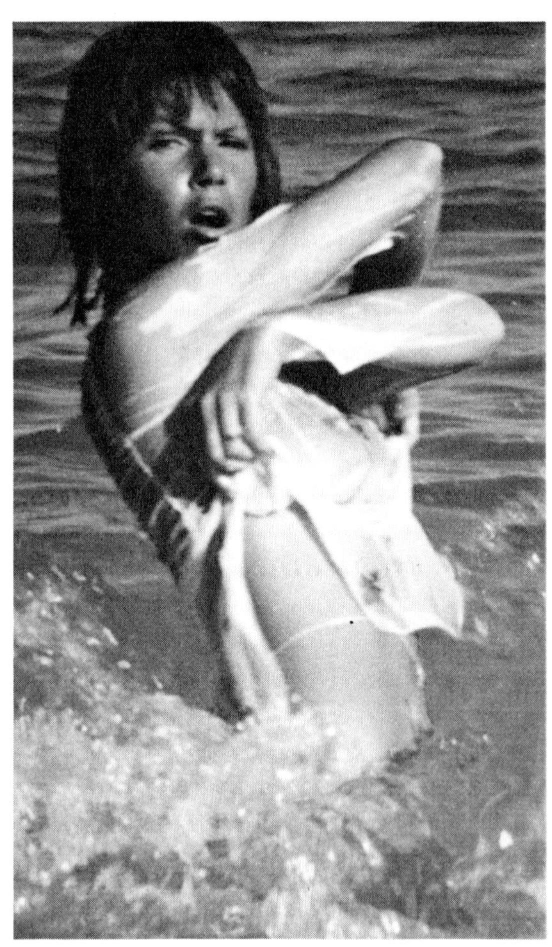
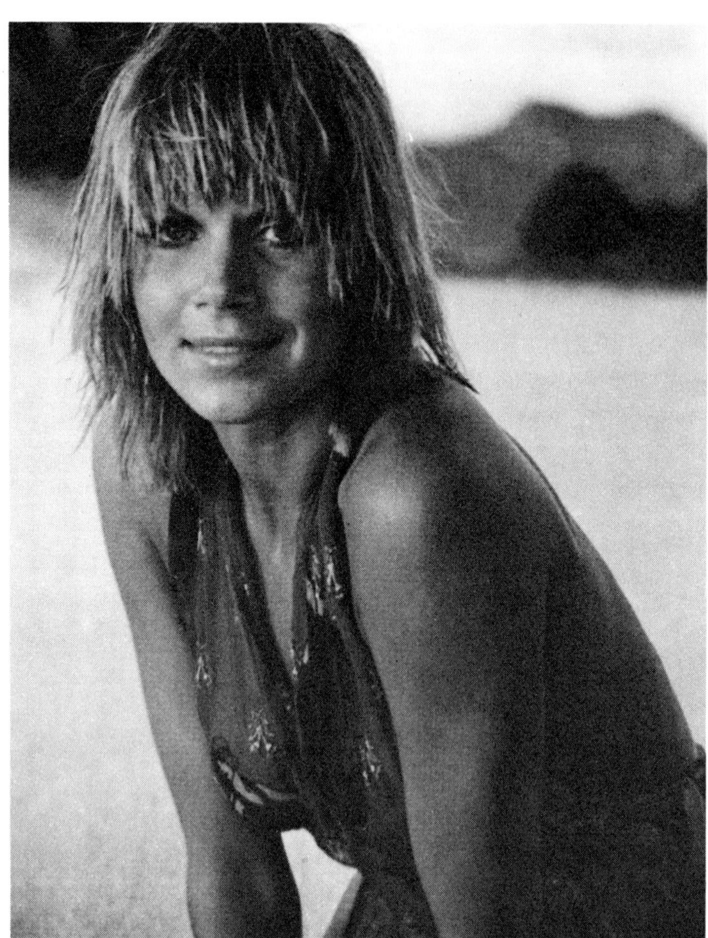
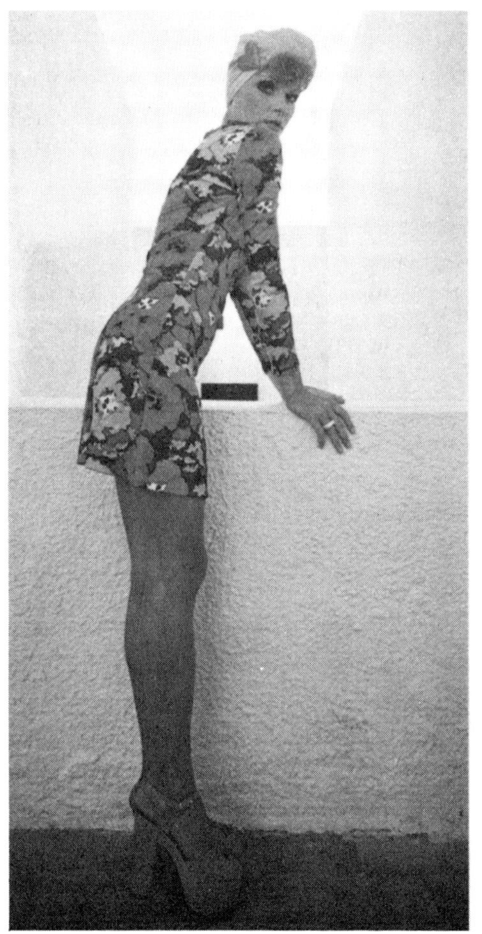
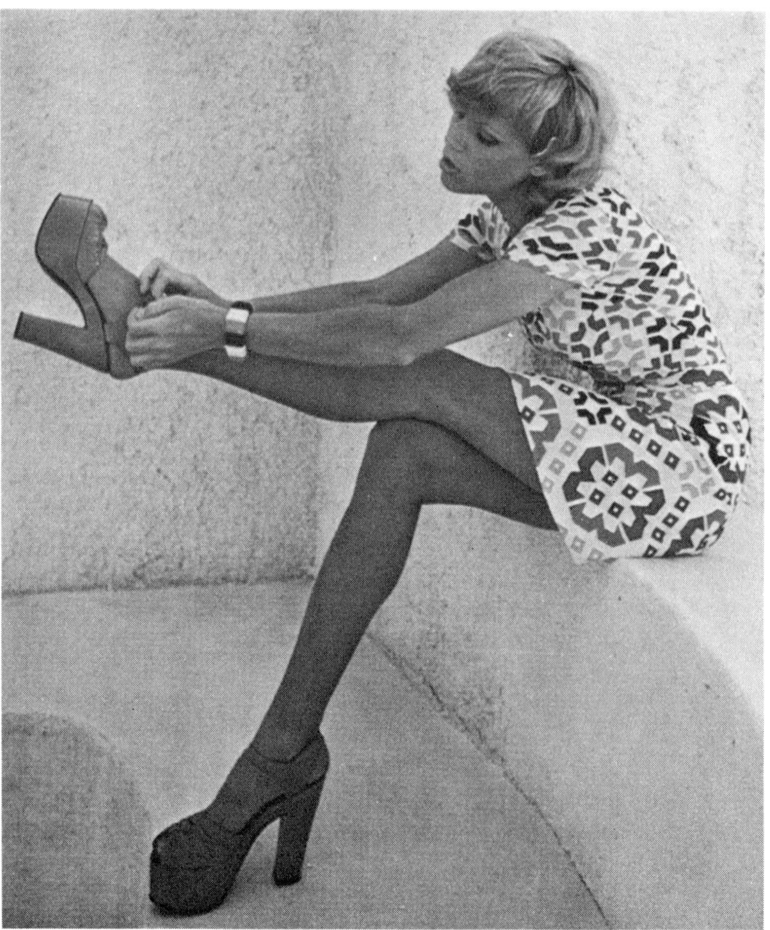

Modelling is a mercurial business in which the brightest stars shine only briefly. There is, however, a selection of high-powered specialists who are essential to the presentation of the model's image to the public for as long as advertisers and the media are interested in her beauty. By the time she reaches thirty, the best years of a model's life are over, but until then the top girls are promoted, pampered, and protected. Whilst the photographer's mighty role in creating the glamorous illusion is well known, there exists another league of silent experts who mould and guide the model on her road to success.

The power behind the glory is immense: model schools, model agencies, public relations companies, producers of fashion shows, printers of index cards, and direct-mailing system are all devoted to bringing a model's existence to the attention of the fashion editors, photographers, and advertisers. In the forties, when the agency system had not begun, models in London were paid a guinea for a photographic sitting, which might have lasted from half an hour to half a day, and hawked their photographs around studios themselves, ever hopeful of work. Fashion houses and photographers, on the other hand, were never sure whether the model would actually appear at the appointed time, until the new model agencies arose, to liaise between model and client on a commission basis. It was Evelyn Spilsbury, Sir Bernard Spilsbury's daughter and a famous model in London in the thirties and forties, who started the first known model agency in London—the Spilsbury–Kent Model Agency.

British model agencies are government controlled, and can only operate under licence from a county council. Models' fees are deposited in separate accounts to protect the models' earnings in case the agency runs into financial difficulties.

But in the London of the late forties and fifties, the stern Jean Bell was perhaps the first serious model agent who commanded respect from client and model alike. If she felt there was little she could do to develop a new young hopeful's career, she would be frank and say so. She retired to live in Spain.

Lucie Clayton was the first model agency to start a model training school in Britain. It is one of the oldest and most respected foundations for models in London, begun by Sylvia Gollidge, who had been a model herself. Now retired to Australia, she called her agency 'Lucie Clayton', a fabricated name. She sold it to the present owners, Leslie and Evelyn Kark, who have added a secretarial college to the empire, and these days they run dressmaking and fashion courses as well. Lucie Clayton's most notable discoveries were Fiona Campbell-Walter in the fifties, and Jean Shrimpton and Celia Hammond in the sixties.

A four-week basic-grooming course at Lucie Clayton costs about £90; Mondays to Fridays, mornings only. Their secretarial courses cost £237 a term, for three terms, and the four-term dressmaking and fashion courses cost £237 a term as well.

Two other highly respected stalwarts of the British model agency business, Peter Hope Lumley and Cherry Marshall, both closed their agencies in 1976, after more than twenty years. Cherry Marshall had become a top model soon after World War II at the age of twenty-three, when modelling was not considered respectable. She opened her agency and charm school in 1954. Her top discoveries were Joy Weston, Nola Rose, the milk girl Zoe Newton, actress Suzy Kendall, former Beatle George Harrison's wife, Patti Boyd, and the late Laurence Harvey's wife, Paulene Stone.

Peter Hope Lumley continues to run a successful public relations business, offering the finest services to the fashion industry.

Entrepreneur Michael Whittaker is another well established London model agent, but his most important work has been in producing fashion shows for television and presenting industrial shows for the fashion industry, promoting fabrics. He designs, mounts, and stages fashion shows, with perhaps sixteen models dancing to pop music. He presents shows all over the world and often employs models in the countries his shows visit. Courtaulds are one of his famous clients.

South African born Gavin Robinson, once a model boy, is one of the most successful young model agents in London. He runs his agency from fashionable Bond Street with Gil Barber, another ex-top model boy. Gavin and Models One in the Fulham Road handle some of the best models in London and Europe. There are many other model agencies in London, such as Askews, Peter Benison, Bobtons, Freddies, Nevs and Promcat.

There are a considerable number of model schools in Britain and America, and many of them need to be examined closely. New young hopefuls take courses in the belief that they will emerge as models, or potential models, but nothing could be further from the truth.

Reputable model schools certainly teach grooming, make-up, hairstyling, figure correction, skin-care, deportment, and dress sense. Specialists give expert advice and tuition, and former models train the youngsters in the technique of modelling, passing on their years of experience. But little can be learnt in four short weeks (working part-time) that will elevate these eager young folk into the realms of high fashion or photographic modelling.

'I've had to retrain every model who has come from a model school', complains Michael Whittaker. At a recent graduation, where some eighty models were put through their paces before an audience of friends and family at the end of their course, each girl showed three fashions: day-wear, evening-wear, and casual clothes. Of the eighty, it is unlikely that any of them had any true model potential. One girl, an Iranian who was as broad as she was short, looked a fright, and ought to have been turned away at the outset. But the model school explained afterwards that she 'might' stand a chance of success in her own country. An unlikely and misleading supposition.

The Image Makers

The centrefold from the composite card of Sliwka, a rising young European model

Sally~Ann Vancliffe

Grosse 1.73
Oberweite 86 Taille 61 Hufte 94
Schuhe 38/40
Haare Blond Augen Grun/Grau

Height 5'8
Bust 34 Waist 24 Hips 37
Shoes 6
Hair Blonde Eyes Green/Grey

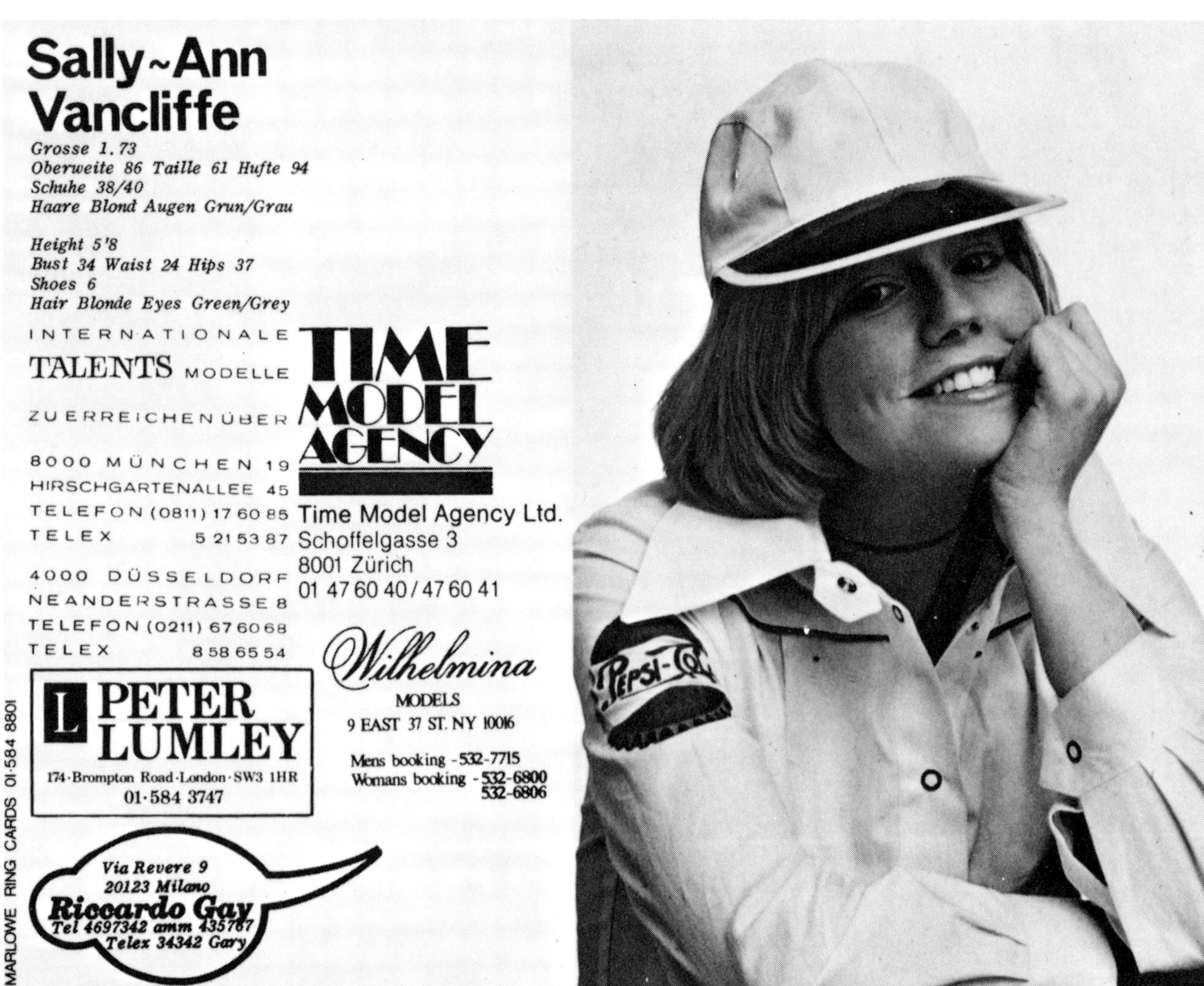

Of the eight model boys who showed their paces, not one of them was over 5ft 9in; far too short to be male models. Unless model schools are going to be brutally honest and let these boys know that their future exists expressly as accessories to the model girls, who, at 5ft 9 or 10in in stockinged feet will tower over them like guardsmen once they have heels and hair on, youngsters will become disillusioned and disappointed, and have wasted money they can ill afford.

Although models do not have the expense of providing their own photographs in New York when contracted to large agencies, it is an added expense in London and Europe. As well as photographs, they will need agency-cards or composites, which, for a new girl who has not yet begun earning money, can be a considerable expense. The composite (which used to be known as the Sed Card because it was devised by Sebastian Sed) consists of two or three poses, including vitally important infor-

mation for fashion editor, photographer, and advertising agency, such as name, height, size, colour of hair and eyes, and name of model agency. These cards are produced in London more economically and at a higher standard than anywhere else in Europe. Models in Paris, Germany, and Scandinavia send to London to have their cards printed, and the two top London companies who produce them are owned by Robert Wheal and his rival Peter Marlow.

'We produce a basic card for £32', says Robert Wheal, 'and this provides a picture on one side, and two pictures on the other side for an extra £3, all in black and white. We provide 750 of these cards for the £35, all told. Of course, colour is more expensive, and as more pictures are added, the price goes up accordingly. But when girls start out, they don't need colour or too many shots. They need to get known. We do all the reproduction on our premises, right up to the printing-plate stage, and then the printing plates are sent fifteen

minutes away to the printing machines.'

As well as the composites, a model will need photographs in order to launch herself. In London, for £40, she could arrange a sitting with a photographer, and choose, say, half-a-dozen poses from thirty or forty shots, at an additional £2 for each print. The index cards are £35, and the mailing list charge is another £11.40. The model needs a portfolio for her photographs—and later on her magazine cuttings, which will cost another £30. 'She could hardly arrive at a photographer or *Vogue* with her pictures in a brown paper bag.' Presentation is important. And so, £125 is the barest minimum for graphic work.

Although Wheal and Marlow provide a service for the model by sending the cards by post to photographers, advertising agencies, fashion editors, newspapers, magazine and casting directors —all the people who regularly book models—the model's agent sends out the cards as well. Many clients work through specific agencies who may or

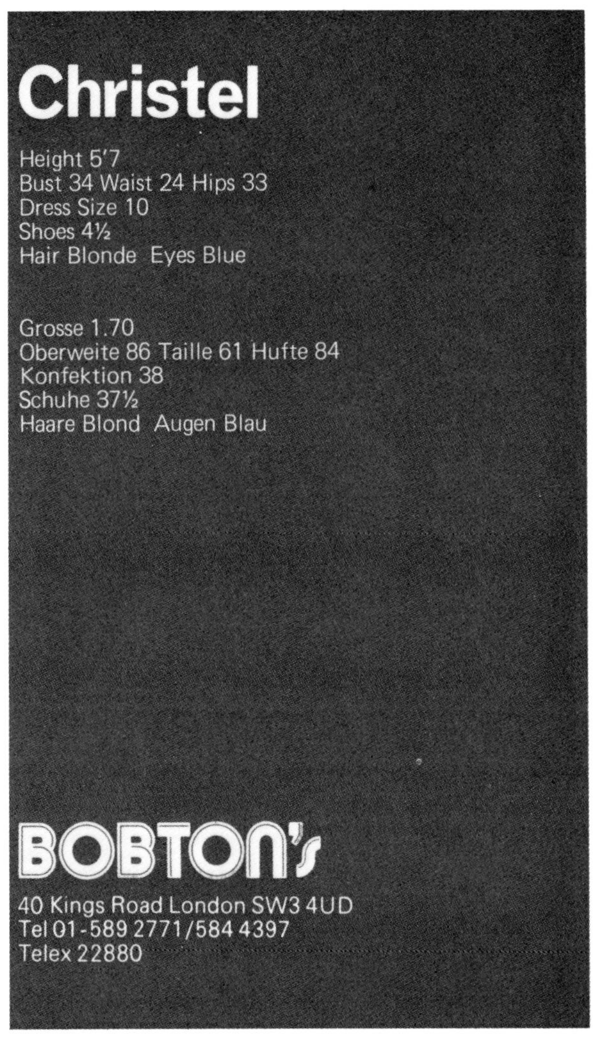

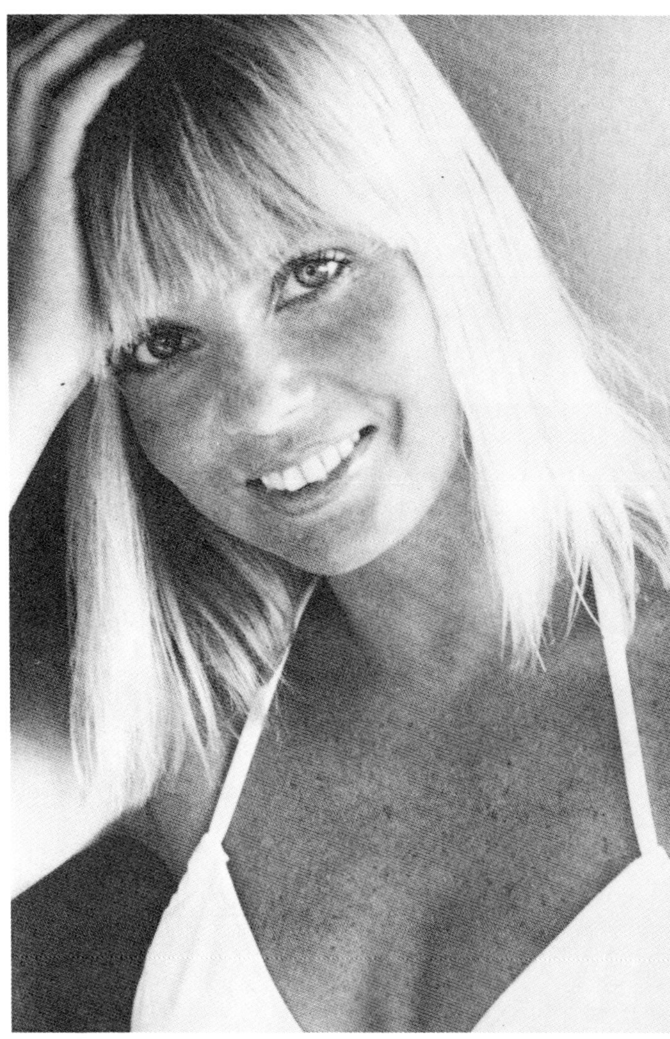

may not be on Wheal's or Marlow's lists; although there might be a certain amount of duplication, it is an added form of advertising.

Wheal and Marlow produce the agency 'head-sheets' as well, consisting of, say, three or four dozen pictures of the agencies' models. Because the British can produce the agency cards and head-sheets so economically and with such good quality, Wheal has been asked to open an office in New York, where it is hoped that his expertise in this field can be offered to models in America at competitive rates.

It is more difficult for a model to start a career in London, as the agencies do not groom the girls in the way the French and, particularly, the American high-powered agencies do, and there are not sufficient glossy magazines or photographers to enable them to build up experience at a reasonable pace. Paris is the best starting point for a new model. There are more glossies with a larger fashion output for which to work, notably *Vogue*, *Elle*, and *Marie-Claire*. There are more photographers from whom to choose; photographers who are creative and who more readily give a new girl a chance. As the output is so great, the search for new faces is ever on.

Model agencies in Paris were forbidden by law until former top American model Dorian Leigh arrived in the fifties, determined to open the first model agency in France. The police, however, protested, believing it to be a cover for prostitution, but Dorian Leigh was determined and went to law. She convinced the authorities that her agency was *bona fide*, a necessity for the protection of the vulnerable young models who were essential to France's lucrative fashion industry.

Today there are many good model agencies in Paris, one of the leading ones being Models International, headed by another former top model, Simone d'Aillencourt-Bénazéraf. She has discovered and promoted many top models

Above and opposite: The fronts of two typical composite cards showing how the vital information about a model should be presented. Christel is photographed by Alex Henderson

her best being Vibéké Knudson—probably the top model in Europe today, Appolonia von Ravenstein, Suzy Quirk (one of Guy Bourdin's favourites), and many others.

Having been a model herself, Simone knows too well what to look for in a new young girl who comes to her for work. As there are no model schools in Paris, the only way to gain experience is through an agency. 'They come to the agency, and I give them advice and a test', says Simone. 'We send them to a good photographer, and if they're lucky, they get taken up right away. We send them to hairdressers; and we have a very good beautician who teaches them how to make-up. They learn a lot in our studio.

'I was very lucky, because I started with *Vogue*, and I learnt a lot by watching what the other girls did with their hair and make-up.' These days the models are groomed by top model agencies who provide expert advice and modern facilities.

John Casablancas heads Élite, another top model agency in Paris. His wife, top model Jeanette Christjansen, is one of the highest paid models in Europe. British-born Christine Lindgren runs Viva, and the top model on her books is Ann Anderson, who, with Vibéké Knudson and Susan Moncur, is rated as one of the top models in Europe today. There are many other leading agencies in Paris, including Pauline's, Christa, Euromodels, and Modelplanning. 'The girls we take on are often fifteen and sixteen years old', says Christine Lindgren, 'and the agent has to mother them. You have to be able to carry them, otherwise you can't get new girls. You have to invest in them, and you're not always lucky; but it's not enough for them simply to be beautiful.

'Fifty per cent is beauty, the rest is talent and the right mental approach to the job.'

In New York, Eileen and Jerry Ford run the biggest and most powerful model agency in the world. Eileen, the high-priestess of models, rules the industry, ever-knowing and greatly respected; yet feared because of the power she wields. 'I always know I'm doing the right things', she says with confidence. 'That's how single-minded I am. I work for my models. I don't

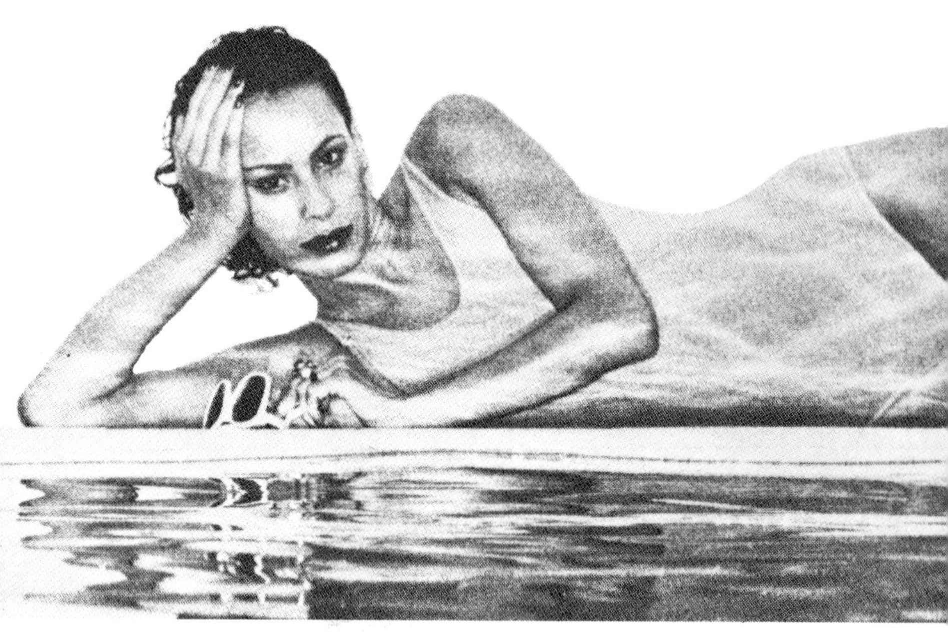

work for anybody else, and if I have to do something for them that somebody else doesn't like, that doesn't concern me at all.'

Eileen Ford started the Ford Agency on 1 October 1946, with twenty-nine models. Today, Fords represent over two hundred people and the agency is made up of a women's division, a men's division, a children's division, and a television section. The Fords success lies in the fact that they are able to find the faces that advertising and editorial people want to see most. Their discoveries have included Suzy Parker, Elsa Martinelli, Ali MacGraw, Jane Fonda, Candice Bergen—and Lauren Hutton, who was turned down by every other agent in New York. Rene Russo is her top girl, who, it is believed, will replace Lauren Hutton.

'You can always tell stars from non-stars', says Eileen. 'You can tell who's going to be a good working model and make $65,000 and $75,000 a year, and who's going to be a star. Stars have an electricity. They light up a room. It's *our business* to find stars.' And they find them with unfailing regularity, travelling the world in their quest.

Eileen and Jerry Ford may feel resented by rivals out of sheer jealousy, or because the Fords built model agency status into what it is today, but they are undaunted by criticism. There is no models *union*, because the Fords *are* the union. Every improvement in the business was made by them, and no other agent can raise the scale of models' fees without looking to the Fords who set the pace. They fought for the increase of model's fees throughout the years, and formulated the first model's contract with top cosmetic companies. Evelyn Kuhn, one of their leading models, was the first model to win such a contract—as Revlon's top girl. The contract was formulated and negotiated by the Fords, and was the forerunner of many such long-term contracts between model and client.

Big-league modelling is tough, competitive, and exciting. The average Ford model will make at least $40,000 a year; at all the major agencies, models who consistently make less than $25,000 annually are advised to look for other employment, which can be tough on a girl in her early twenties without any specific training. Of the five thousand young hopefuls who pass through the Ford door each year, only one or two out of every five hundred will make it. But this does not discourage the girls from trying. The gamble is worth taking. But interviewing the eager beauties can be wasted energy; there are few Patti Hansens or Rene Russos who reach the top, seen regularly on *Vogue* and *Harpers Bazaar* covers.

Rio, photographed by Niel Kirk

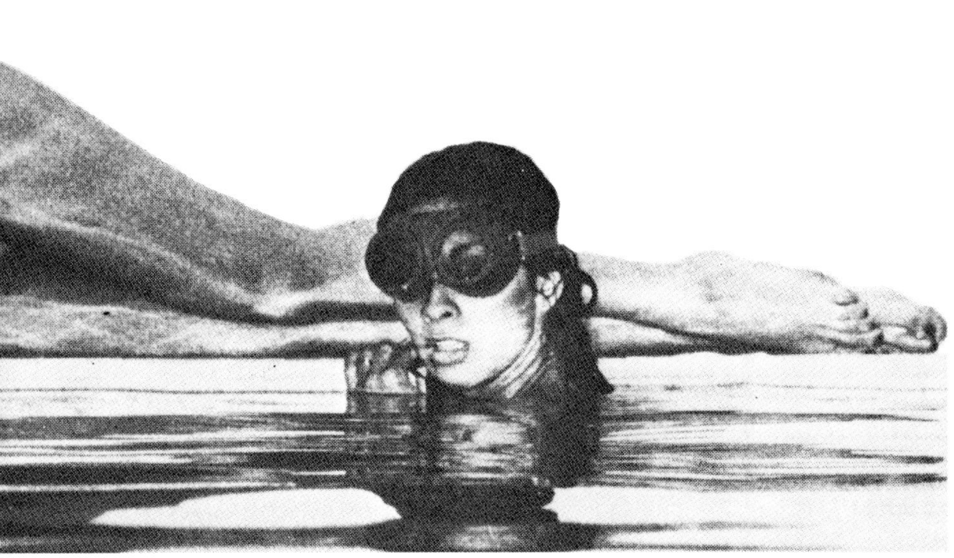

Among the Ford stars of the past was Wilhelmina, who now, with her husband Bruce Cooper, has run her own model agency, the Wilhelmina Agency, successfully for the past ten years. They are the second largest model agency in New York, after Fords, with three others in the same league: the Stewart Agency, Barbara Stone, and Zoli.

'Newcomers are placed under contract when they come to us', says Wilhelmina, 'because we put a tremendous amount of public relations, training, and money behind them. I put three employees behind them for the first six months, who do nothing else but hold their hand and improve them. I personally give them modelling classes for nothing. We provide television training too, and because of these added services and facilities that we put at their disposal, a contract is necessary to safeguard our investment. At the moment it has a get-out clause on either side, but I'm trying to change that.'

Model agencies cannot guarantee income on the contract because the agency is employed by the model, but the *client* employs the model.

The Wilhelmina Agency is situated on the top floor of a modern building on East 37th Street, the hub of the business activity. The seventh-floor studio downstairs, like the Fords agency, has a ramp for show model training, and a full set-up for television video-tape recording, which the models can see themselves after doing readings for television commercials. Although the studio is often rented out to clients, it is available to the models for test-photography sessions. Any test-photographer who doesn't have a studio knows that he can use our studio', says Wilhelmina. 'We have a sort of house photographer who works for the magazines, which automatically makes life easier for us, because once he discovers somebody, it clicks very quickly.'

Models under contract at Wilhelmina's are able to join the voice-production classes, which take place four nights a week, under the tutelage of Dr Jaegar, a professor of the University of Carolina. 'We've had tremendous results from these classes, because we've discovered talent in models; talent they didn't know they had. Because of this, our television commercial income has increased. Our calibre of models and their talent has increased too. Instead of a hot twelve, we now have a hot eighteen or twenty; when I say hot, I mean that they get every job they go for, and I think it has a lot to do with the training we give. Dr Jaegar is tough on them; he rips their guts out, and puts them back in one by one. It's a tough course to go through and I have a tremendous fallout. Out of forty-five girls, you end up with perhaps fifteen at the end because the others just couldn't cope with it. But that's the business. It's tough one way or another.'

Wilhelmina does the make-up guidance herself. The models sit in front of her in her office and do their own make-up. Though there are facilities downstairs, it is too far from the telephone, and Wilhelmina prefers to be accessible at all times. 'I watch them make-up while I carry on with my work. I say, "No. No. You're going down, and I want the line to go up." I let them do it themselves, because I find that if I do it for them, they wash it off at night, and in the mornings they've forgotten how it was done. And then they get more creative; they see other models come in, and try out new ideas. And then they come to me for confirmation.'

'When we started the agency', Bruce Cooper puts in, 'we did not pirate models from other agencies. We found our own, new, young girls and trained them. We were the ones who started the black models in this country. If you run into a black community and ask them about an agency in New York, they'll always say Wilhelmina first. Wilhelmina became the idol in the black community.' She discovered the black models Naomi Sims and Beverly Johnson, and among the others, Pat MacGuire, Jane Hitchcock, and Margaux Hemingway. They found Elsa Peretti in London, and brought her over to New York. 'She had one pair of black jeans, one pair of Indian moccasins, a cowboy hat and thirteen dollars in her pocket. She had the most fabulous legs, and a wonderful flair.' They helped her financially, got her into *Vogue;* and now she is one of the most famous jewellery designers in America. Lois Chiles is another top girl on Wilhelmina's books, but she is seldom available for modelling assignments as her movie career has taken over.

Although there is frequent grumbling about the rates they can now charge, most people on the advertising and editorial ends of the glamour business agree that powerful agencies are both good and necessary. They find the faces that industry needs to sell its products. For the men and women who make their living from their faces and bodies, the agencies offer great financial protection.

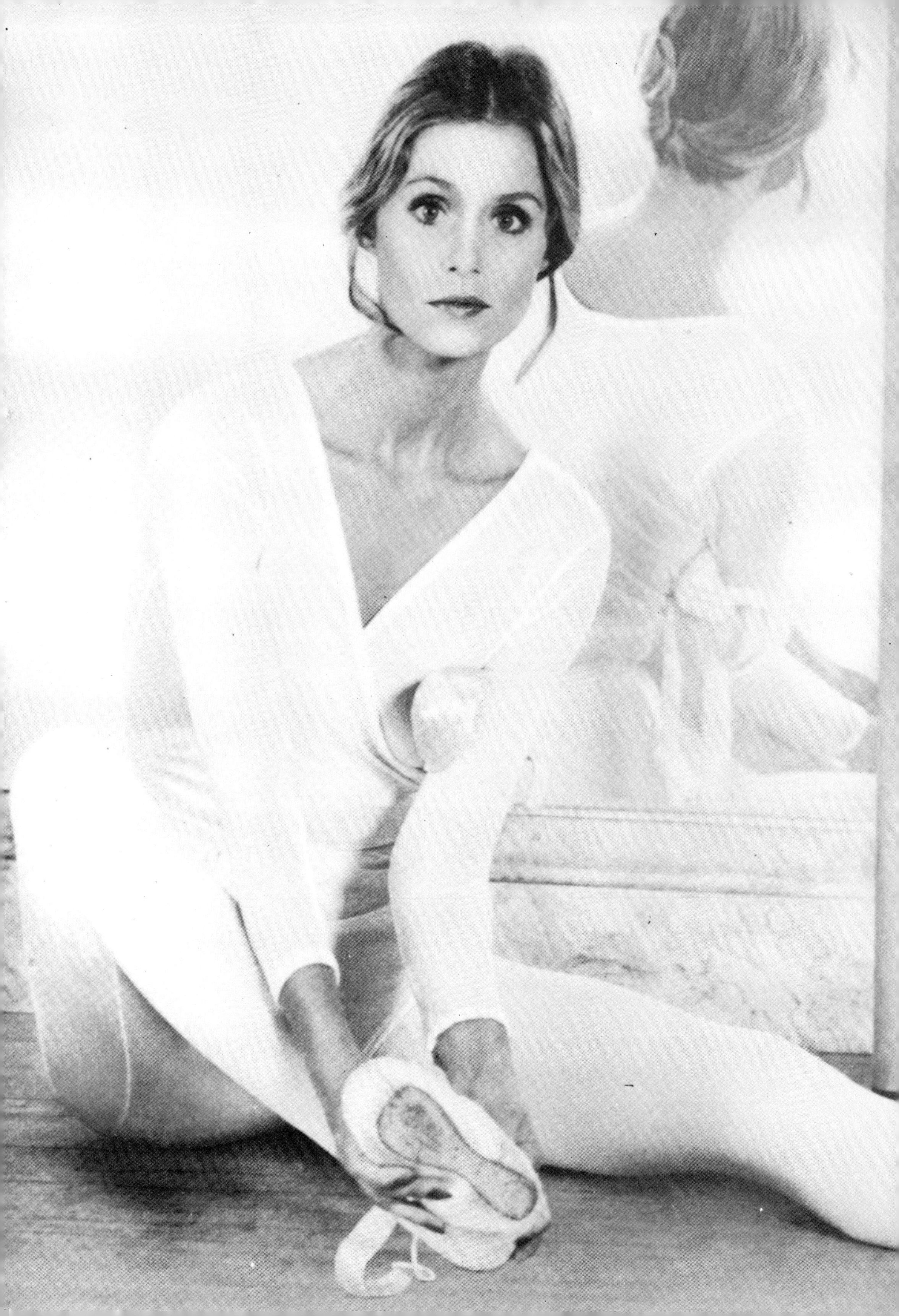

Where do you go to my lovely?

By the very nature of their work, models tend to live an unreal existence, in an artificial world orientated to the media. The vanity that surrounds their daily lives is not conducive to marital harmony because their partners find the preoccupation with their health and looks claustrophobic.

Models live the short, frenzied existence of a butterfly, subjected to highs and excessively low downs. They are idolised and petted for weeks on end, and then, after being out of work for four or five days, rejection starts setting in, and a brittle, edgy personality emerges. Like actors, they become insecure and feel unloved and unwanted.

By the time she is thirty to thirty-five, the best years are behind a model and she is ready to be put out to grass. But this method is simpler with horses who have had a long and successful run than with once-glamorous and high-earning young beauties. It is for this reason that young girls who are launching themselves into a modelling career are advised to be equipped with a solid educational background before setting out for the bright lights, so that, when the time comes, they have something on which to fall back as a means of earning a living, and getting themselves into daily routine. Having a second career running concurrently with modelling is a vital necessity, although not always practical because of the disciplines and long hours imposed on the modelling profession. But a hobby, for instance, that might turn into a second profession when the telephone stops ringing and models are no longer sought after for their looks and limbs is a wise thought.

Jean Shrimpton, for instance, who tried stills-photography, now runs an antique shop in Devon. Many models are prudent enough to save some of their earnings whilst they are in the high-yielding bracket. They invest wisely either in property, or else they form conglomorates. Buying annuities and life-assurances is another form of saving for the future. Naturally enough, a great many girls marry and, with the support of an affluent husband, raise a family, starting a second career as wife and mother. Witness Jean Patchett and Dolores Hawkins, once New York's top models, and Barbara Goalen and Shelagh Wilson, London's top girls of the

Lauren Hutton as she appears for Revlon's Ultima II beauty cream. Courtesy Revlon

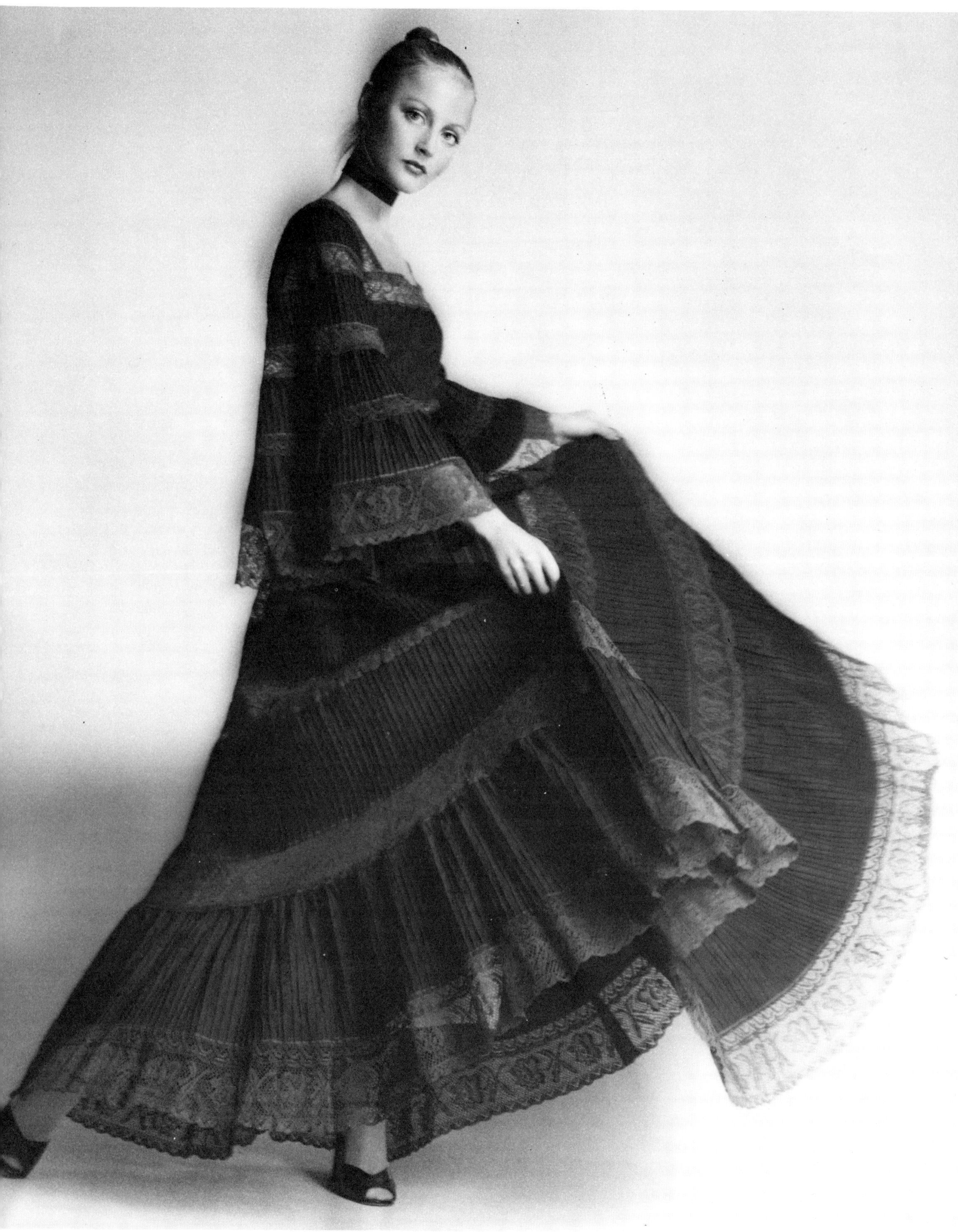

fifties, who have settled for happily married lives, with children on whom they dote. Shelagh Wilson started with *She* magazine, as fashion editor, when she first gave up modelling, and remained there for eight years.

Various other models joined top glossies as fashion editors when they retired from modelling. In London, former top models Sheila Whetton and Grace Coddington both work as fashion editors for *Vogue*. Enik Munik works for *Elle* in Paris. Jean Dawnay, who became Princess Galitzine, is involved in the promotion of Prince George Galitzine beauty products, and American top model Sunny Griffin has become Avon's beauty and fashion director, travelling the United States, advising and helping Avon girls to improve the brand image of the multi-million dollar product.

Aside from the many models who have made the successful transition from model to movie actress—and they are in the minority when it is considered how many girls throughout the world earn a living modelling—the most popular choice of second vocation is the model school or model agency business. Here, models put into practice knowledge acquired through years of experience in applying their craft and industry. They offer good business sense and professionalism to the beauty business. Having built up contacts on both sides of the fence throughout the years, working with fashion editors, photographers, advertising agents, advertisers, fashion designers, *and* other models, they amass countless contacts, and have an all-round knowledge and understanding of the highly lucrative modelling industry.

The first American model to venture into this field was Dorian Leigh, who began the first model agency in Paris, breaking new ground in France. Before

Opposite: Ingrid Boulting, photographed by Francesco Torres

Left: Shaun Casey, one of the up-and-coming models of the seventies. Photograph by Patrice Cassanova

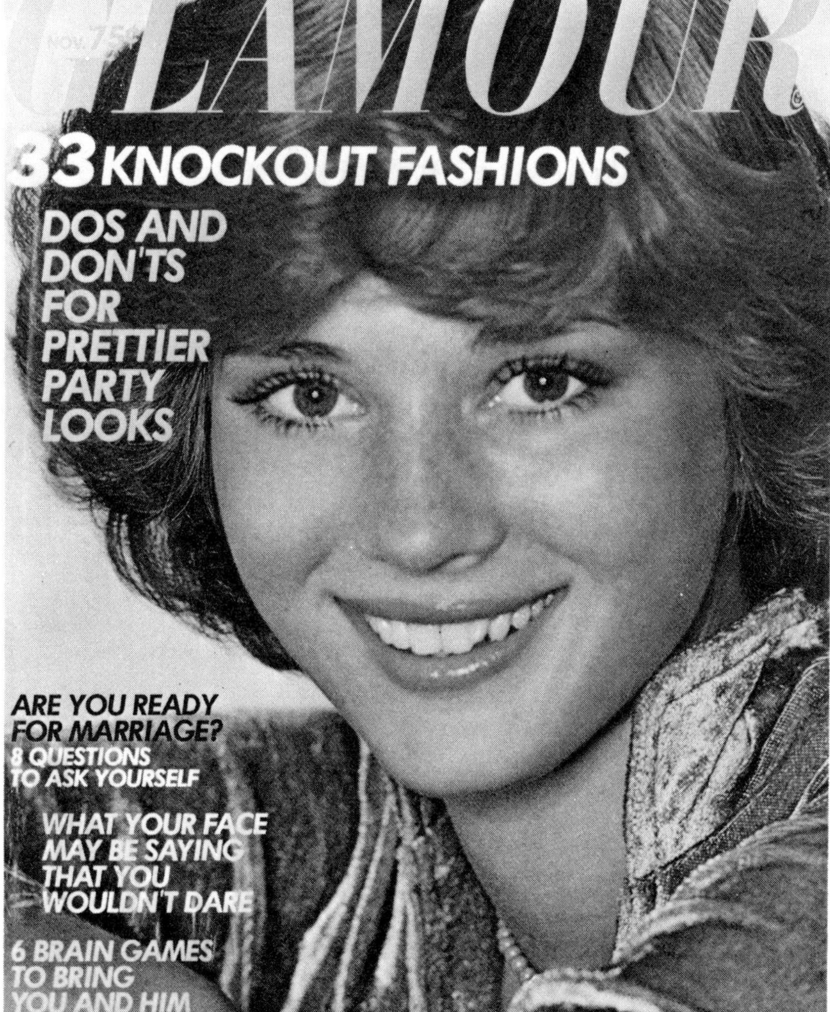

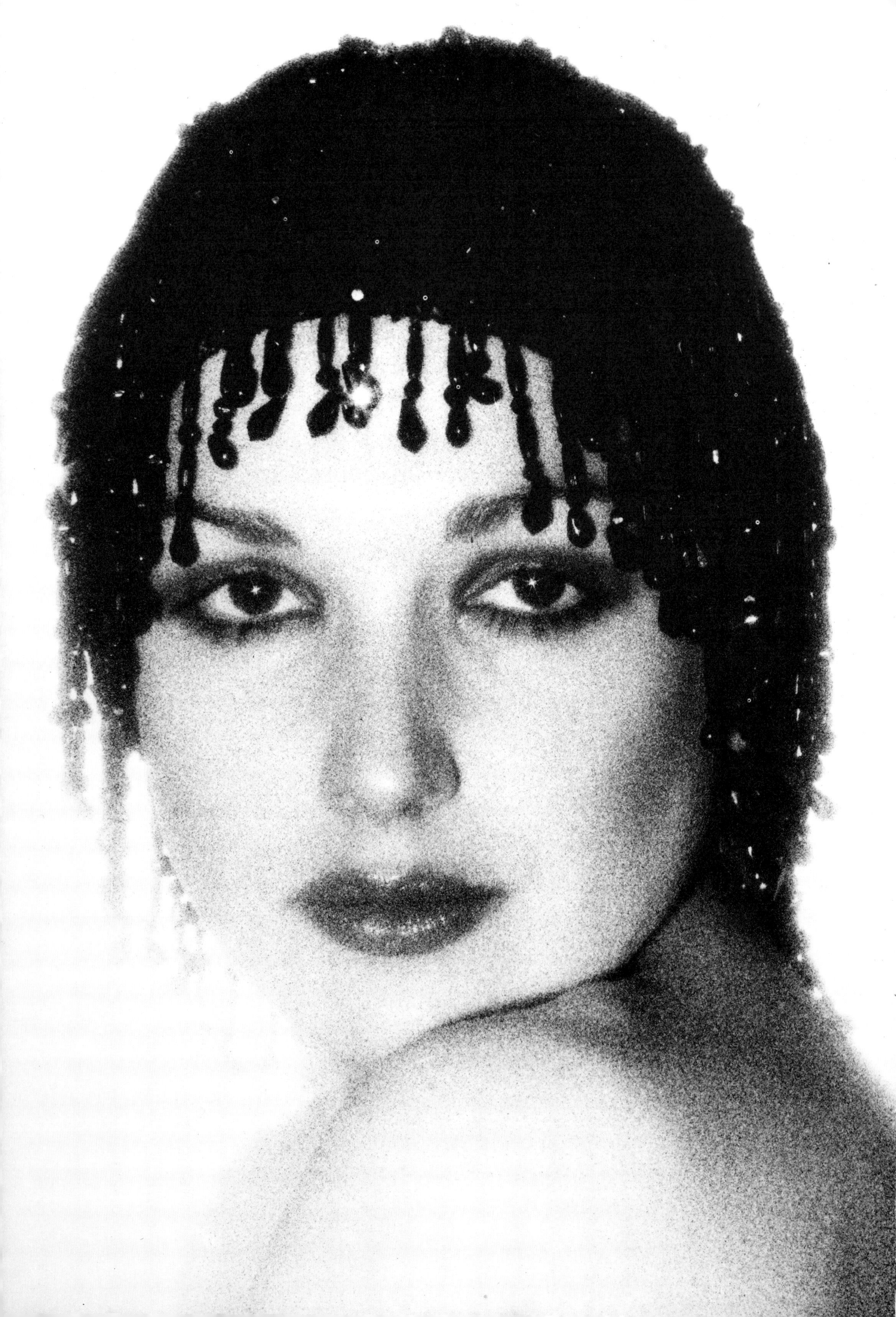

her, Eileen Ford had modelled for a short while before pioneering what has become the largest model agency in the world. In London, in the forties, Evelyn Spilsbury, a former top model, also went into the model agency business. One of the finest French models of all time, Simone d'Aillencourt, married film director José Bénazéraf. These days she heads Models International, one of the top model agencies in Paris. Dutch-born Wilhelmina, the phenomenon of the sixties, runs the Wilhelmina Agency, the second largest model agency in New York, with her husband, Bruce Cooper. Sir Norman Hartnell's top model, Dolores, opened a model school in South Africa, where she trains aspiring young hopefuls, and many other models are employed by model schools in Britain and America to instruct girls in deportment, make-up, face and hair-care, and general presentation.

Many show models remain with the top fashion houses where they once worked, as vendeuses, or saleswomen, in the ready-to-wear showrooms. The head of the *cabine* at Nina Ricci's, the Russian-born Nadine, is in charge of fourteen models. She used to be a model herself.

But not all who have once been beautiful and successful continue thus. Nina Dyer was once married to the steel millionaire Baron Heini Thyssen. After her divorce from him, she became Princess Sadruddin, wife of Prince Aly Khan's brother. She was found dead after an overdose of drugs in France, following her divorce from him.

The deaths of models, either accidental, or self-inflicted, are almost legendary in the world of modelling. The great model, Praline, Pierre Balmain's exquisitely beautiful top girl, was killed in a car crash. Another remarkable French model, Nicole de la Margé, was also killed in a car crash.

Others, like Anna, committed suicide when they got too old and could not come to terms with time. Anna was a beautiful Swedish girl who must have been in her late forties at the time of her death. She came to Paris from Sweden and modelled for Jacques Fath, and had been around for quite a while by the time she began modelling for Nina Ricci, but she was marvellous looking in spite of her age. Jules-François Crahay, the designer at Nina Ricci, designed a collection for Anna, aimed at women of her age. He chose beautiful pastel colours and produced very distinguished-looking clothes for her to show.

She never talked about herself, and nobody knew much about her private life. However, it was known that she had been married and divorced. She went on a trip to Germany with several other models to show the Nina Ricci collection. When they got to passport control at the German border, an immigration officer stopped Anna because the date of her birth on her passport had been altered. The rest of the entourage was delayed, and time was running short. Anna gave a thousand excuses about how her passport came to be damaged, but the officer wouldn't let her through. The *directrice* of the house was absolutely furious and created quite a scene about the delay. 'How dare you do this?' she reproached Anna. 'What are we going to do? We will arrive in Germany with not enough models for the collection!' And so poor Anna was sent back to Paris, but the rumpus was overheard and the incident reported in the German newspapers the next day.

Unfortunately, by the time she got back to Paris, everyone at the salon knew what Anna had done, and so she went to the Swedish Embassy and said: 'I'm out of a job. I've got no money. Please, can you get me back to Sweden?' It was late on a Friday afternoon, and she was told to return the following Monday morning when her request would be considered.

Anna didn't appear at work on the Monday morning, and she didn't arrive at the Swedish Embassy either. Her body was discovered in her room, with her wrists cut.

She had been romantically involved with a young man and feared that through the discovery of her birthdate being altered, her young lover would realise that she had lied about her age. Her humiliation was so great that rather than face him, she decided to end it all. The distraught young man admitted after the funeral that he had always known her true age, but had concealed his knowledge of it from her, realising her sensitivity about it.

Patricia Gibbs in a photograph by Ray Duffurn

Despite the pitfalls, disappointments and heartbreaks suffered by many models, young girls are, however, encouraged to enter this glamorous and highly lucrative profession. It provides not only self-improvement, self-analysis, chances to travel and meet interesting people from various walks of life, but opportunities to earn more than in any other respectable profession. It enables girls to be independent and, by saving and investing wisely, the money earned from their hard work and industry provides for them secure futures.

Memories and scrap-books of fashion covers and breathtaking photographs when their youth, health, beauty and earning powers were at their peak are satisfying reminders of their abilities and determination to succeed in their chosen field; the most highly paid and glamorous a young girl can enter.

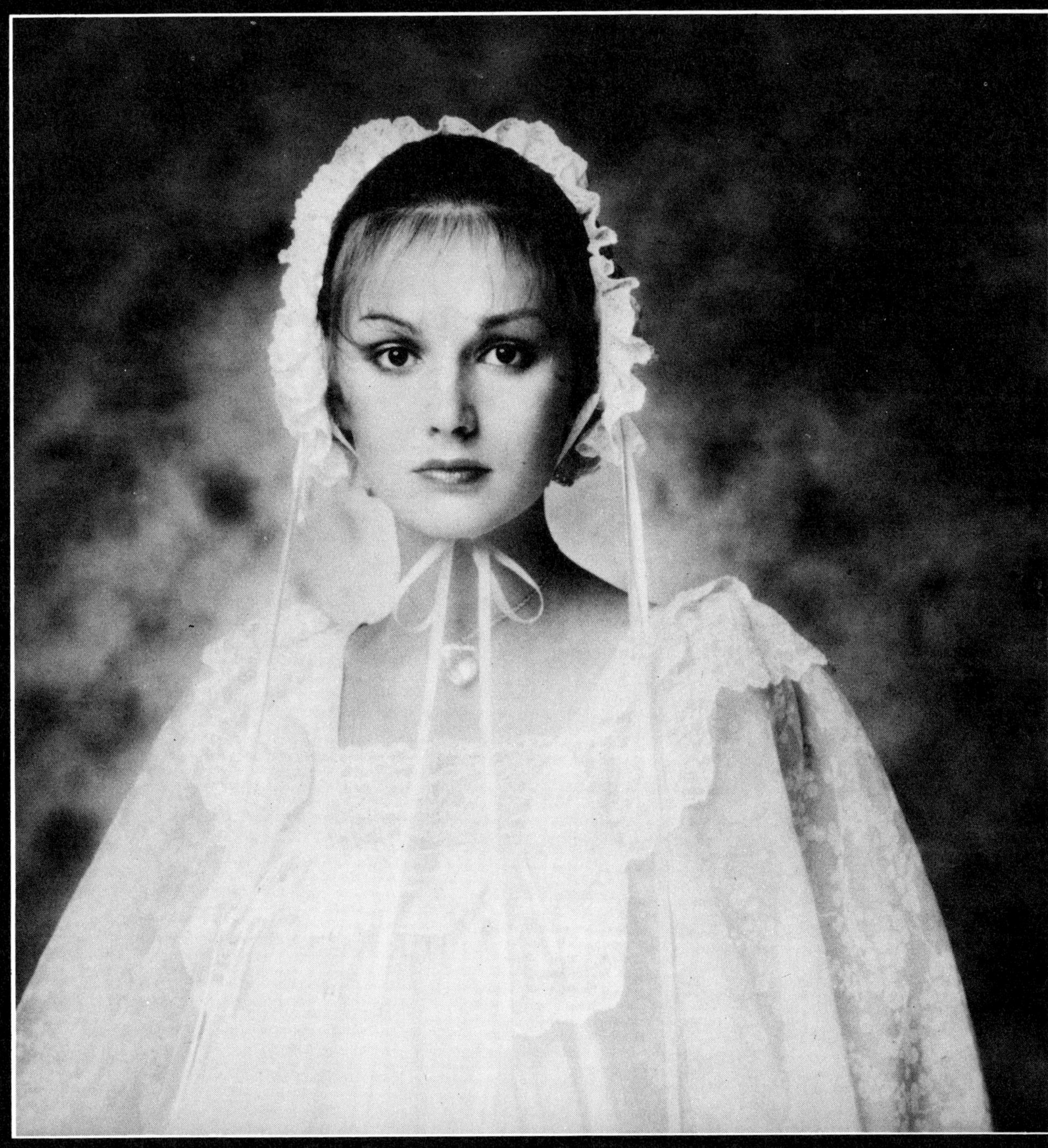

Sue Purdy, photographed for *Brides* magazine, by Barry Lategan. Courtesy Condé Nast Publications

Models' Beauty Secrets

A special guide for enthusiastic young hopefuls

In order to succeed as a model you must have the correct basic essentials in bodily frame and proportions, good bone structure, height, appealing features and the right mental approach. Good hair and the overall appearance of radiant good looks are vital—the healthy bloom on the peach. Beauty comes from within, and many a striking model succeeds without the classical features of great beauty, relying instead on physical appeal and individual personality.

To acquire this desired beauty and glamour you need to be healthy. A healthy body provides the healthy mind so necessary for success in order to withstand the arduous hours of demanding work and concentration.

When embarking on a modelling career, most girls are about 16lb too heavy, even though they consider themselves to be slim.

The ideal model's measurements are 116lb in weight, 34in bust, 22in waist, 34in hips, and a preferred height of between 5ft 7in and 5ft 9in—though shorter models have certainly made the grade.

Under the heading of figure and the condition of your skin, hair and teeth, consider diet and nutrition, as well as exercise, concentrating on the legs, arms and hands, posture and movement.

When examining your face, study its shape and sculpture. Excess fat can be reduced (remember, though, that when you diet your face is the first place to lose weight; when you put weight back on, your face is last in line). Good features can be highlighted and bad or irregular features cleverly disguised with make-up and shading. The neck and shoulders are invariably ignored and many a model's age has been betrayed by the lines on her neck and hands.

Your hair reflects good health. Dry, dull hair is unforgivable, and unnecessary. Hair on legs, arms and body is unattractive, and facial hair need not be a problem.

Although diet alone may bring you down to the required weight, daily exercise is vitally important in order to rid yourself of that bulging stomach, flabby thighs and upper arms, and loose skin where it shows most.

There is no short-cut to beauty and therefore concentration, discipline and routine, although tedious, are necessary in order to achieve successful results. A half-hearted approach will achieve half-hearted results.

Your diet will depend largely on your present weight condition and this can be modified accordingly. For good health, you need enough sleep. Six to eight hours seems adequate for many, but you yourself may need more in order to feel fresh and energetic. Lack of sleep reveals itself in the loss of skin tone and colour, loss of hair lustre, and eyes without that bright, lively glint.

Too much smoking and drinking leaves its mark on your looks. Cut it out, or reduce your intake. The body's function depends on neither, and gains nothing from them.

For healthy looks, choose healthy foods. Eat what you *need*, not what you *desire*. Models eat to live, they do not live to eat. Buy lean meat instead of fatty cuts. Avoid fried foods, and stick to grilled or boiled meats. Vegetables that are steamed are better than vigorously boiled servings, when the water containing all the goodness is invariably thrown away—besides, vegetables boiled for too long in too much water lose their calorie content. Choose fresh fruit and vegetables in preference to the frozen varieties. Fresh fruit and poultry are necessities for a healthy diet.

Your calorie intake will decide how much you should eat each day. A good average is 2,000 a day, but this depends on your height. If you are over 5ft 5in you need more; under that height, less. But a lot depends on the amount of energy you burn up each day. Energy burns up calories, so if you do more, simply eat more; if you do less, eat less.

But eat little and often. Small intakes, at, say, three-hourly intervals, are better than one hefty meal when you get home from a tiring day's work. A good breakfast starts the day right, while a large luncheon is preferable to a large evening meal because you burn up the calories as the day progresses. A large meal at night hardly has the chance of being burnt up as you relax and sleep afterwards. All animals sleep after their meals; models need to burn up the sugar in their systems by keeping active.

Liquids should be taken between meals rather than during them. Stick to non-sugar drinks and beware of alcohol. Gin and Scotch, for instance, contain 100 calories per $1\frac{1}{2}$ fluid ounces. The tonics, ginger ales and bitter lemons normally consumed with spirits are laced with sugar, and their calorie content is between 70 and 95 per 8 fluid ounces. Gin or vodka taken with grapefruit juice or plain soda water is infinitely better for you.

A top model's daily diet consists of:

Breakfast	Calories
Half a fresh grapefruit (or small glass of unsweetened orange or grapefruit juice)	55
One large boiled egg	80
Black coffee (no sugar, use concentrate or saccharin)	

Mid-morning	
Raw tomatoes, carrots or mushrooms	20 ea

Lunch	
Half a fresh grapefruit (or fruit juice)	55
Small, lean steak or lamb chop (4oz)	400
Salad (two lettuce leaves, 10 calories, one tomato, 35) say,	90
Black coffee (no sugar, use concentrate or saccharin)	

Late afternoon	
A cup of bouillon	30

Dinner

Soup (tomato or vegetable) (cupful)	90
Fish or chicken (4oz)	200
Two vegetables (carrots or string beans)	40
Salad with fresh lemon dressing	45
Black coffee (no sugar, use concentrate or saccharin)	
	1,135

To bring her calorie content up to 2,000 a day she might choose from any of the following: a glass of milk (16c); a slice of bread (60); a tablespoon of butter (100); a tablespoon mayonnaise (110); a tablespoon jam (50); a teaspoonful sugar (15); a slice of chocolate cake with icing (445!); ice-cream ($3\frac{1}{2}$ fluid ounces) (130); a fresh peach (35); one baked potato (90); ten French fries (115); two tablespoons gravy (35); half a cup of cheese sauce (245).

If you over-eat at one meal, balance your calorie intake by eating less at the next. If you've got a date and know you're going out to a restaurant, don't be a bore about your diet. Learn about calorie content and choose from the menu wisely. Start with a half a grapefruit or clear consommé, for instance. Your choice of main courses need not be made dull by selecting the right calories. Ask the head waiter for the *fresh* vegetables of the day. The choice is not so easy when dining with family or friends, however, as the food is invariably dished up without thought of diet. In that case, eat less beforehand, during the day, or balance your diet by eating less the following day.

With a good, balanced diet, strictly speaking, you don't need vitamin pills. With so many prepared and frozen foods, however, it is a good idea to boost the vitamin intake. Keep vitamin pills in reserve in case you are unable to obtain the fresh foods containing these vital health-giving compounds, perhaps through illness, work, or whilst on holiday, but, remember, there is no substitute for fresh foods. Freezing or defrosting vegetables, or allowing fresh vegetables to wilt or grow old, is another known method of vitamin loss.

If you are nervy or edgy, tired or quarrelsome, no doubt you lack thiamine in your diet—vitamin B1. This can be remedied by including in your diet bacon or pork, oatmeal, wheat germ and wholemeal bread, lentils and peas.

A lack of vitamin B2 (Riboflavin) can cause scaling and skin flaking and cracking around the corners of the mouth. Avoid this by remembering meat and yeast extracts, oatmeal, herrings and milk, together with the vitamin B1 foods. It will work wonders for your nerves and restore that brightness to your eyes.

The most important of all is vitamin C, lacking in most diets and required to be taken every day as the body does not store it. Vitamin C provides healthy blood and gums and protection from infection. It is to be found in fresh citrus fruits, such as oranges and lemons, and vegetables, such as cabbage, cauliflower, Brussel sprouts, watercress, blackcurrants and new potatoes.

Minerals such as calcium are needed for strong bones and teeth and healthy gums, and are found in milk, yoghourt, cheese, broccoli and turnip greens. Iron will put colour into your lips and zip into your general condition. You'll find iron in eggs, yeast, liver, lentils, avocados and oysters.

Vitamin D is needed for good teeth and bones. It is known as the sunshine vitamin because your body manufactures it when exposed to the sun's rays. But, remember, the sun is a killer to any good skin, scorching off the fine layers of tissue, leaving a dry, hardened texture concealed only by heavy make-up, a telltale sign of many a bad skin. A dark suntan may look wildly attractive, adding to your sparkling beauty, but you will suffer later on when heavy lines and a coarse texture form as the inevitable consequence. For vitamin D, rely on fish such as tuna, mackerel, salmon, herring and sardines, and you can't go wrong.

Apart from proteins and vitamins, carbohydrates are the principle source of energy, vitally important to a model's health. Without enough carbohydrates, the body burns up too much of the protein needed for tissue repair. Carbohydrates are found in foods containing starches and sugars, fruits and juices, and should be taken in moderation. Consuming more carbohydrates than the body needs results in the carbohydrates being stored away in the body, turning into the great enemy—fat.

Balanced intakes of protein provide energy and help to maintain skin health. Proteins are the most concentrated source of calories and, therefore, remember to include in your diet corn, soya beans, peanuts and the oils of seafood.

Exercise

Ballet dancers acquire exquisite figures by constantly exercising before they learn their dance steps and routines. To lose that flabby tummy, bulging diaphragm, and achieve shapely arms and legs, a minimum of ten minutes' exercise *every day* is required of models. Exercise helps the blood's circulation, improves breathing and reduces unwanted flab, but take care not to replace that flab with muscle. Even though your weight may be down to the desired requirement, exercise is essential to maintain your shape and form. Exercise won't lose weight; your diet will do that—but it can change your shape and dimensions. These are a few simple, elementary exercises to be carried out daily.

General exercises These tone up body and muscle in general, improve balance and co-ordination and help posture and carriage. Other *specific* exercises are designed for arms, legs, neck and other areas such as waist, hips, arms and legs.

If you have not exercised regularly before, take it gently at first, building up each day. If you feel pain or your muscles straining, stop at once and relax a while.

Running and swimming are the best general exercises for all-round body condition, providing exercise for all muscles and joints. Jumping and skipping are also very good for you, but start off slowly, building up each day.

Another very good general exercise is touching your toes ten times a day, but start off with, say, five times and work your way up. Stand upright in bare feet and loose, comfortable clothing—or naked. Lift your arms high above your head and touch your toes without bending your knees. Breathe out heavily as your arms descend, and take a deep breath as you lift them above your head again.

Waistline. Good waistline exercises are the 'windmills'. Stand with legs apart and arms outstretched horizontally. Swing your arms around, first to the left and then to the right, as far as your trunk will allow them to go. Do this ten times. Next, stand upright, legs apart, your arms outstretched above your head in a V-shape. Swing your left arm down to touch your right foot with your fingers, and then the fingers on your right arm to touch your left foot, keeping knees stiff and swinging in rhythm to touch your toes ten times. Remember to breathe out when you swing your arms down, and in when you swing them up.

Diaphragm The most effective diaphragm exercise is touching your toes whilst lying flat on the floor with legs outstretched together and arms extended above your head. But take care—this can be extremely painful if done to excess and you will not be aware of the pain until the next day. Start with two movements a day, building up to three, four, five, etc, until you get to fifteen or twenty. Swing your arms and trunk forward until your head touches your knees—but remember not to bend the knees nor the arms. Then, very slowly, lift the trunk and arms and lie back on the floor without bending arms or knees, keeping the back upright. Breathe out as you swing forward and take a long, deep, slow breath in as you lie back. Muscles can be easily strained if this is done too long or too vigorously, so please be cautious.

Legs Leg exercises are easier. Get hold of a chair and then, supporting yourself by holding on to the back of it with one arm, the other arm outstretched horizontally to keep your balance, swing one leg forwards and backwards as high as it will go, without bending either leg. Do this twenty times, then turn around and do it with the other leg.

Next, stand facing the chair in a 'ballet fifth position', with legs apart and feet turned out, and hold on to the chair with both hands. Slowly bend your knees, keeping your back upright, feet flat on the floor, tummy and buttocks tucked in. Gradually lower yourself without bending your back, as far as you can go. Then, slowly stretch

Below: An exercise for the waistline

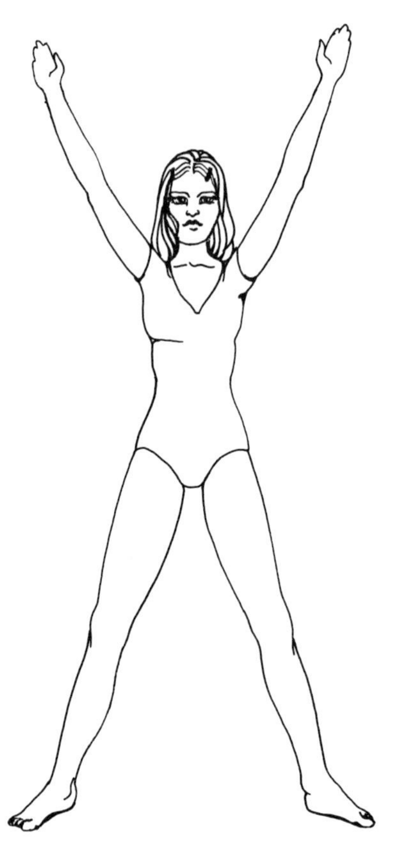

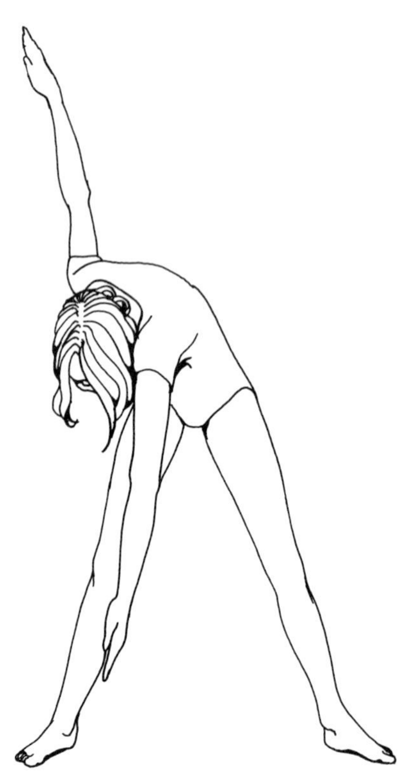

Below: Exercising the legs

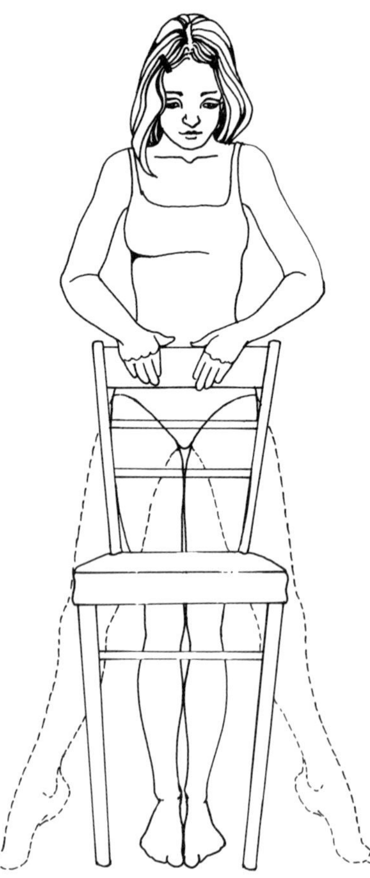

upright, keeping your tummy and buttocks tucked in under you, and raise yourself up on to your toes. Next time, lower yourself whilst standing on your toes, holding your balance.

Hips For a good hip exercise, sit on the floor with your legs stretched out and apart, back straight, tummy tucked in, and arms stretched out behind you, with hands on the floor. Swing your left leg over your right leg, without bending it, to touch the floor on the other side as far over as it will go, and then your right leg over your left. Do this ten times with each leg.

Another good hip exercise is 'riding a bike in the air'. Lie on your back with arms stretched out beside you. Raise your body off the floor until your shoulders support you with your outstretched arms on the floor holding your balance. Rotate your legs in the air as though riding a bicycle. Ride hard and fast.

Arms In order to keep arms toned and

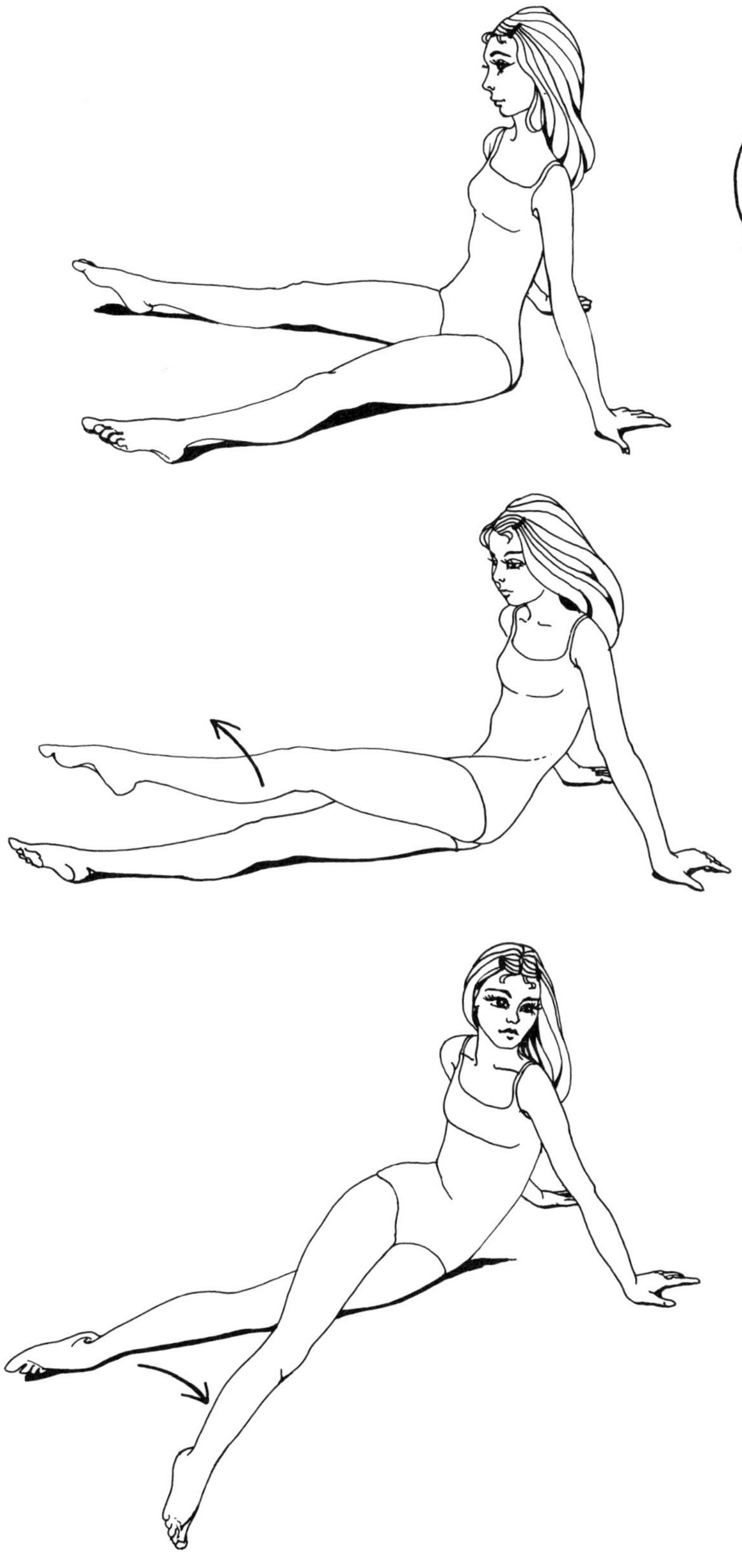

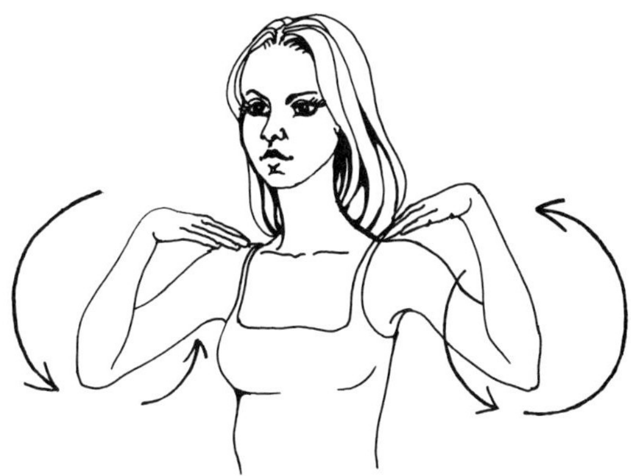

Below: How to exercise the arms

firm, stand upright with shoulders well back, tummy and buttocks tucked in. Stretch arms and hands out horizontally, and then, with palms outstretched upwards, touch your shoulders with your fingertips. Swing arms back out again and touch shoulders again. Do this twenty times in quick, rhythmical movements.

Another effective arm exercise is to remain in the same position with one hand on your hip, and swing the other outstretched arm round and round in a 360-degree movement from the shoulder a dozen times. Repeat with the other arm.

Neck and shoulders

Your neck is the continuation of your face and an integral part of your stature. It supports your head and helps to give you graceful posture. These exercises will prevent drooping and wrinkling of the neck and keep the skin firm, tightening up any superfluous under-chin flab.

Stand upright with your arms at your sides. Keeping your chin up, swing your head to the left then to the right, back to the left, to the right again, as far as it will go. Next, throw your head backwards then forwards until your chin touches your chest. Do each exercise ten times.

Just as your neck is an extension of your face and helps to improve posture, your shoulders are important for good carriage and elegant stance. Always keep your shoulders well back and never forward unless you want to end up with rounded shoulders and a hunched back.

Above: A good exercise for the hips

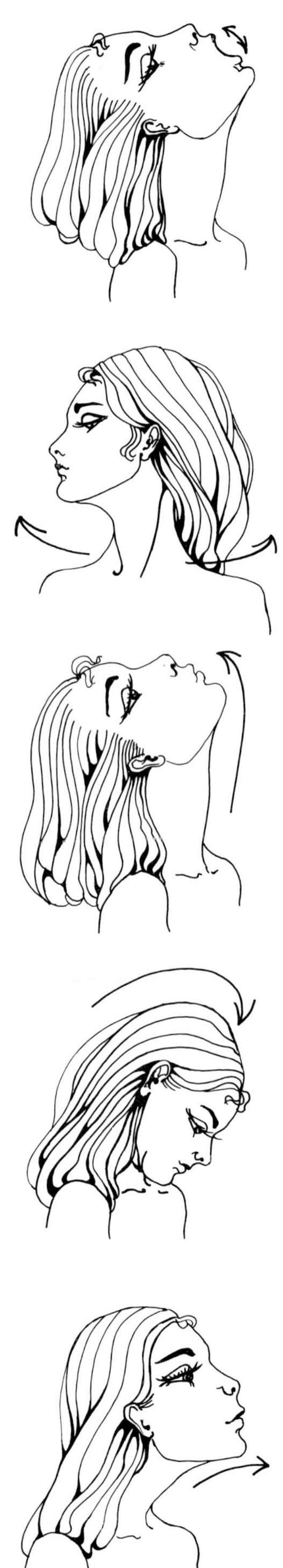

Above: An exercise for the neck

Moreover, keep your shoulders relaxed at all times. You will find that your neck and back will automatically straighten as you sit and stand upright keeping your shoulders back.

A good shoulder exercise is to sit flat on the floor with your back upright, keeping your shoulders pinned against the wall. With your legs outstretched in front of you and your chin flopped

Below: Exercising the shoulders

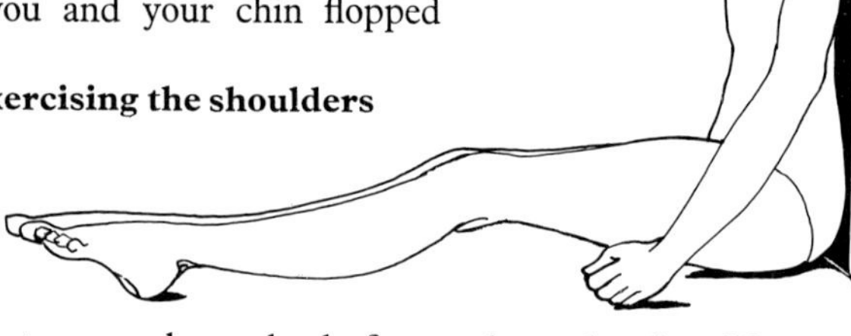

forward on to your chest, slowly force your spine up the wall, supporting yourself with your hands on the floor at the end of outstretched arms. When you have gone up as far as possible, push the back of your neck against the wall, hold it there, count to ten, then sink back on to the floor and start all over again.

These simple exercises practised by top models are elementary guides to deportment and posture. Only by constant daily routine and concentration on the exercises will they help to improve your figure, circulation and general healthy condition.

Skin care

The art of make-up is acquired through continual practice and experiment, during which time you get to know about your face, the way it moves and the effects you can achieve with your new-found artistry. Your entire personality can change with a different eye make-up, for instance, and, as fashion itself changes continually, you have to be adaptable.

Models in Paris, however, are spoiled because highly-paid make-up artists and hairdressers visit *Vogue* and *Elle* and many of the top photographic studios to apply the models' make-up and style their hair. In New York and London, however, models are more self-sufficient and this helps them immensely with assignments on location throughout the world.

Before make-up can be applied, care of the skin has to be considered.

Good skin should be clear, soft and smooth. Skin can be kept younger and fresher for longer by taking care of it,

but only a face-lift can remove lines and wrinkles deeply imbedded. Skin care is a preventive, not a cure.

Before deciding about make-up, consider whether your skin is dry, oily, sensitive or normal. Whatever the type of skin you have, there are four rules for its care: to cleanse, tone, moisturise and lubricate. Although you can get away without moisturising because so many foundations have moisturisers nowadays, cleansing the skin is essential.

Whether you use make-up or not, it is likely that a thin layer of oily dirt from actual dirt, diesel fumes and air pollution will form on the skin's surface. Soap and water is a splendid method, but a creamy cleanser for dry skin and a less greasy cleanser for greasy skin is recommended. Depending on the texture of your skin, match up with a tonic or astringent to remove the cleansing traces, remembering to start at the base of the neck, working upwards and outwards in gentle strokes. *Never* use downward and inward strokes on the face and neck, and remember to be very gentle on your skin when handling it.

The skin needs moisture and, as it does not produce or hold sufficient water, it is important to apply a moisturiser when removing make-up before going to bed at night, or every time your clean your face.

Lubricating or nourishing the skin is necessary because, as you grow older, your glands slow down and fail to produce sufficient oil, or *sebum*. The latest skin creams are less oily than before, so you need not go to bed with an oily face.

Remember to treat your neck as part of your face; lines on the neck are an easy giveaway, as are uncared-for hands. So treat your hands with the same care you lavish on your face and neck. A model's hands are an extension of her beauty, an accessory to her craft, often photographed near to her face.

Make-up

The foundation is the basis of good make-up. It conceals flaws and skin blemishes, giving the face a clear canvas for the application of make-up. Choose a daytime foundation, in the daylight outside the store, to match the texture of your skin. If you are choosing a foundation for evening wear, select it under the shop's artificial light to be in accord with the evening's artificial light when you will be wearing it, but take care not to choose under fluorescent light, which has a blue tone. Although foundations are normally tested on the back of the hand, remember hands are usually rougher and redder than faces, so be cautious in matching tones.

Face Once you have discovered your skin type—dry, oily, etc—find out the shape of your face. Is it oval, round, square, long or oblong, triangular or heart-shaped? The ideal shape is oval and this effect is created by high-lighting and shading. High-lighting brings a feature forward into promi-nence with a lighter application and shading with a darker base produces the opposite effect, 'pushing into the shadow' features you do not want accentuated.

High cheek-bones and sunken cheeks are the most desirable look and, to achieve this, the cheek-bones are high-lighted, and the cheeks shaded.

Chin Double-chins are carefully con-cealed by applying a darker foundation underneath the chin along the full area, but take care to blend into the neck. Never forget to apply the same make-up to your neck as to your face. Nothing looks worse than a painted face with a bright white neck. But take care not to leave marks on collars and scarves. The opposite technique, ie a lighter founda-tion, is applied to receding chins.

Shadows under the eyes are con-cealed by high-lighting rather than shading them away! Use a lighter base, blending into the line of the shadow, and powder over lightly.

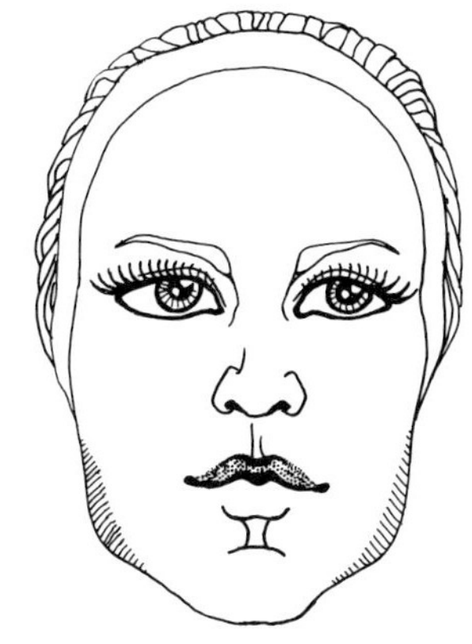

How to shade a square face for the oval look

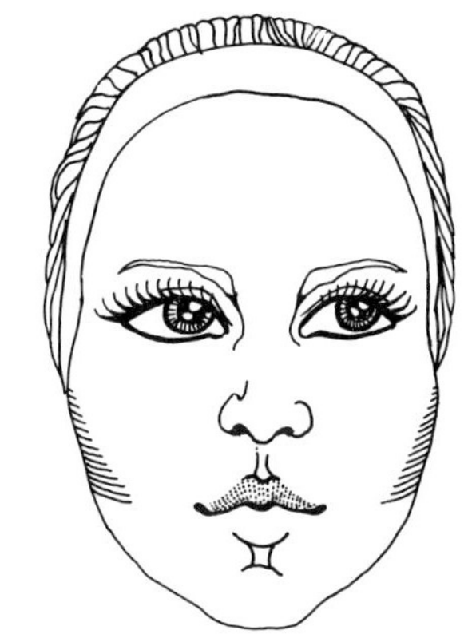

A round face is shaded under the cheek bones

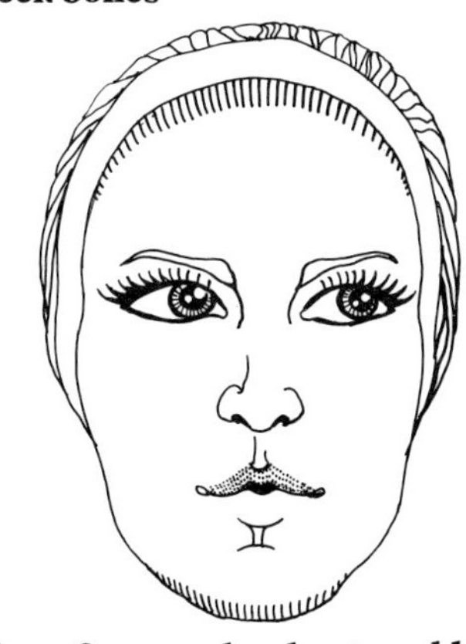

A long face can be shortened by shading below the hairline and above the chin

Nose If your nose is long and thin, shade the tip. If it is broad, run a thin light line down the centre, from the bridge to the tip, and shade the sides from the eyebrows to the nostrils. Do not use shiny make-up on a big nose. It will appear larger. Apply matt make-up instead.

The old-fashioned rouge is called blusher these days, and helps to add warmth to the face. It also helps in the shading and sculpting of the face when correctly applied.

Lips A lip-brush is the vital tool for

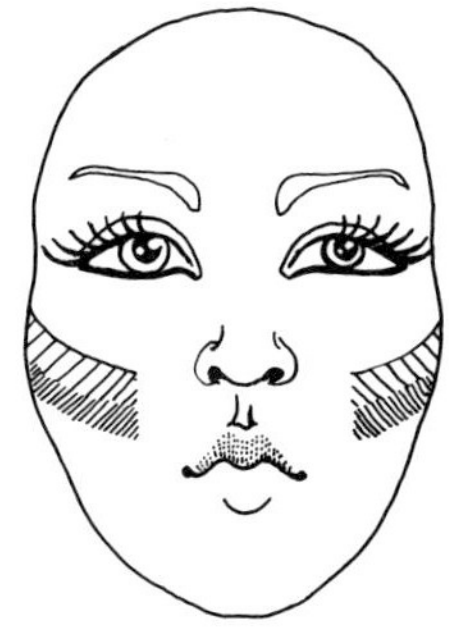

Oval face shading

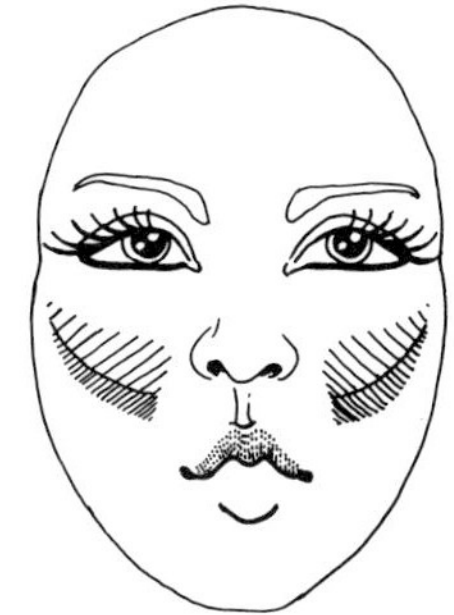

Round face shading

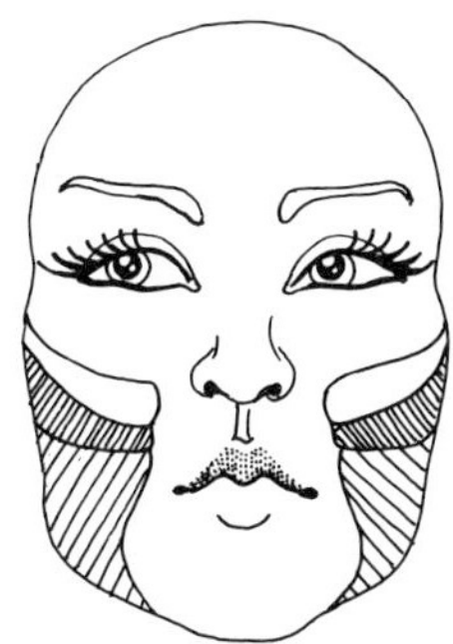

Square face shading

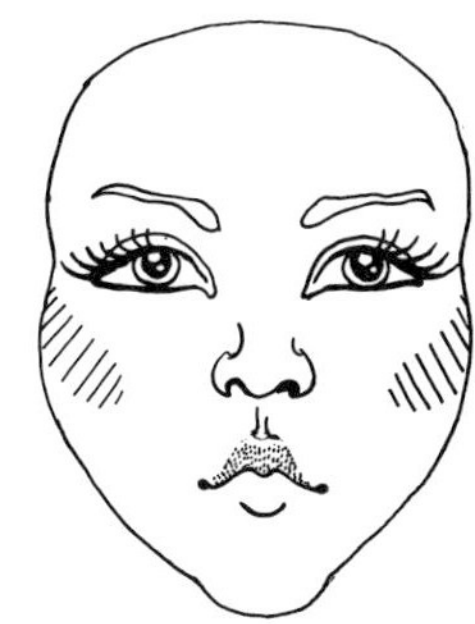

Heart-shaped face shading

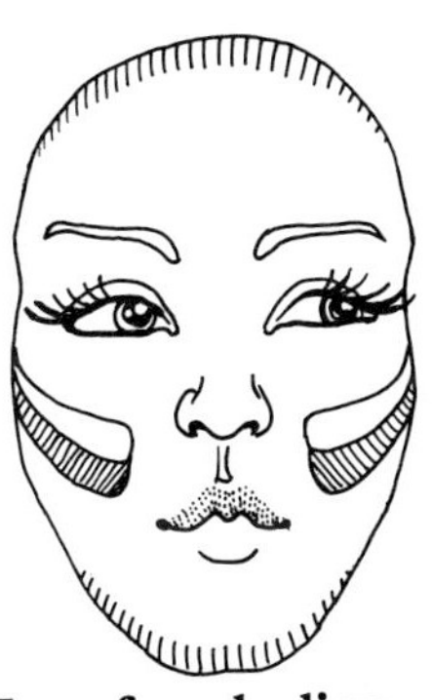

Long face shading

lips. Don't take the quick, easy way by using a stick; it merely glides across the lips and comes off rather quickly. The lip-brush enables you to paint into the grain of the lips. But make sure your lips are free from dry make-up, and are dry before applying the lip-brush.

For full lips, keep the lipstick just inside the natural lip-line, avoiding pale lipstick, which will have the effect of high-lighting, therefore enlarging a full mouth, bringing it into prominence.

Models with a thin lip-line are inclined to apply the lipstick *over* the natural lip-line in an endeavour to enlarge the mouth, but this looks messy and fools no-one. Simply apply a *light* coloured lipstick and add a shiny pearlised colour on top.

However well made-up the face may be, or immacuately applied the lipstick, if, once the mouth is opened, a rush of uneven, yellowing, or decaying teeth reveal themselves, then the game is up. Although it is not advocated that models should fly out for cosmetic dentistry and tooth-capping at the drop of a hat, if there *are* imperfections either to teeth or gums, they will show up in photographic modelling and therefore action should be taken.

Teeth Models should retain their individual look and try not to copy the look of others. They should not yearn for two rows of perfectly capped teeth, but rely on their own individuality. One internationally known top model has a gap of about a quarter of an inch between her front teeth and earns a quarter of a million dollars a year. If she or the advertisers do not want the gap to show, she simply shuts her mouth and smiles through closed lips!

However, preventive care of teeth is essential for clean, healthy looks. Avoid eating sweet, sugary stuff and brush your teeth after every meal. Eat apples, fresh celery and carrots, and good results will be your reward.

Eyes The basic necessities for eye make-up are to discover whether your eyes are too small (in which case eyebrows have to be plucked away to give more space, and be made thinner, neater and finer), large, upward-slanting, downward-slanting, or at irregular heights. A pale high-light is applied *under* the brow for small eyes, and a deeper shadow just slightly above the eye-crease. Keep the liner fine, extending to outer corners. Apply a touch of white between the two lines at the outer corner. False eyelashes above and below the eye will help to open up the eye, as will mascara applied to your own lashes.

Eye make-up requires considerable skill and this can only be achieved through practice, experiment and impartial criticism.

Hair

Once you are confident of the way your face has emerged, concentrate on your hairstyle, which must match the shape of your face. Almost any style can be worn with an oval face, but if you have a round face, do not add to it by having a bouffant hairdo, emphasising your moon shape. Keep the hair flat on the sides, cut in a bob, shaped in at the sides of your cheeks, or wear it up, in a chignon. Long faces need fringes and fullness on the sides. Steer clear of hair piled up or hanging long and loose if you have a long face.

Heartshaped faces can take a centre-parting and wide foreheads need a soft, side-swept fringe. Sweep the hair up and away from your face if you have a narrow or short forehead.

If you have a large nose, balance your profile by fullness of hair on the crown, flattened down to the nape to emphasise the shape of your head. Small, neat noses can take small, neat hairstyles without overbalancing the profile.

Wigs and hairpieces

Because of the more natural and less complicated-looking hairstyles these days, wigs and hairpieces aren't used as frequently as before. However, top models still tend to carry at least three different hairpieces around with them to ring the changes. They are particularly useful away on location when there is little or no time to get to hairdressers, or to reset your own hair for different styles. Many a model can appear completely different with an inventive, different hairstyle and make-up; it is this adaptability and versatility that helps to make the model much sought after.

The most popular hairpieces are the backfalls, mounted on to a frame, with a small comb in the front which helps to anchor the piece on to the head. They can be long, short, curly or straight and are placed on the head half-way, with the hair falling to the sides and the back.

But take care to select only the best hair when buying. The best hair comes from Italy and it is heavy and 'swinging'. It photographs well. Avoid coarse and bleached hair which will tangle up and become unmanageable, resulting in waste of time and money. Good hair costs more, but it is a wise investment. Be extra careful to match the piece exactly to your own hair tone and texture, and when tinting or recolouring your hair take the piece along to an expert for matching.

Treat the hairpiece as though it were your own hair. Ask the expert how to clean or carefully shampoo it. It should be pinned to a soft wig-block, and set on rollers or in pincurls in the normal way. Do not drench the base on to which the piece is woven otherwise it will loosen the weave or the knots and fall apart.

Take care to conceal the join between the hairpiece and your own hair by

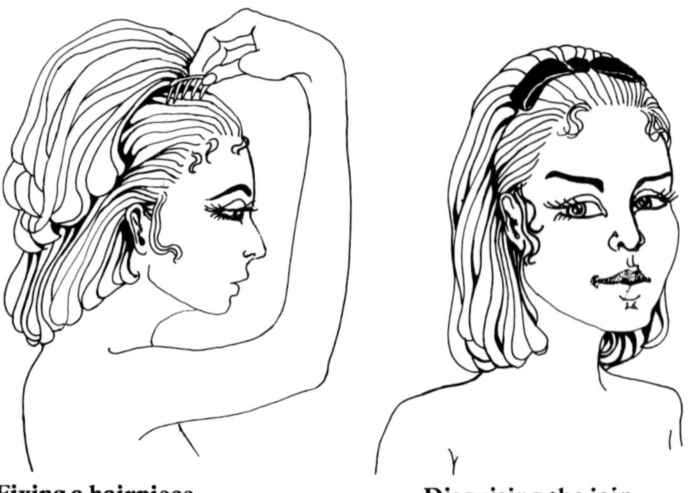

Fixing a hairpiece   **Disguising the join**

brushing some of your own hair over the join, or by slipping a bandeau or pretty ribbon across the top.

Hair care

Lustrous, rich-looking hair with a healthy, natural appearance is vital to a model's presentation. This can only be achieved by care and attention, continual brushing, shampooing, conditioning and, above all, good health.

Consider whether you have oily, dry or natural hair and choose a shampoo to suit your needs. The labels on the bottles will guide you. Dandruff cannot be cured, but it can be kept under control by frequent use of anti-dandruff shampoos. A greasy scalp can produce dandruff, so guard against it.

For oily hair, avoid greasy or fatty foods, and eat fresh fruit, vegetables, fish and poultry. Wash your hair once every five days with a mild shampoo. Do not brush too much and avoid using water too hot or over-heated rollers.

Dry hair needs washing once a week with a mild, emollient shampoo. Use a conditioner to stimulate the oil glands in the scalp. Brush regularly and avoid back-combing and hair lacquer, which will only add to the dryness—perhaps the very reason for its present dry condition. In your diet, include plenty of butter, cream, eggs and fresh fruit.

Setting lotions give the hair body and crispness, but select carefully from the many on the market, depending on whether your hair is dry, oily, fine, wiry or floppy.

Hair colouring is an expert's craft, and so is styling. Consult a reputable hair stylist who will advise on tones and cut, and discuss style and shape to suit your face and the current fashion. Models who have developed an expertise with their own hair, shampooing, conditioning, setting and combing out, soon learn to restyle and to colour it themselves, but cutting is an expert's job and should be left to them.

Because of limited space, these suggestions are only the foundation of helpful beauty secrets revealed by top models. There are many publications on the market in which diet, nutrition, exercises, skin, make-up and hair are dealt with more comprehensively, giving a fuller account of the essentials and disciplines employed by models after many years of experience.

Appendix B
Recommended Model Schools and Agents

Model schools do not make fashion models out of hopeful young girls, no matter how much they may insist that they do. However, they do advise on deportment, make-up, diet, exercises and clothes-sense. They can put you on the right road to self-improvement. They will also suggest photographers and models' agents who might help your modelling career. Many model schools run a separate model agency division, but the reputable ones are just as selective about the girls they have trained as the ones that come from outside.

If you are in doubt about the model school of your choice, simply go along to see them and listen to their sales pitch. If they promise to make a model out of you, you are wasting your time and money. If they charge exorbitant fees for their courses, think again. The safest path to travel is by choosing a model agency that provides tuition for its models, such as The Ford's Agency and Wilhelmina Models Inc in New York. Here, the largest modelling schools are John Powers and Barbizon but, as mentioned, it is advisable to consult initially the two top model agencies, The Ford's and Wilhelmina. The Mary Webb Davis Agency in Los Angeles is a highly recommended model school and agency, and Nina Blanchard is another one of the best. In Detroit, Auston Enterprises covers the mid-West. Gary Grizzelle, who heads Auston, has four modelling schools in the Detroit area.

There are no modelling schools in Paris, but the most highly recommended agencies who advise and mould their models are Elite, headed by John Casablancas, and Models International run by former top international model, Simone D'Aillencourt. In London, an agency with a reputable modelling school which can be recommended by the author, is the Lucie Clayton Fashion School and Model Agency.

The following is a selected list of reputable model agencies, some with their own schools, throughout the world, but bear in mind that new ones start up regularly, whilst others often close down. In all instances the agencies will suggest photographers who will provide you with good photographs. Some of the top model agencies bear the cost of your promotional photographs themselves, others ask you to pay for them yourself. The photographs are vitally important to your modelling career, and required to show to prospective employers. The composite cards made from the photographs, however, are more important as they are extremely economical and more effective. In America, the best company is in New York, Bad Flyers Design Inc. In London, Robert Wheal provides composites for models throughout Britain and Europe.

Composite Cards

Michael Kerns
Bad Flyers Design Inc
30 East 42nd Street, Room 1007
New York, New York 10017, USA
Telephone (212) 682-1705

Robert Wheal Promotion Consultants
23 Redan Place
London W2
Telephone 01-727 3828

Model Agencies and Schools

New York City

Ford Models Inc
344 East 59th Street
New York, New York 10022
Telephone (212) 688-8538

Stewart Models Corp (*no school*)
405 Park Avenue
New York, New York 10022
Telephone (212) 753-4610

Barbizon School of Modelling
689 5th Avenue
New York, New York 10022
Telephone (212) 826-0440

Wilhelmina Models Inc
9 East 37th Street
New York, New York 10016
Telephone (212) 532-7141

Zoli (*no school*)
121 East 62nd Street
New York, New York 10021
Telephone (212) 758-5959

John Robert Powers (Modelling)
  School
8 West 58th Street
New York, New York
Telephone (212) 421-3920

USA

Arizona

Fosi's Modeling-Talent Agency and
  School
2777 North Campbell,
Tucson 85719
Telephone (602) 795-3534
Owner/Director: Fosi Costello Burritt
SAG Franchise

Plaza Three Model Agency-Talent
  Agency
4343 North 16th
Phoenix 85016
Telephone (602) 264-9703
Cast: Darlene Wyatt, Specialist in TV
  Commercial talent
SAG Franchise. Convention and top
  fashion models

California

Nina Blanchard Agency-Artists
  Manager
1717 North Highland Avenue, 901
Los Angeles 90028
Telephone (Printing) 462-7274;
  (TV) 462-7341

Brebner Agency
1615 Polk
San Francisco 94109
Telephone (415) 775-1802, 771-3488

Commercial Talent Agency
6922 Hollywood Boulevard
Hollywood 90028
Telephone (213) 466-6433
Contact: Joan Mangum (Print and
  Photography)

Mary Webb Davis Agency
515 North La Cienega
Los Angeles 90048
Telephone (213) 655-6747, 652-6850
TV Department: Pacific Artists
Telephone (213) 657-5990

Grimme Agency
41 Grant Avenue
San Francisco 94108
Telephone (415) EX 2 9175

La Belle Agency
Artists' Manager-Model and Talent-
  Represents SAG Actors
El Paseo, Studio 111
Santa Barbara 93102
Telephone (805) 965-4575

Joan Mangum at Bernard Sandler's
  Commercial Talent Agency
6922 Hollywood Boulevard
Hollywood 90028
Telephone (213) 466-6433

Pacific Artists, TV Commercials
515 No. La Cienega
Los Angeles 90048
Telephone (213) 657-5990, 652-6850
Printing: Mary Webb Davis
Telephone (213) 655-6747

Sabina Model Agency
Merchant Street Center
Merchant and Battery Streets
San Francisco 94111
Telephone (415) 788-3939
Director: Sabina Roberts

Ann Wright Associates, Ltd
8422 Melrose Place
Los Angeles 90069
Telephone (213) 655-5040
Bob Lloyd

Canada

See Canada section

Connecticut

The Connecticut Modeling Agency
  Inc
1326 Shippan Avenue
Stamford 06902
Telephone (203) 325-1538 and
  (212) 828-4050

District of Columbia

Barbizon Model Agency
5530 Wisconsin Avenue
Chevy Chase, MD 20015
Telephone (301) 656-5996
Printing, Fashion, TV, Trade Shows,
  Conventions

Cappa Chell Models
1739 Connecticut Avenue
NW 20009
Telephone (202) NO 7-6171
Fashion Shows and Photography and
  Conventions, Television, AFTRA
  and Films
also at
One Tysons Corner Office Building
Suite 101
McLean, VA 22101
Telephone (703) 893-9500
President: Gladys Davis

Detroit

Auston Enterprises
302 South Main Street
Royal Oak, Michigan 48067
Director: Gary Grizzelle

Florida

Eva Kovacs Modeling and Finishing
  Academy
404 Fifth Avenue
Indialantic, Florida 32903
Telephone (305) 727-1734

Sunny Talent
4814 Vincennes
Cape Coral 33904
Telephone (813) 542-7836

Joann Torretta's Modeling School
  and Agency
566 Riviera Drive
Tampa 33606
Telephone (813) 253-3986

Ann Wright, Florida Casting
333 Alcazar Avenue
Coral Gables, Florida 33134
Telephone (305) 445-2505

Hawaii

Patricia Stevens Modeling Agency
2895 Kalakaua
Honolulu
Telephone (808) 922-5511

Indiana

Act I Model and Talent Agency
3843 North Meridian
Indianapolis 46208
Telephone (317) 926-2324

Iowa

Corrine Shover Model Agency
4030 First Avenue NW
Cedar Rapids 52401
Telephone (319) 362-1347

Kentucky

Alix Adams Agency
404 Speed Building
Louisville 40202
Telephone (502) 587-0765
Owner/Director: Ruth Devine

Ohio

The Cincinnati Modeling Agency
7784 Montgomery Road
Cincinnati 45236
Telephone (513) 791-5523

Norma Sharkey Agency Inc
41 East First
Dayton 45402
Telephone (513) 274-3971

Wright Modeling Agency
4435 North High Street
Columbus, Ohio 43214
Telephone (614) 261-7262, 7466

Oregon

Cinderella Models Casting and
  Referral Agency
610 Broadway SW
Portland 97205
Telephone (503) 227-6619
Owner: Susan Ferguson MAA

Pennsylvania

Caldwell Models
100 Park Avenue
Swarthmore 19081
Telephone (215) 521-1095
Director: Patt Caldwell

Charming Models School and Agency
6 Scottsdale Plaza
Harrisburg 17111
Telephone (617) 533-3400
Director: Fay Sherman MAA

Models' Guild of Philadelphia, Inc
The Drake, Suite 412
Philadelphia 19102
Telephone (215) 735-4067, 5606
Director: Ann Bacher
SAG, AFTRA: Fashion, Printing,
  Promotion, Talent

The Wheeler School
William Penn Hotel
Pittsburgh 15219
Telephone (412) 261-6848

Texas

Kim Dawson
1143 Apparel Mart
Dallas 75207
Telephone (214) 638-2414

Joan Frank Productions
Suite 228, 2 Turtle Creek Village
Dallas 75219
Telephone (214) 522-3240

Ben Shaw Studios (*models only*)
403 Westheimer
Houston 77006
Telephone (713) JA 6 4301
Ben Shaw Studios (*models only*)
815 Brooklyn Avenue
San Antonio 78215
Telephone (512) CA 3 6231

Utah

Barbizon School of Modeling
22 South Main Street
Salt Lake City 84101
Telephone (801) 322-2597
Director: Dorothy Mitchell

Washington

Lola Hallowell Model and Talent
  Agency
158 Thomas Street 14
Seattle 98109
Telephone (206) 623-7311

The Carolyn Hansen Agency
1516 - 6th Avenue
Seattle 98101
Telephone (206) 622-4992
Owner/Director: Carolyn Hansen

Maryland

Patricia Stevens, AFTRA
Westview Mall Prof. Offices
Baltimore 21228
Telephone (301) 744-0900
Fashion Shows, Conventions, TV,
  Photography

Taylor Models
Baltimore
Telephone (301) 685-5454

Minnesota

Eleanor Moore Agency, Inc
1610 - B West Lake
Minneapolis 55408
Telephone (612) 827-3823

Nevada

Lenz Model Agency, Inc and
  Convention Service
1454 East Charleston Boulevard
Las Vegas 89104
Telephone (702) 382-3245

Joyce Conover Model and Casting
Main Street
Millburn, NJ
Telephone (201) 232-0908

National Talent Associates
280 Park Avenue
Rutherford 07070
Telephone (201) 935-0330
Offices in:
New York. Telephone (212) 343-6730
Chicago. Telephone (312) 531-8575
California. Telephone (213) 462-6777
Specialising in children only

Serendipity Models and Casting
  Agency
92 Broadway
Denville, NJ 07834
Telephone (201) 625-2125

New York State

John Robert Powers School
300 Delaware Avenue
Buffalo 14202
Telephone (716) 856-1500
Director: Nancy Volkert

North Carolina

Jan Thompson Talent Agency
2621 Croydon Road
Charlotte 28209
Telephone (704) 377-5987

Trim (Troyanne Ross) Talent Agency
600 Queens Road
Charlotte 28207
Telephone (704) 376-4271

For additional information about modelling agencies or schools in America, consult:

The Modelling Association of America
c/o Ms Margaret Cornell, President
Flair College
9301 Candelaria, North East
Albuquerque
New Mexico 87112

The Madison Avenue Handbook
Peter Glenn Publications
Obtainable: 17 East 48th Street
New York, New York 10017
Telephone (212) 688-7974

London

Andy's People
152 Shaftesbury Avenue
London WC2
Telephone 01-836 2528

Askew Team (Model Agency)
18 Bruton Place
London W1
Telephone 01-493 0631

Bobtons Model Agency
40 King's Road
London SW3
Telephone 01-584 4397

Elisabeth Smith Model Agency
148 College Road, Harrow
Telephone 01-863 2331

Ena Holloway Agency
60 Neal Street
London WC2
Telephone 01-836 0449

International Model Agency
2 Hinde Street
London W1
Telephone 01-486 3312

The Model Agency
48 Crawford Street
London W1
Telephone 01-724 3322

Lucie Clayton Fashion School and
Model Agency
168 Brompton Road
London SW3
Telephone 01-581 0024

Nevs Model Agency
18 Coulson Street
London SW3
Telephone 01-581 2295

Penny Personal Management
146a Brompton Road
London SW3
Telephone 01-584 8577

Pretty Ugly
6 Windmill Street
London W1
Telephone 01-580 4882

Ashton Laraine
IFM
82 Park Street
London W1
Telephone 01-629 3176

Beauchamp Promotions
14 Beauchamp Place
London SW3
Telephone 01-589 3338

Carian Agency
17 Henrietta Street
London WC2
Telephone 01-373 2238

Norman Hartnell School of
Deportment
26 Bruton Street
London W1
Telephone 01-629 0992

Freddie's
2 Lowndes Street
London SW1
Telephone 01-235 8778

The London Academy of Modelling
143 New Bond Street
London W1
Telephone 01-499 4751

London Casting and Management
(as The London Academy of
Modelling)

Models One (*agency only*)
200 Fulham Road
London SW10
Telephone 01-351 1195

Paul's People
61 Chandos Place
London WC2
Telephone 01-836 2503

Petal Model Agency
28 Walpole Street
London SW3
Telephone 01-730 7284

Gavin Robinson
30 Old Bond Street
London W1
Telephone 01-499 5440

Sarah Cape (Inc Blackboys)
233a Portobello Road
London W11
Telephone 01-229 1436

Suzannah-Jon Model Agency
1a Hinde Street
London W1
Telephone 01-935 9129

Annie Walker Agency
44 Parkway
London NW1
Telephone 01-485 1058

Snapshot Ltd
61 Blandford Street
London W1
Telephone 01-486 4538

Top Models
37 Percy Street
London W1
Telephone 01-636 8771

Whittaker Enterprises
33 Brook Street
London W1
Telephone 01-629 0770

Paris

Elite Model Management (and
L'Agence)
(John Casablancas)
7 Rue d'Artois
75008 Paris
Telephone 359 0396

Paris Planning (François Lano)
29 Rue Tronchet
Paris Ville
Telephone 265 0483

Catherine Harlé
38–42 Passage Choiseul
Paris 2
Telephone 742 2523

Pauline's Agency (and Prestige)
47 Rue de l'Arbre Sec
Paris 1
Telephone 260 3929

Look Models
19 Rue de la Pompé
Paris 75016
Telephone 870 9546

Models International
(Simone d'Aillencourt)
3 avenue Victor Hugo
Paris 16e
Telephone 704 7900

Viva
33 Champs Elysees
Bureau 603, 6th Floor
Paris
Telephone 359 9171

Europlanning
19 Rue de la Reynie
Paris 75004
Telephone 278 5527

Flash
30 Rue Godot de Mauroy
Paris 75009
Telephone 073 1140

Karin Models
1 Square de la Tour Maubourg
Paris 75007
Telephone 705 6710

Australia

Vivien's
566 St Kilda Road
Melbourne
Victoria 3004
Telephone 510673

Vivien's
46 Gurner Street
Paddington
Sydney, New South Wales 2021
Telephone 334151

Belgium

Lambraun International
87 Avenue Louise
1050 Brussels
Telephone 02 38 88 72

Canada

Audrey Morris and Assoc
Place Bon Aventure
Suite 34, East Floor
Montreal
Telephone (514) 866 1167

Constance Brown
3465 Cote des Neiges
Montreal
Telephone (514) 934 0393

Eleanor Fulcher Model Agency
667 Yonge Street
Toronto
Telephone (416) 924 9233

Denmark

Copenhagen Models
(Trice Tomsen)
2 Toldbodgade
DK 1253 Copenhagen
Telephone 01 11 22 86

Germany

Gunther Models
8 Munich 40
Ausbacherstrasse 4
Telephone 089 37 84 51

Gunther Models
2 Hamburg 20
Mansteinstrasse 18
Telephone 040 491 35 93

Umbrella Models
(Kristin Hagge)
200 Hamburg
Neuer Wall 48
Telephone 040 36 76 46

Holland

The Agency (and Modelplanning)
Prinsengracht 720
Amsterdam
Telephone 220456

Euromodel
Herengracht 160
Amsterdam
Telephone 231011

Italy

International Model Agency
Via Sardegna 29
Rome
Telephone 4755178

Riccardo Gay
via Revere 9
20123 Milan
Telephone 4694 395

Top Life
via Paolo Giovio 11
20144 Milan
Telephone 485610

South Africa

Stella Robinson (Model Agency)
404 Merbook House
123 Commissioner Street
Johannesburg
Telephone 22 1375

Mannequins Incorporated
210 Loop Street
Cape Town
Telephone 43 2861

Matty Reid Modelling School
7th floor, Regent House
87 Market Street
Johannesburg 2000
Telephone 23 2867

Dominique (Modelling School)
241 Voortrekker Road
Belville
Cape Town 7530
Telephone 97 0398

La Vogue Studios (Modelling School)
Suite 4510
320 West Street
Durban

Spain

Top Planning (Model Agency)
Balmes 191
Barcelona
Telephone 218 6995

Sweden

Västsvenska Modellgruppen
Kristinelundsgatan 18
41137 Gothenburg
Telephone 031 20 89 36

Silvia Stjern-Larner
Formskäraregatan 5
S-41261 Tothenburg
Telephone 031 13 15 45

Switzerland

Foto Gen
Bahnofplatz 5
8001 Zurich
Telephone 01 27 11 70

Time Model Agency
Schoffelgasse 3
8001 Zurich
Telephone 01 47 60 40

Index